Dairy Products

Dairy Products

Special Issue Editors

Beth Rice Bradley
Therese O'Sullivan

MDPI • Basel • Beijing • Wuhan • Barcelona • Belgrade

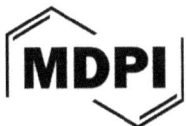

MDPI

Special Issue Editors
Beth Rice Bradley
Foodsense, LLC
USA

Therese O'Sullivan
Edith Cowan University
Australia

Editorial Office
MDPI
St. Alban-Anlage 66
4052 Basel, Switzerland

This is a reprint of articles from the Special Issue published online in the open access journal *Nutrients* (ISSN 2072-6643) from 2017 to 2018 (available at: https://www.mdpi.com/journal/nutrients/special_issues/Dairy_products)

For citation purposes, cite each article independently as indicated on the article page online and as indicated below:

LastName, A.A.; LastName, B.B.; LastName, C.C. Article Title. *Journal Name* **Year**, *Article Number*, Page Range.

ISBN 978-3-03897-368-3 (Pbk)
ISBN 978-3-03897-369-0 (PDF)

Contents

About the Special Issue Editors

Beth Rice Bradley is an adjunct lecturer in the Department of Nutrition and Food Science at the University of Vermont (UVM). In addition to teaching at UVM, Dr. Bradley consults directly with the food industry as owner of Foodsense, LLC. Dr. Bradley's strength is in translating nutrition science to help companies to meet their health and wellness goals. Prior to founding Foodsense, LLC, Dr. Bradley was Director of Scientific Affairs at National Dairy Council (Dairy Management, Inc.), where she led the scientific outreach strategy for translating dairy science for industry, academic, government, and health professional thought leaders at a global level. For her graduate work at the University of Vermont, Dr. Bradley investigated the effects of industrially produced and naturally occurring trans-fatty acids on coronary heart disease risk.

Therese O'Sullivan is an Accredited Practicing Dietitian of 15 years and has worked in both clinical and university settings. She is a senior lecturer at Edith Cowan University (ECU), where she teaches in the Masters of Nutrition and Dietetics and supervises PhD students. Therese is currently leading a double blind randomized control dietary trial in children at ECU, investigating the effects of full fat and reduced fat dairy products on body composition, along with heart and gut health. This project was underpinned by extensive community consultation, which involved focus groups with parents and consultation with a parenting expert. She is a firm believer in the value of community consultation and producing useful and translatable research.

Preface to "Dairy Products"

Dairy foods, including milk, cheese and yogurt, are key contributors of energy and essential nutrients in the human diet. Dairy food consumption is associated with nutrient adequacy, bone health, and a reduced risk of chronic disease.

Recently, bioactive components in dairy foods have become of interest for their role, beyond basic nutrition, in health. While dairy contributes saturated fat to the diet, it is not associated with increased risk for cardiovascular disease. Further, specific types of fat within dairy fat have been linked with improved metabolic health and immune function, and the amount of milk fat globule membrane enclosing the fat may be important in cardiac and muscular outcomes. Dairy proteins, casein and whey, mitigate muscle loss, particularly after exercise. Other bioactive components in dairy, such as probiotic bacteria, have been implicated in beneficial effects on the microbiome.

In a time when overnutrition is just as detrimental to human health as undernutrition, the health effects of foods beyond basic nutrition are of interest to the scientific community. Dairy components have become of special interest for their roles in nutrition, cardiometabolic health, and immunity. In this book, experts address the effects of dairy components on health and immunity. Mechanisms of action are also explored.

Beth Rice Bradley, Therese O'Sullivan

Special Issue Editors

nutrients

MDPI

Article

Gastric Emptying and Gastrointestinal Transit Compared among Native and Hydrolyzed Whey and Casein Milk Proteins in an Aged Rat Model

Julie E. Dalziel [1,2,*], Wayne Young [1,2,3], Catherine M. McKenzie [4], Neill W. Haggarty [5] and Nicole C. Roy [1,2,3]

1   Food Nutrition & Health Team, Food & Bio-Based Products Group, AgResearch,
    Grasslands Research Centre, Palmerston North 4442, New Zealand;
    wayne.young@agresearch.co.nz (W.Y.); nicole.roy@agresearch.co.nz (N.C.R.)
2   Riddet Institute, Massey University, Palmerston North 4442, New Zealand
3   High Value Nutrition, National Science Challenge, Liggins Institute, The University of Auckland,
    Auckland 1142, New Zealand
4   Bioinformatics and Statistics, AgResearch, Grasslands Research Centre, Palmerston North 4442,
    New Zealand; catherine.mckenzie@agresearch.co.nz
5   Fonterra Co-Operative Group, Palmerston North 4442, New Zealand; neill.haggarty@fonterra.com
*   Correspondence: julie.dalziel@agresearch.co.nz; Tel.: +64-6-351-8098

Received: 9 November 2017; Accepted: 7 December 2017; Published: 13 December 2017

Abstract: Little is known about how milk proteins affect gastrointestinal (GI) transit, particularly for the elderly, in whom digestion has been observed to be slowed. We tested the hypothesis that GI transit is faster for whey than for casein and that this effect is accentuated with hydrolysates, similar to soy. Adult male rats (18 months old) were fed native whey or casein, hydrolyzed whey (WPH) or casein (CPH), hydrolyzed blend (HB; 60% whey:40% casein), or hydrolyzed soy for 14 days then treated with loperamide, prucalopride, or vehicle-control for 7 days. X-ray imaging tracked bead-transit for: gastric emptying (GE; 4 h), small intestine (SI) transit (9 h), and large intestine (LI) transit (12 h). GE for whey was 33 ± 12% faster than that for either casein or CPH. SI transit was decreased by 37 ± 9% for casein and 24 ± 6% for whey compared with hydrolyzed soy, and persisted for casein at 12 h. Although CPH and WPH did not alter transit compared with their respective intact counterparts, fecal output was increased by WPH. Slowed transit by casein was reversed by prucalopride (9-h), but not loperamide. However, rapid GE and slower SI transit for the HB compared with intact forms were inhibited by loperamide. The expected slower GI transit for casein relative to soy provided a comparative benchmark, and opioid receptor involvement was corroborated. Our findings provide new evidence that whey slowed SI transit compared with soy, independent of GE. Increased GI transit from stomach to colon for the HB compared with casein suggests that including hydrolyzed milk proteins in foods may benefit those with slowed intestinal transit.

Keywords: colon; fecal output; motility; opioid; serotonin; elderly

1. Introduction

Milk is a widely consumed natural beverage renowned as a nutritious protein source [1]. Research has revealed additional health properties that may be conferred via the pharmacological actions of digested milk peptides on cardiovascular function, regulation of food intake, and metabolism [2–4]. Milk proteins make up 3.5% of cows' milk, consisting of 80% caseins and 20% whey proteins [5]. Casein and whey are used in different food products for specific uses; for example, casein is the major component of cheese. Whey protein in the concentrated form is used as a dietary supplement for those needing an easily digestible nutritious protein source including, the elderly, infants, and athletes.

During gastrointestinal (GI) digestion, the behaviour of milk proteins differs, with casein considered as a slowly digestible protein and whey a rapidly digestible protein [6]. Whey is rapidly expelled from the stomach, whereas caseins precipitate in the low pH of the stomach and coagulate, slowing gastric emptying (GE). Size, structure, and solubility of casein micelles in the stomach affect digestibility and alter GI transit. Although casein has long been known to slow both GE (due to curd formation) and small intestinal (SI) transit, these effects may be altered by specific hydrolysis methods. Casein is a rich source of peptides released upon hydrolysis or during GI digestion that include angiotensin-converting enzyme inhibitors, opioids, and antimicrobial peptides [2]. Some of these peptides have been shown to affect GI transit (due to the presence of opioid peptides) [7–9]. Modulation of GI transit rate by peptides has the potential for functional benefits through slower small intestine transit, allowing greater absorption time for nutrients, or increased transit to reduce constipation.

The effect of the hydrolysis of dairy proteins on GI motility to influence the transit of contents is not well understood. By determining how hydrolysis of different types of dairy protein affects GE and GI transit will provide better information on health effects of potential functional foods. A number of GI disorders that affect gastric and colonic motility occur more frequently in the aging population [10], including slowed gastric emptying [11] and constipation [12,13]. Slowed gastric emptying with aging can affect regulation of appetite, postprandial glycemia, and blood pressure [11]. More generally, delayed GE can result in early satiety, bloating, pain or discomfort, malnutrition, and weight loss [14,15]. Functional dairy foods may assist self-management of mild dysmotility, as occurs in functional gastrointestinal disorders, to increase or decrease transit of intestinal contents. For example, in the elderly, slower small intestine transit might assist nutrient uptake, whereas faster colonic transit may help reduce constipation.

While whey reaches the jejunum faster than casein, hydrolysis is slower, which is thought to allow for greater absorption over the length of the SI [16]. Whether this is due to increased digestibility of whey or slower for casein GE is unknown [17]. The ability of whey to alter transit throughout the GI tract is also less understood than for casein. Whey protein hydrolysate (WPH) protein has a nutritionally available amino acid composition. Both WPH and intact whey are used as protein supplements for the elderly. This is because whey affects a range of biological processes associated with aging in humans: antimicrobial activity, immune modulation, improved muscle strength and body composition [18], as well as protection against cardiovascular disease, osteoporosis, cancer, hypertension. It also has cholesterol-lowering and mood-enhancing properties [2,16,19–21]. Despite the widespread use of whey and casein milk proteins, studies directly comparing the effect of their hydrolysis on GI transit and their modes of action via receptor pathways with aging are lacking.

Because composition and processing of milk proteins has an impact on their digestion and absorption [22–24], combining specific milk protein components provides a way to potentially maximize benefits for digestive health. In addition, milk proteins are digested during the various stages of human GI tract digestion to give rise to an array of peptides that can elicit a variety of physiologic effects that affect the rate of digestion and transit for casein and whey proteins [2,22,25,26]. Some of these peptides modulate opioid [26–29] or serotonin receptors [30]. Whey supplementation may confer benefits for modulation of GI motility in the elderly. As an example, slowed GI transit resulting in constipation affects 25–30% of people over 65 years of age [12,13], and foods which target this will be of considerable benefit. Because large intestine (LI) transit is slower in aged than in young [31,32] rats, they are used as a model for mature to elderly humans. Gastric emptying also slows with age in rats [33,34], which matches the changes that occur in elderly humans [10,35].

The aim of this study was to investigate how whey and casein milk proteins affect GE and GI transit in an aged rat model [36] and whether this differs when the proteins are pre-hydrolyzed. We hypothesized that GI transit is faster in response to whey than for casein, and that this effect is enhanced with hydrolyzates. We therefore compared the effect of casein, whey, CPH, and WPH, on the rate of GI transit of solids in an aged rat model, using hydrolyzed soy as an example of rapid transit and intact casein an example of slow transit. We also wanted to compare casein and whey with their hydrolyzed counterparts, CPH and WPH, as protein sources to discriminate GE and GI transit differences. We also compared a combination formula composed of partially hydrolyzed 60:40 whey/casein, renowned for its nutritional properties and ease of digestion, to determine its potential as a supplement for the elderly by investigating its actions on GI transit [37]. We also wanted to determine whether casein would slow GE and GI transit in this model as expected and therefore provide a benchmark for measuring other milk proteins in this aged animal model.

The ability of specific modulators to reduce the transit changes induced by the milk proteins was investigated using loperamide (a mu opioid agonist which inhibits GI transit) and prucalopride (a serotonin type 4 receptor agonist which increases GE and colonic transit) [36]. This was to show whether any milk-protein-induced changes detected for GI transit were reversible and to suggest the neural pathways involved.

Rats were the animal model of choice because many dietary preclinical studies are done in this species and pharmacological modulatory doses have been determined [36]. To track the transit of solid contents along the GI tract, we measured the movement of six metallic beads over 12 h from the stomach to the large intestine by high resolution X-ray imaging [36,38]. This technique utilises a barium slurry providing a mix of solid and semi-solid gastric contents, similar to human measurement techniques [15]. This method using metallic beads as markers for transit of solid contents has been validated in two previous studies in which the beads were found in the fecal pellets [36,38].

2. Materials and Methods

2.1. Animals

This study was conducted following ethical approval (AE12933) by the AgResearch Grasslands Animal Ethics Committee (Palmerston North, New Zealand (NZ)) in accordance with the Animal Welfare Act, 1999 (NZ). Male Sprague Dawley rats were bred at the AgResearch Ruakura Small Animal Unit (Hamilton, New Zealand) and raised in group housing with littermates to 18 months of age (804 ± 13 g). The animals were housed at a constant temperature of 21 °C and maintained under a light/dark cycle (06:00/18:00) in sawdust-lined plastic or stainless steel cages, with food and water provided ad libitum. They were fed a normal rat chow pellet soy-based diet (Prolab® RMH 1800, LabDiet, St. Louis, MO, USA) until seven days prior to the study when they were individually caged and switched to a hydrolyzed soy-based diet (OpenStandard Rodent Diet, Research Diets, Inc., New Brunswick, NJ, USA) in powdered form, for compatibility with metabolic cage requirements. The animals were monitored three times weekly for weight, food intake, and General Health Score (1–5; NZ Animal Health Care Standard). Cages and feeding and drinking containers were cleaned and sterilized weekly. Twenty-eight out of 226 rats were excluded from the study and euthanized due to age-related health issues including: weight loss, lethargy, excessive drinking, swollen or inflamed tissue not cured with antibiotic treatment, or invasive tumours. At the end of the study, all remaining rats were euthanized using carbon dioxide inhalation overdose.

2.2. Study Design

This study was designed to include one control group and five test diet treatment groups that were also treated with modulatory drugs, either 4 mg/kg/day prucalopride or 1 mg/kg/day loperamide or dimethyl sulfoxide (DMSO) control carrier (Figure 1). The study was carried out as a block design as six blocks of ~36 animals, with age and weight balanced among treatment groups (i.e., 18 groups × 12 animals per group), which resulted in 9–13 animals for each diet plus the drug treatment group.

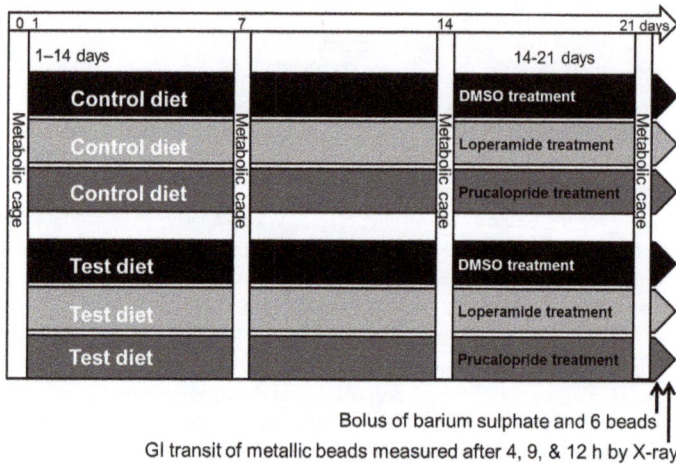

Figure 1. Study design shown for the dietary control (hydrolyzed soy) and one of the five milk protein test diets. GI, gastrointestinal; DMSO, dimethyl sulfoxide.

The drug doses were previously determined to be effective over seven days [36]. Rats were fed the powdered treatment diet for three weeks (day 0 to day 22) and treated with modulatory drugs over the third week (days 15–22). Four days prior to the start of the study, the rats were acclimatized to metabolic cages for 1 h to reduce possible stress symptoms. Rats were individually placed in metabolic cages for 24 h (from 10 am to 10 am) on days 0, 7, 14, and 21, after which food intake and fecal and urine output, were measured.

2.3. Dietary Protein

Milk proteins were provided by Fonterra Co-operative Group. Animals were treated with diets in which protein was 20% of the diet (energy) provided as hydrolyzed soy for the control treatment group, and the following milk protein products for the five test diet treatment groups: casein (sodium caseinate 1800), whey (lactic whey protein concentrate WPC7009), partially hydrolyzed CPH (MPH948, degree of hydrolysis (DH) 7.6%), partially hydrolyzed WPH (WPH917, DH 5.0%), partially hydrolyzed HB of 60:40 whey/casein (MPH942, DH 12–17%). The protein was added to a nutritionally balanced protein-free base diet (OpenStandard Modified Rodent Diet, Research Diets, Inc. New Brunswick, NJ, USA) of final composition (kcal %): 15% fat (soybean oil), 65% carbohydrate (cornstarch, maltodextrin 10, dextrose), cellulose, BW200, inulin, minerals, and vitamins.

2.4. Pharmacological Treatments

Loperamide hydrochloride (S2480) and prucalopride (S2875) were from Selleck Chemicals (Houston, TX, USA). Animals were administered 4 mg/kg/day prucalopride or 1 mg/kg/day loperamide (in 100% DMSO) or DMSO vehicle only (control) for seven days via a subcutaneous 2 mL capacity slow release osmotic mini-pump (Durect Corporation, Alzet Osmotic Pumps, Cupertino, CA, USA), while controls received DMSO vehicle only via the same delivery method. The surgical implantation procedure has been described previously [36]. Continuous dosing overcame rapid metabolism of prucalopride in rats [39] and avoided frequent subcutaneous injections for loperamide (half-life 9–14 h). Each compound was dissolved in DMSO to give stocks of 20 mg/mL that were diluted in DMSO to give the correct concentration in the mini-pump to deliver the appropriate dose per weight of rat at a flow rate of 10 µL/h.

2.5. GI transit Procedures and Measurements

Non-fasted rats were used to maintain normal digestion and transit, and to avoid retention of beads in the stomach as has been reported for solid capsules in fasted rats [40]. The methods used for measuring GI transit have been described previously [36,38]. Briefly, each rat received six solid stainless steel beads, d = 1.4 mm (Bal-tec, Los Angeles, CA, USA), via oral gavage in 2 mL of 15% barium sulfate (E-Z-HD 98% *w/w*, Cat. No. 764, E-Z-EM Canada Inc., provided by Palmerston North Hospital, Palmerston North, New Zealand). Isoflurane anesthesia was induced in a chamber and persisted for 5 min, during which gavage was performed upon recovery of the swallow reflex.

2.5.1. X-ray Imaging

GI transit was tracked at three time points by X-ray imaging under brief isoflurane anesthesia to monitor: exit from stomach (4 h), SI transit (9 h), and LI transit (12 h). The 12 h time point was carried out post-mortem. The metallic beads were visualized by X-ray and the relatively opaque barium sulfate outlined the GI, enabling identification of bead location. Ventral and right lateral views were taken using a portable X-ray unit (Porta 100 HF 2.0 kW High Frequency, Job Corporation, Yokohama, Japan) including: camera and digital cassette (Canon 55G DR sensor panel, Melville, NY, USA) in conjunction with a laptop computer (Lenovo ThinkPad W530, Morrisville, NC, USA). Image files (DICOM) were visualized using MicroDicom DICOM Viewer v8.7 (Simeon Antonov Stoykov, Sofia, Bulgaria).

2.5.2. Gastric Emptying

Comparative measures of GE were obtained by determining the proportion of animals in which all six beads had exited the stomach for a given treatment over time.

2.5.3. GI transit Score

The rating scale used to classify GI bead location comprised six beads, each given a numeric score depending on its location within the GI tract: (0) stomach; (1) proximal SI; (2) distal SI; (3) cecum; (4) colon; or (5) expelled. The total transit score was the sum of the individual bead scores (maximum = 30 if all expelled). The experimenter was blinded to treatment. A transit score of 3–4 means that on average half of the beads were in the proximal SI. Scores of 10–14 place most of the beads in the distal SI, whereas 16–20 places most in the cecum and 20–22 places half of them as distal as the colon [36,38].

2.5.4. Colonic Transit

The number of beads per rat that had moved from the cecum to the colon or rectum over 3 h was compared. The movement of beads between 9 h (when the majority were in the cecum or distal SI) and 12 h (when a proportion had moved to the colon or rectum) was measured to assess possible differences between treatments in the probability that a bead had transited into the colon by 12 h.

2.5.5. Bead Transit through Colon

The average bead distance travelled along the colon for the beads that had transited from the cecum to the colon over 9–12 h was calculated as a percent of the LI length from the cecum or colon junction to the anus.

2.6. Statistical Analysis

All analyses were carried out using GenStat version 17 (VSN International Limited, Hemel Hempstead, UK) or Minitab 17 Statistical software (Minitab Inc., State College, PA, USA). Results are expressed as the mean ± standard error of the mean (SEM).

2.6.1. Animal Metrics

Data were analysed using a Linear Mixed Model via restricted maximum likelihood (REML) for the effect of 14 days of diet treatment only on the difference in the response variable of interest (weight, feed intake, urine output, or fecal output) between day 0 (pretreatment) and day 14 (prior to commencement of pharmacological treatments). To compare among all diet × drug treatments, data were analysed using a Linear Mixed Model (via REML) for the response variable of interest (weight, feed intake, urine output, or fecal output) on day 21, using treatment as factor (18 combinations of drug and diet) and the relevant value on day 14 as covariate. Fisher's least significant differences were used for the post hoc test.

2.6.2. Transit from Stomach

Logistic regression analyses were carried out at each time point (4, 9, and 12 h) using treatment as the factor, separately to compare differences in the proportion of rats with zero beads in the stomach (0/1).

2.6.3. Transit Score

Changes in GI transit were measured relative to the DMSO/control-treated rats. Due to the expected correlated nature of the data, a linear mixed model (via REML) using drug treatment and diet as factors was used to analyze the data. Fisher's least significant differences were used for the post hoc test.

2.6.4. Cecum to Colon Transit

Differences in cecum to colon transit were compared using a linear mixed model (via REML) using treatment as factor (18 combinations of drug and diet) and Fisher's least significant difference post hoc test.

2.6.5. Bead Transit through Colon

Differences in percent distance of bead transit through the colon were compared using a linear mixed model (via REML) using treatment as factor (18 combinations of drug and diet) and Fisher's least significant difference post hoc test.

3. Results

3.1. Dietary Effects

Changes in animal metrics are summarized in Table 1.

Table 1. Animal food intake and fecal output.

Protein	Food Intake (g)	*n*	Fecal Output (g)	*n*
Control				
Hydrolyzed soy	23.5 ± 2.0 [a]	16	3.3 ± 0.6 [a]	15
Casein	21.8 ± 1.8	10	3.9 ± 0.4	10
Whey	22.2 ± 1.8	10	3.5 ± 0.4 [b] [(*a)]	10
CPH	22.4 ± 1.8 [b]	9	2.8 ± 0.4 [c]	8
WPH	24.5 ± 1.8 [c]	9	4.9 ± 0.4 [d] [(**a)] [(*b)] [(**c)]	9
HB	25.5 ± 1.8 [d]	9	4.3 ± 0.4 [e] [(*c)]	9

Table 1. *Cont.*

Protein	Food Intake (g)	n	Fecal Output (g)	n
Loperamide				
Hydrolyzed soy	20.0 ± 1.8 (*a)	15	2.9 ± 0.4	15
Casein	20.4 ± 1.8	9	3.1 ± 0.4	9
Whey	19.5 ± 1.8 (*a)	12	2.2 ± 0.4 (*a) (*b)	12
CPH	18.2 ± 1.8 (**a) (*b)	9	2.7 ± 0.4	9
WPH	18.4 ± 1.8 (***a) (***c)	11	3.2 ± 0.5 (**d)	11
HB	20.4 ± 1.8 (**d)	9	3.0 ± 0.5 (*e)	9
Prucalopride				
Hydrolyzed soy	24.1 ± 1.8	15	3.6 ± 0.4 f	15
Casein	21.3 ± 1.5	7	3.5 ± 0.4	7
Whey	23.6 ± 1.8	8	3.7 ± 0.4	8
CPH	23.6 ± 1.8	8	4.1 ± 0.4 (*c)	8
WPH	22.8 ± 1.8	7	4.1 ± 0.3	5
HB	23.2 ± 1.8	8	4.8 ± 0.4 (*f)	8

Data shown after 21 days on protein diet with drug treatment over last 7 days. CPH, casein protein hydrolysate; WPH, whey protein hydrolysate; HB, 60:40 whey/casein hydrolyzed blend. Data show mean ± SEM. Asterisks in brackets indicate statistical significance (* $p < 0.05$, ** $p < 0.01$, *** $p < 0.001$) of the differences among diet and drug treatments compared with those indicated by the superscript letters.

3.1.1. Body Weight

No physiologically significant differences in body weight (more than 10% difference) occurred from that of 818 ± 14 g on the hydrolyzed soy diet ($n = 50$) between days 0 and 14. However, body weight decreased by 2.2% (18 g) on the casein diet, $p < 0.01$, although only a small change is notable for aged rats where body weight among the other diets varied by less than 1%.

3.1.2. Food Intake

When on the control hydrolyzed soy diet (day 14), food intake was 26.4 ± 0.7 g/day ($n = 50$). When pre-treatment food intake was compared between days 0 and 14 on the test diets, intake of the casein diet was 11.4% less than the hydrolyzed soy control and less than all the other diets ($p < 0.05$). However, this effect was not detected by day 21.

3.1.3. Fecal Output

Fecal output was not altered between days 0 and 14 on the test diets. By 21 days for control animals receiving DMSO treatment, however, fecal output for WPH was increased by: 50.3% compared with the hydrolyzed soy diet, 42.0% compared with the whey diet, and 74.1% compared with the CPH diet. Fecal output for the HB was increased by 51.0% compared with CPH.

3.1.4. Urine Output

No differences in urine output were detected with any diet × drug treatment between days 0 and 14.

3.2. Pharmacological Modulation of Dietary Effects

To determine the effect of the pharmacological treatments on food intake, this was compared among treatments at day 21 (Table 1).

3.2.1. Food Intake

Loperamide reduced food intake by 15.1% on the hydrolyzed soy diet, by 25.0% on the WPH diet, and by 20.2% on the HB diet, by 18.6% on the CPH diet.

3.2.2. Fecal Output

Loperamide did not alter fecal output on the hydrolyzed soy diet. Loperamide reduced fecal output for WPH by 34.7%. Loperamide reduced fecal output for the whey diet by 35.5% and reduced that for the HB diet by 29.9%. For animals on the CPH diet, prucalopride increased fecal output by 45.4%. It is notable that for animals receiving prucalopride treatment, fecal output was increased for animals on the HB diet by 32.0% compared with those on hydrolyzed soy (also receiving prucalopride).

Twenty-one animals across 14 of the 18 treatment groups (21/198) were excluded from further analysis because no meaningful transit measurements were possible due to GE being substantially delayed over 12 h, as previously reported to occur in 10% of animals using this method [36]. Notably, 13 animals across all loperamide treatment groups were affected but only five were DMSO treated and three were prucalopride-treated animals.

3.3. Dietary Effects on Bead Transit (DMSO/Control Treated)

3.3.1. Gastric Emptying

For DMSO/control-treated animals on the hydrolyzed soy diet, all beads had exited the stomach in 7% of animals at 4 h post-gavage, 64% at 9 h, and 80% at 12 h (Figures 2 and 3). At 4 h, any delays in GE would be evident. For the casein and CPH, beads remained in the stomach of most animals, indicating a prolonged delay in GE. In contrast, GE at 4 h was 33% more likely to have occurred for whey than for either casein or CPH, yet was similar by 9 h. At 9 h, GE was increased for the HB by 116% compared with casein, 230% compared with CPH, and 80% compared with whey. An 80% difference persisted at 12 h between the HB and casein only. Thus the effect of the proteins on GE may be approximately ranked from rapid to the most delayed: whey > HB > (WPH = hydrolyzed soy) > (casein = CPH).

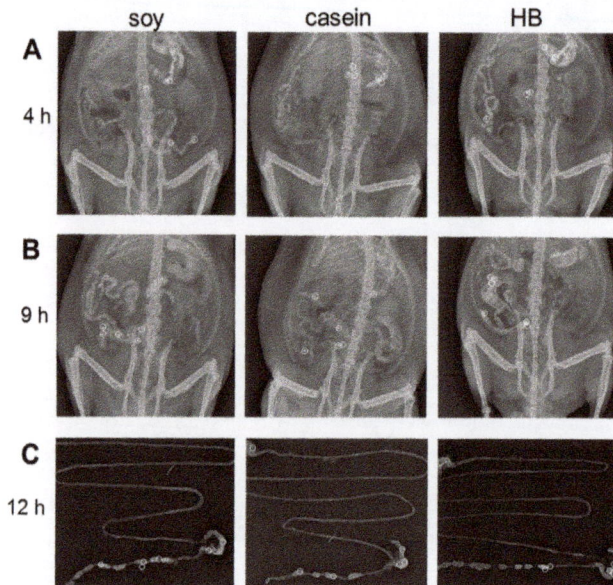

Figure 2. Location of six metallic beads tracked over time for animals treated for soy or milk protein diets. Representative examples of bead location are shown at: (**A,B**) 4 h and 9 h in vivo and (**C**) post-mortem GI tract at 12 h of X-ray images in ventral view for animals on soy, casein, and hydrolyzed blend (HB) diets (treated with DMSO).

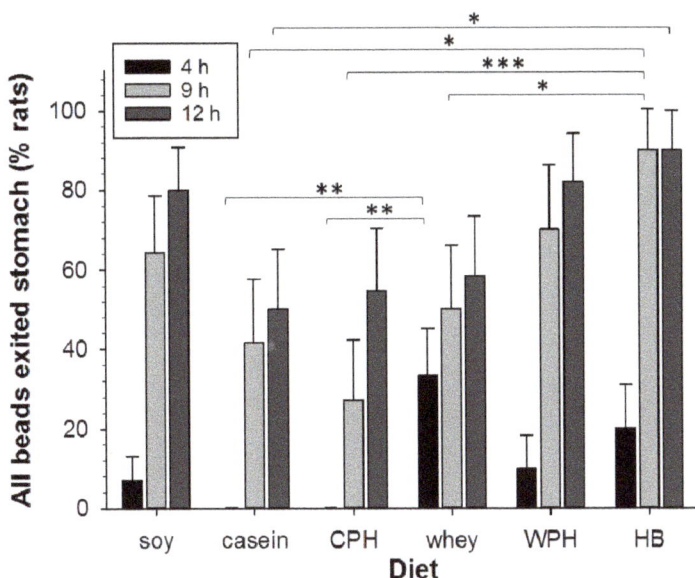

Figure 3. Comparison of gastric emptying (GE) of beads over 12 h for animals treated with soy or milk protein diets (n = 8–15 animals per group). The percentage of rats in which all beads had exited the stomach (mean per treatment) is shown at 4 h (black), 9 h (light grey), and 12 h (dark grey) for: soy, casein, hydrolyzed casein (CPH), whey, hydrolyzed whey (WPH), and hydrolyzed blend (HB). Asterisks indicate the significance of each treatment relative to controls (* $p < 0.05$; ** $p < 0.01$; *** $p < 0.001$). Data show mean ± SEM.

3.3.2. GI Transit

At 9 h, the transit score was decreased by 37% for casein and decreased by 24% for whey compared with hydrolyzed soy, and a 22% difference persisted at 12 h for casein but not whey (Figure 4). CPH and WPH did not alter transit compared with their intact protein counterparts, respectively. However, when casein was used as a benchmark, transit at 9 h was increased by 55% for WPH and 68% for the HB. Transit for the HB was increased by 38% compared with whey at 9 h. The effect of the proteins on transit score at 9 h may be approximately grouped and ranked from rapid to slowest transit: (hydrolyzed soy = HB = WPH) ≥ CPH ≥ (whey = casein). Similar to our previous studies, the beads were always found in fecal pellets, providing further validation for this method in monitoring GI transit of solids [36,38].

3.3.3. Caecum to Colon Transit

Bead movement from the cecum at 9 h to the colon at 12 h was compared and no significant differences found. Once in the colon, the percent bead distance travelled along the colon for the beads that had transited from cecum to colon by 12 h did not reveal any diet effect.

3.3.4. Pharmacological Modulation of Bead Transit

GE for the DMSO–hydrolyzed soy diet was not altered by the pharmacological modulators (Figure 5A). Transit was slowed by loperamide for the DMSO–hydrolyzed soy control diet treatments at 9 h and 12 h (Figure 5B). Slowing of GI transit for casein was reversed by prucalopride (9 h), but slowing for whey was not affected by prucalopride. Loperamide affected transit for neither casein nor whey treatment conditions. Rapid GE for the HB (9 h and 12 h) was slowed 80–90% by loperamide

(Figure 5A). Furthermore, the relatively shorter transit (9 h) for the HB compared with the intact proteins was also inhibited by loperamide (Figure 5B). No significant drug effects were detected for cecum to colon transit. The modulatory drugs did not alter bead transit through the colon on any of the diets.

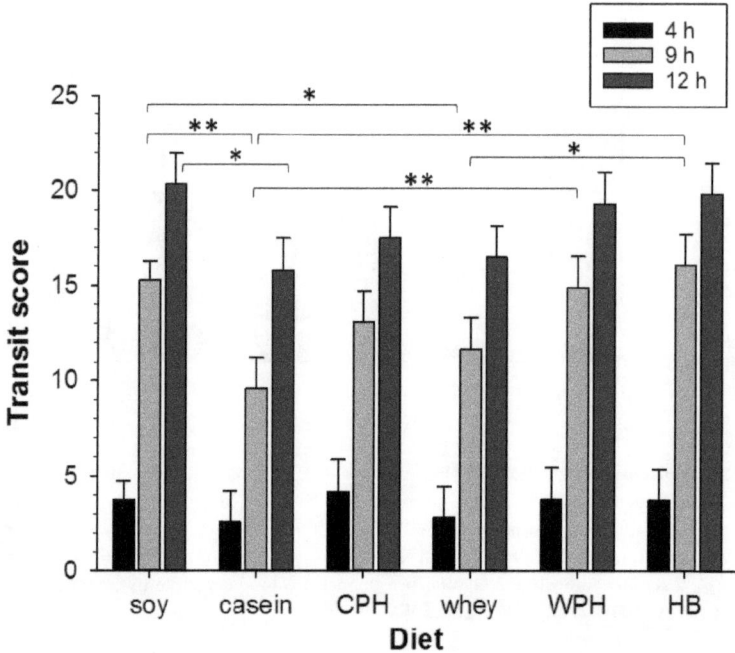

Figure 4. Comparison of GI transit tracked over 12 h for animals treated with soy or milk protein diets (*n* = 1–14 animals per group). Transit scores are shown at 4 h (black), 9 h (light grey), and 12 h (dark grey) for: soy, casein, hydrolyzed casein (CPH), whey, hydrolyzed whey (WPH), and hydrolyzed blend (HB). Asterisks indicate the significance of each treatment relative to controls (* $p < 0.05$; ** $p < 0.01$). Data show mean ± SEM.

Overall changes in movement of GI contents induced by the dietary and pharmacological treatments are summarized in Table 2.

Table 2. Summary of altered GI function.

Protein	GE	SI Transit	LI Transit	Fecal Output
Hydrolyzed soy	fast	fast (↓LP)	fast (↓LP)	ND
Casein	slow	slow (↑PC)	slow	ND
Whey	>casein	<soy	mid	(↓LP)
CPH	slow	mid (↓LP)	mid	(↑PC)
WPH	fast	fast (↓LP)	fast (↓LP)	>whey & soy (↓LP)
HB	fast	fast (↓LP)	fast (↓LP)	>CPH

GI, gastrointestinal; GE, gastric emptying; SI, small intestine; LI, large intestine; CPH, casein protein hydrolysate; WPH, whey protein hydrolysate; HB, 60:40 whey–casein hydrolyzed blend; LP, loperamide; PC, prucalopride; ↓, slowed by; ↑, accelerated by; ND, not determined.

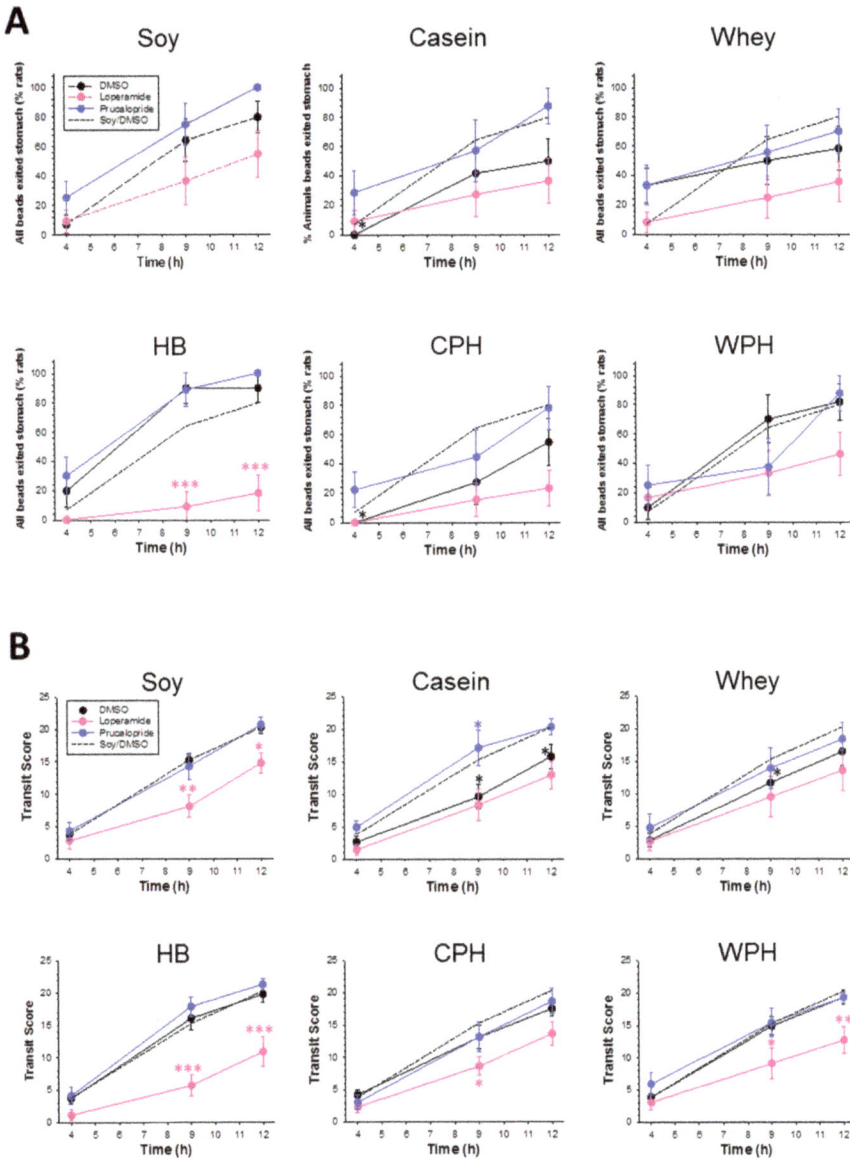

Figure 5. Effect of pharmacological modulators on dietary changes in GE and GI transit for animals treated with soy or milk protein diets. (**A**) The percentage of rats in which all beads had exited the stomach, and (**B**) transit scores for: soy, casein, hydrolyzed casein (CPH), whey, hydrolyzed whey (WPH), and hydrolyzed blend (HB). Asterisks indicate the significance of each treatment relative to controls (* $p < 0.05$; ** $p < 0.01$; *** $p < 0.001$). Data show mean ± SEM.

4. Discussion

The initial finding of this study was that casein (intact) slowed GI transit compared with hydrolyzed soy, as expected, and set a comparative benchmark with the other milk proteins.

The slowed GI transit by casein can be largely attributed to delayed GE. The slowed GI transit for whey, however, was not due to delayed GE but rather is likely to be localised to slower bead movement through the SI. Contrary to our hypothesis, CPH and WPH proteins did not reduce GI transit time relative to their intact counterparts (or hydrolyzed soy) and once in the colon, the transit was not different from the other proteins studied.

4.1. Hydrolyzed Soy Protein

GE and GI transit and fecal output measurements for the hydrolyzed soy treatment were similar to those previously reported using this method in aged rats [36]. Because loperamide was effective at inhibiting GI transit, this suggested that mu opioid receptors were available, arguing against any dietary soymorphins specific to these receptors having a strong inhibitory influence on motility. The corresponding decrease in food intake detected for soy by loperamide was also reported previously [36].

4.2. Casein Protein

Delayed GE of solids and SI transit for casein compared with hydrolyzed soy is consistent with a previous rat study on the effect of casein relative to soy protein isolate on transit of the liquid phase of chime, in which GE was slowed at 1 h and SI transit slower after a further h [41]. Our finding that GE is slower for casein than for whey or WPH is consistent with decreased food intake on the casein diet (at 14 days) compared with the other diets.

Reversal of slowed GI transit for casein (compared with soy) by prucalopride suggests that peptides with pharmacological actions are present in the casein and that these likely inhibited neural control of GI motility. Because transit by casein was not further inhibited by loperamide, this implicates endogenous opioid agonist peptides such as the β-casomorphins in the slower SI and LI transit with casein (compared with soy). Such peptides would have been released from the casein during gastric digestion and might therefore also have contributed to the delayed GE for casein. The decrease in food intake could be due to delayed GE or opioid antagonist peptide release during digestion [42,43].

4.3. Whey Protein

The GE of solids for whey was markedly faster than for casein, but SI transit was slower for whey than that for either hydrolyzed soy or the HB. The relatively slower GI transit for whey was therefore not due to delayed GE as for casein, but rather was localised to the SI. This provides new evidence that whey did in fact slow SI transit compared with casein and demonstrates this as independent from GE.

The lower GI effect of loperamide in decreasing fecal output indicates that an opioid agonist was able to slow fecal movement for whey in the distal colon–rectum region. It is possible that the altered fecal output by loperamide for whey in vivo involved additional effects on fluid and electrolyte secretion [44].

4.4. Hydrolyzed Casein

Similarly to casein, GE was also slowed for CPH. This may be attributed to it only being 7.6% hydrolyzed such that significant peptide release could still occur during digestion. GI transit was not altered by CPH, compared with soy or casein, but unlike casein, loperamide was effective at inhibiting GI transit for animals fed the CPH diet. This suggests that the CPH lacked sufficient opioid agonist activity to significantly slow transit. This was likely due to the partial hydrolysis used to generate the CPH, resulting in partial release of some small peptides (e.g., opioid agonist) that are then lost during processing. The remaining peptides released during digestion would then be insufficient to elicit a significant transit slowing effect. Although hydrolysis of the casein protein did not increase GE or GI transit compared with the casein overall, prucalopride increased fecal output, suggesting that it had been slowed on this diet in the distal colon–rectum region. The ability of the serotonin agonist to further increase fecal output suggests that it reversed a partial inhibitory effect of the CPH on colonic motility. Our results differ from those previously reported for CPH (DH 27%), in which hydrolysis increases transit compared with casein in rats [8], although trended similarly over 12 h. The degree of casein hydrolysis was positively associated with slowed GI transit. CPH is considered a rich source of opioid receptor ligands, in particular the beta casomorphins which activate the mu receptor [45], slowing GI transit in the rat compared with whey [7]. However, an effect of hydrolysis on GE and transit in our study was not detected under normal conditions. However, when challenged using pharmacological modulators, differences in responsiveness to these became evident, suggesting different bioactive peptides between the two casein forms. This suggests that during digestion, peptides with mu opioid receptor activity were released from casein, but fewer from CPH.

4.5. Hydrolyzed Whey

GE and GI transit effects of WPH were similar to those for hydrolyzed soy, rather than being slowed as for casein. No delay in GE occurred as a result of whey hydrolysis. This is consistent with the knowledge that casein aggregates in the stomach where it is digested by physiological enzymes, whereas being soluble proteins, whey and soy pass rapidly through the stomach and undergo digestion by pancreatic enzymes [3].

Despite the apparent similarity between GI transit effects of the WPH diet compared with soy, fecal output was increased compared with soy (and native whey). There was no corresponding increase in food intake for whey, possibly due to the short term satiating effect attributed to whey proteins in some studies [46]. Taken together, the rapid GE and increased fecal output in response to WPH suggest that this would be a useful ingredient in a functional food or beverage for the elderly to enhance GE and reduce constipation.

Loperamide was effective at inhibiting overall GI transit only if the whey was hydrolyzed. This suggests that the WPH lacked mu opioid agonist activity to inhibit transit. Loperamide did however decrease fecal output to a similar extent for both intact and WPH forms (both by 35%). The effect on fecal output being common to both forms of whey suggests an alternative mechanism was involved, probably localised to the rectum.

4.6. Hydrolyzed Whey–Casein Blend

The HB produced the most rapid GI transit of the milk proteins studied with rapid GE a contributing factor. This is consistent with these proteins having undergone a greater degree of hydrolysis compared with CPH and WPH. The HB was similar to soy in transit attributes imparted, in particular that both had increased SI transit compared with casein (and whey). The rapid SI transit rate and increased fecal output (compared with CPH) attributes of the WPH component appear to dominate. We recognise that this might also be due to relative higher level of hydrolysis for the HB. Relative to casein, the HB produced the greatest increase in transit through the SI of the proteins studied, an effect partly attributed to more complete GE. Our results suggest that the HB might also be a useful ingredient in a functional food or beverage for the elderly to enhance GE, which can slow with healthy aging [11].

Our findings agree with a study in which a partially hydrolyzed 60:40 whey–casein-based formulae accelerated transit of milk and stools compared with its non-hydrolyzed cow milk protein counterpart [9].

4.7. Modulators and Mechanisms

All three hydrolyzed ingredients studied were sensitive to opioid agonist modulation in slowing transit. This suggests that they either do not contain significant milk-derived opioid peptide concentration or contain alternate components that speed transit. The heightened sensitivity of HB-fed rats to a mu opioid agonist suggests that milk-derived opioid peptides that inhibit GI transit via the mu opioid receptor are not present in significant amounts. The greater degree of hydrolysis for the whey and casein in the blend compared with the CPH or WPH means that different peptides are likely present that confer pro-motility actions. These findings are consistent with the idea that industrial hydrolysis of milk proteins precludes subsequent release of peptides that occurs during the normal digestive process in the GI tract [17].

The shortened GI transit for the HB suggests absence of motility slowing peptides possibly together with additive pro-motility actions of peptides in the mixture. This is supported by the greater fecal output for the HB compared with soy when both received prucalopride treatment. In contrast, casein was sensitive to a serotonin agonist (5-HT$_4$) in reversing the slowed transit.

5. Conclusions

In summary, the expected slower GI transit for casein relative to hydrolyzed soy provided a comparative benchmark. Lack of loperamide modulation of the slowed casein effect corroborated opioid agonist activity for casein peptides in the SI. Reversal of the casein-induced slow transit by prucalopride showed that a 5-HT$_4$ agonist could counter this effect. Our findings provide new evidence that whey protein slows SI transit compared with hydrolyzed soy and indicate that this is independent of GE. This suggests that whey protein may slow small intestine transit to allow time for increased nutrient absorption to occur without slowing GE, which would be helpful for improved nutrition in the elderly. Further studies would be required to verify whether nutrient uptake has been affected. Despite the inability of the CPH or WPH to shorten transit compared with their intact counterparts, fecal output was increased upon whey hydrolysis. Furthermore, opioid agonist inhibition of transit on CPH or WPH diets suggests little opioid agonist activity by peptides in these hydrolysates. The increased the rate of GI transit from stomach to colon relative to casein by WPH and the HB suggests that their incorporation in dairy formulations may be beneficial in treating functional GI disorders involving constipation, particularly for the aged.

Acknowledgments: This research was supported by funding from the Ministry of Business Innovation and Employment, New Zealand (C10X1003), with co-funding from Fonterra Co-operative Group Ltd. We thank the following AgResearch staff for their assistance: L.J. Ryan, K.E. Dunstan, and S.E. Burton for carrying out the animal study and J.S. Peters for technical assistance, R. Broadhurst and B. Smith for animal breeding, H. Gillespie and M. McArthur for animal care, and I. Steffert for veterinary advice. We thank N. Moffatt and L.M. Shaw for carrying out the X-rays (Institute of Veterinary, Animal and Biomedical Sciences, Massey University, Palmerston North, New Zealand).

Author Contributions: J.E.D. analysed the data, interpreted the results and wrote the paper; W.Y. contributed to animal study design and analysis; C.M.M. contributed statistical design and analysis; J.E.D., W.Y., N.W.H. and N.C.R. designed the study and critically revised the manuscript.

Conflicts of Interest: The authors declare no conflict of interest. All authors had complete access to the data that supports the publication. N.W.H. is an employee of Fonterra Co-operative Group Ltd. who provided the milk protein ingredients and partially funded the research.

References

1. Visioli, F.; Strata, A. Milk, dairy products, and their functional effects in humans: A narrative review of recent evidence. *Adv. Nutr.* **2014**, *5*, 131–143. [CrossRef] [PubMed]
2. Boutrou, R.; Henry, G.; Sanchez-Rivera, L. On the trail of milk bioactive peptides in human and animal intestinal tracts during digestion: A review. *Dairy Sci. Technol.* **2015**, *95*, 815–829. [CrossRef]
3. Jahan-Mihan, A.; Luhovyy, B.L.; Khoury, D.E.; Harvey Anderson, G. Dietary proteins as determinants of metabolic and physiologic functions of the gastrointestinal tract. *Nutrients* **2011**, *3*, 574–603. [CrossRef] [PubMed]
4. Nongonierma, A.B.; FitzGerald, R.J. The scientific evidence for the role of milk protein-derived bioactive peptides in humans: A review. *J. Funct. Foods* **2015**, *17*, 640–656. [CrossRef]
5. Cerbulis, J.; Farrell, H.M., Jr. Composition of milks of dairy cattle. I. Protein, lactose, and fat contents and distribution of protein fraction. *J. Dairy Sci.* **1975**, *58*, 817–827. [CrossRef]
6. Mahé, S.; Roos, N.; Benamouzig, R.; Davin, L.; Luengo, C.; Gagnon, L.; Gaussergès, N.; Rautureau, J.; Tomé, D. Gastrojejunal kinetics and the digestion of [15N]β-lactoglobulin and casein in humans: The influence of the nature and quantity of the protein. *Am. J. Clin. Nutr.* **1996**, *63*, 546–552. [PubMed]

7. Daniel, H.; Vohwinkel, M.; Rehner, G. Effect of casein and β-casomorphins on gastrointestinal motility in rats. *J. Nutr.* **1990**, *120*, 252–257. [PubMed]
8. Mihatsch, W.A.; Franz, A.R.; Kuhnt, B.; Högel, J.; Pohlandt, F. Hydrolysis of casein accelerates gastrointestinal transit via reduction of opioid receptor agonists released from casein in rats. *Biol. Neonate* **2005**, *87*, 160–163. [CrossRef] [PubMed]
9. Mihatsch, W.A.; Högel, J.; Pohlandt, F. Hydrolysed protein accelerates the gastrointestinal transport of formula in preterm infants. *Acta Paediatr. Int. J. Paediatr.* **2001**, *90*, 196–198. [CrossRef]
10. Soenen, S.; Rayner, C.K.; Jones, K.L.; Horowitz, M. The ageing gastrointestinal tract. *Curr. Opin. Clin. Nutr. Metab. Care* **2016**, *19*, 12–18. [CrossRef] [PubMed]
11. Soenen, S.; Rayner, C.K.; Horowitz, M.; Jones, K.L. Gastric emptying in the elderly. *Clin. Geriatr. Med.* **2015**, *31*, 339–353. [CrossRef] [PubMed]
12. Morley, J.E. Constipation and irritable bowel syndrome in the elderly. *Clin. Geriatr. Med.* **2007**, *23*, 823–832. [CrossRef] [PubMed]
13. Roque, M.V.; Bouras, E.P. Epidemiology and management of chronic constipation in elderly patients. *Clin. Interv. Aging* **2015**, *10*, 919–930.
14. Pasricha, P.J.; Parkman, H.P. Gastroparesis: Definitions and diagnosis. *Gastroenterol. Clin. N. Am.* **2015**, *44*, 1–7. [CrossRef] [PubMed]
15. Abell, T.L.; Camilleri, M.; Donohoe, K.; Hasler, W.L.; Lin, H.C.; Maurer, A.H.; McCallum, R.W.; Nowak, T.; Nusynowitz, M.L.; Parkman, H.P.; et al. Consensus recommendations for gastric emptying scintigraphy: A joint report of the American Neurogastroenterology and Motility Society and the Society of Nuclear Medicine. *Am. J. Gastroenterol.* **2008**, *103*, 753–763. [CrossRef] [PubMed]
16. Abrahão, V. Nourishing the dysfunctional gut and whey protein. *Curr. Opin. Clin. Nutr. Metab. Care* **2012**, *15*, 480–484. [CrossRef] [PubMed]
17. Vandenplas, Y.; Alarcon, P.; Fleischer, D.; Hernell, O.; Kolacek, S.; Laignelet, H.; Lönnerdal, B.; Raman, R.; Rigo, J.; Salvatore, S.; et al. Should partial hydrolysates be used as starter infant formula? A working group consensus. *J. Pediatr. Gastroenterol. Nutr.* **2016**, *62*, 22–35. [CrossRef] [PubMed]
18. Ha, E.; Zemel, M.B. Functional properties of whey, whey components, and essential amino acids: Mechanisms underlying health benefits for active people (review). *J. Nutr. Biochem.* **2003**, *14*, 251–258. [CrossRef]
19. Krissansen, G.W. Emerging health properties of whey proteins and their clinical implications. *J. Am. Coll. Nutr.* **2007**, *26*, 713S–723S. [CrossRef] [PubMed]
20. Madureira, A.R.; Tavares, T.; Gomes, A.M.P.; Pintado, M.E.; Malcata, F.X. Invited review: Physiological properties of bioactive peptides obtained from whey proteins. *J. Dairy Sci.* **2010**, *93*, 437–455. [CrossRef] [PubMed]
21. Sreeja, V.; Jana, A.; Aparnathi, K.; Prajapati, J. Role of whey proteins in combating geriatric disorders. *J. Sci. Food Agric.* **2013**, *93*, 3662–3669.
22. Barbé, F.; Le Feunteun, S.; Rémond, D.; Ménard, O.; Jardin, J.; Henry, G.; Laroche, B.; Dupont, D. Tracking the in vivo release of bioactive peptides in the gut during digestion: Mass spectrometry peptidomic characterization of effluents collected in the gut of dairy matrix fed mini-pigs. *Food Res. Int.* **2014**, *63*, 147–156. [CrossRef]
23. Barbe, F.; Menard, O.; Le Gouar, Y.; Buffiere, C.; Famelart, M.H.; Laroche, B.; Le Feunteun, S.; Remond, D.; Dupont, D. Acid and rennet gels exhibit strong differences in the kinetics of milk protein digestion and amino acid bioavailability. *Food Chem.* **2014**, *143*, 1–8. [CrossRef] [PubMed]
24. Boirie, Y.; Dangin, M.; Gachon, P.; Vasson, M.P.; Maubois, J.L.; Beaufrère, B. Slow and fast dietary proteins differently modulate postprandial protein accretion. *Proc. Natl. Acad. Sci. USA* **1997**, *94*, 14930–14935. [CrossRef] [PubMed]
25. Chabance, B.; Marteau, P.; Rambaud, J.C.; Migliore-Samour, D.; Boynard, M.; Perrotin, P.; Guillet, R.; Jollès, P.; Fiat, A.M. Casein peptide release and passage to the blood in humans during digestion of milk or yogurt. *Biochimie* **1998**, *80*, 155–165. [CrossRef]
26. Sanchon, J.; Fernandez-Tome, S.; Miralles, B.; Hernandez-Ledesma, B.; Tome, D.; Gaudichon, C.; Recio, I. Protein degradation and peptide release from milk peptides in human jejunum. Comparison with in vitro gastrointestinal simulation. *Food Chem.* **2018**, *239*, 486–494. [CrossRef] [PubMed]
27. Meisel, H.; Bockelmann, W. Bioactive peptides encrypted in milk proteins: Proteolytic activation and tropho-functional properties. *Antonie Van Leeuwenhoek* **1999**, *76*, 207–215. [CrossRef] [PubMed]

28. Yoshikawa, M.; Tani, F.; Yoshimura, T.; Chiba, H. Opioid peptides from milk proteins. *Agric. Biol. Chem.* **1986**, *50*, 2419–2421. [CrossRef]

29. Fernández-Tomé, S.; Martínez-Maqueda, D.; Girón, R.; Goicoechea, C.; Miralles, B.; Recio, I. Novel peptides derived from α_{s1}-casein with opioid activity and mucin stimulatory effect on HT29-MTX cells. *J. Funct. Foods* **2016**, *25*, 466–476. [CrossRef]

30. Nongonierma, A.B.; Schellekens, H.; Dinan, T.G.; Cryan, J.F.; Fitzgerald, R.J. Milk protein hydrolysates activate 5-HT_{2c} serotonin receptors: Influence of the starting substrate and isolation of bioactive fractions. *Food Funct.* **2013**, *4*, 728–737. [CrossRef] [PubMed]

31. Munakata, A.; Iwane, S.; Todate, M.; Nakaji, S.; Sugawara, K. Effects of dietary fiber on gastrointestinal transit time, fecal properties and fat absorption in rats. *Tohoku J. Exp. Med.* **1995**, *176*, 227–238. [CrossRef] [PubMed]

32. Varga, F. Transit time changes with age in the gastrointestinal tract of the rat. *Digestion* **1976**, *14*, 319–324. [CrossRef] [PubMed]

33. Horiuchi, A.; Tanaka, N.; Sakai, R.; Kawamata, Y. Effect of age and elemental diets on gastric emptying in rats. *J. Gastroenterol. Hepatol. Res.* **2014**, *3*, 1340–1343. [CrossRef]

34. Smits, G.J.M.; Lefebvre, R.A. Influence of aging on gastric emptying of liquids, small intestine transit, and fecal output in rats. *Exp. Gerontol.* **1996**, *31*, 589–596. [CrossRef]

35. Brogna, A.; Ferrara, R.; Bucceri, A.M.; Lanteri, E.; Catalano, F. Influence of aging on gastrointestinal transit time an ultrasonographic and radiologic study. *Investig. Radiol.* **1999**, *34*, 357–359. [CrossRef]

36. Dalziel, J.E.; Young, W.; Bercik, P.; Spencer, N.J.; Ryan, L.J.; Dunstan, K.E.; Lloyd-West, C.M.; Gopal, P.K.; Haggarty, N.W.; Roy, N.C. Tracking gastrointestinal transit of solids in aged rats as pharmacological models of chronic dysmotility. *Neurogastroenterol. Motil.* **2016**, *28*, 1241–1251. [CrossRef] [PubMed]

37. Sánchez-Hidalgo, V.M.; Flores-Huerta, S.; Matute, G.; Serrano, C.; Urquieta, B.; Espinosa, R. Whey protein/casein ratio and nonprotein nitrogen in preterm human milk during the first 10 days postpartum. *J. Pediatr. Gastroenterol. Nutr.* **1998**, *26*, 64–69. [CrossRef] [PubMed]

38. Dalziel, J.E.; Fraser, K.; Young, W.; McKenzie, C.M.; Bassett, B.A.; Roy, N.C. Gastroparesis and lipid metabolism-associated dysbiosis in Wistar Kyoto rats. *Am. J. Physiol. Gastrointest. Liver Physiol.* **2017**, *313*, G62–G72. [CrossRef] [PubMed]

39. Buiter, H.J.C.; Windhorst, A.D.; Huisman, M.C.; de Maeyer, J.H.; Schuurkes, J.A.J.; Lammertsma, A.A.; Leysen, J.E. Radiosynthesis and preclinical evaluation of [^{11}C] prucalopride as a potential agonist pet ligand for the 5-HT_4 receptor. *Eur. J. Nucl. Med. Mol. Imaging Res.* **2013**, *3*, 1–13. [CrossRef] [PubMed]

40. Saphier, S.; Rosner, A.; Brandeis, R.; Karton, Y. Gastro intestinal tracking and gastric emptying of solid dosage forms in rats using X-ray imagining. *Int. J. Pharm.* **2010**, *388*, 190–195. [CrossRef] [PubMed]

41. Hara, H.; Nishikawa, H.; Kiriyama, S. Different effects of casein and soyabean protein on gastric emptying of protein and small intestinal transit after spontaneous feeding of diets in rats. *Br. J. Nutr.* **1992**, *68*, 59–66. [CrossRef] [PubMed]

42. Duraffourd, C.; De Vadder, F.; Goncalves, D.; Delaere, F.; Penhoat, A.; Brusset, B.; Rajas, F.; Chassard, D.; Duchampt, A.; Stefanutti, A.; et al. Mu-opioid receptors and dietary protein stimulate a gut-brain neural circuitry limiting food intake. *Cell* **2012**, *150*, 377–388. [CrossRef] [PubMed]

43. Yeomans, M.R.; Gray, R.W. Opioid peptides and the control of human ingestive behaviour. *Neurosci. Biobehav. Rev.* **2002**, *26*, 713–728. [CrossRef]

44. Ruppin, H. Review: Loperamide—A potent antidiarrhoeal drug with actions along the alimentary tract. *Aliment. Pharmacol. Ther.* **1987**, *1*, 179–190. [CrossRef] [PubMed]

45. Silva, S.V.; Malcata, F.X. Caseins as source of bioactive peptides. *Int. Dairy J.* **2005**, *15*, 1–15. [CrossRef]

46. Bendtsen, L.Q.; Lorenzen, J.K.; Bendsen, N.T.; Rasmussen, C.; Astrup, A. Effect of dairy proteins on appetite, energy expenditure, body weight, and composition: A review of the evidence from controlled clinical trials. *Adv. Nutr.* **2013**, *4*, 418–438. [CrossRef] [PubMed]

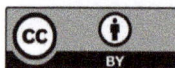

nutrients

Article

Enrichment of Probiotic Fermented Milk with Green Banana Pulp: Characterization Microbiological, Physicochemical and Sensory

Carolina de Oliveira Vogado [1], Eliana dos Santos Leandro [1,*], Renata Puppin Zandonadi [1], Ernandes Rodrigues de Alencar [2], Verônica Cortez Ginani [1], Eduardo Yoshio Nakano [3], Sascha Habú [4] and Priscila Araújo Aguiar [1]

[1]   Faculty of Health, Department of Nutrition, University of Brasília, Distrito Federal CEP 70910-900, Brazil; carol_vogado@yahoo.com.br (C.d.O.V.); renatapz@yahoo.com.br (R.P.Z.); vcginani@gmail.com (V.C.G.); priscilla01araujo@gmail.com (P.A.A.)
[2]   Faculty of Agronomy and Veterinary Medicine, University of Brasília, Distrito Federal CEP 70910-900, Brazil; ernandesalencar@unb.br
[3]   Department of Statistic, University of Brasília, Distrito Federal CEP 70910-900, Brazil; eynakano@gmail.com
[4]   Department of Environmental Technology, University Technological Federal of Paraná, Paraná CEP 80230-901, Brazil; sashabu@yahoo.com.br
*   Correspondence: elisanleandro@yahoo.com.br; Tel.: +55-613-107-1747; Fax: +55-613-273-3676

Received: 5 February 2018; Accepted: 19 March 2018; Published: 29 March 2018

Abstract: The aims of this study were (i) to evaluate the growth kinetic of *L. paracasei* LBC 81 in fermented milks enriched with green banana pulp (GBP); (ii) to evaluate the effect of the incorporation of GBP on the chemical composition and the sensory acceptance; and (iii) to study the viability of the probiotic and technological properties during refrigerated storage. The amount of GBP used were 3.0, 6.0 and 9.0 g/100 g. The results show that the higher the concentration of GBP added, the shorter the time taken to reach pH 4.6. It was observed that the incorporation of GBP did not affect negatively the viability of *L. paracasei* LBC 81 during storage. The fermented milk elaborated with 6.0 g/100 g of GBP was the most accepted. The present study indicates that the enrichment of fermented milk with GBP favors the stability of the probiotic strain, *L. paracasei* LBC 81 during storage.

Keywords: probiotic; green banana pulp; fermented milk; dairy

1. Introduction

Probiotics are live microorganisms that are capable of colonizing the gastrointestinal tract (GIT) and, when consumed in adequate amounts, confer benefits to human health, such as prevention against some types of cancer, intestinal regulation, improvement of digestibility, reduction of lactose intolerance, reduction of side effects of antibiotics, and reduction of the symptoms of irritable bowel syndrome [1,2]. The lactic acid bacteria (LAB) group is composed of several probiotic strains. The *Lactobacillus* genus is the most representative of the probiotics [3] and it is widely used in foods.

Dairy products are the most important group of foods that carry probiotics, in which fermented milk is the most traditional group in this category. To obtain health benefits, it is recommended that a product contains at least 10^6 Colony Forming Units (CFU)/g of the probiotic strain at the time of consumption [4]. Therefore, it is very important to study the growth and the viability of probiotic strains on food.

The viability of probiotic microorganisms is an important parameter in the development of probiotic foods, such as fermented milk. Several factors can affect the viability of probiotic strains in fermented milks, including their formulation ingredients [5], the presence of fruits pulp on formulation [6], the pH of the medium, water activity, oxygen content, and storage conditions of the product (i.e., temperature) [3].

Several ingredients have been added during the elaboration of yoghurts and fermented milks, with different objectives: to improve the nutritional value; to stimulate growth; and to accentuate the survival of the probiotic strain during the refrigerated storage period. Among these ingredients, studies have highlighted prebiotic substances (i.e., inulin) [7], quinoa flour [8] and fruit flours [9].

Another ingredient that has aroused interest in the elaboration of yogurts is green banana pulp [10,11]. The green banana is rich in several nutrients and bioactive compounds, such as resistant starch, phenolic acids, minerals and vitamins that are important to human health [12]. In addition to the health benefits of the consumer, it has been observed that the incorporation of green banana pulp does not affect the technological or sensory characteristics of the yoghurts.

The incorporation of green banana pulp (GBP) in the elaboration of yoghurt increases the growth of probiotic strains, such as *Lactobacillus acidophilus* and *Bifidobacterium bifidum* [10]. However, there are no related studies in the literature showing the effect of the incorporation of GBP on the growth kinetics of probiotic strains and in survival during refrigerated storage. Furthermore, it is important to evaluate the effect of the incorporation of GBP into other technological variables during storage, such as syneresis and color of the product.

To the best of our knowledge, there are no studies that have evaluated the effect of GBP on fermented milk characteristics. Furthermore, considering that GBP is a nutrient source that helps the growth of lactic bacteria, the characterization of the product regarding the survival of probiotic strains and technological parameters during refrigerated storage must be performed. Thus, the aims of this study were (i) to evaluate the growth kinetics of *L. paracasei* LBC 81 in fermented milks enriched with different amounts of green banana pulp; (ii) to evaluate the effect of the incorporation of green banana pulp on the chemical composition and the sensory acceptance of fermented milk; and (iii) to study the viability of the probiotic strain and the technological properties of fermented milks during refrigerated storage.

2. Materials and Methods

2.1. Microorganisms

The dehydrated culture of *Lactobacillus paracasei* subsp. *paracasei* LBC 81 was cultivated in a medium containing Reconstituted Skim Milk Powder (RSMP) (Nestlé, Araçatuba, São Paulo, Brazil) in an amount of 10 g/100 g to water weight. The culture of microorganism was immediately incubated in a bacteriological oven at 37 °C for 14 h. A second activation of the culture was performed under the same conditions. All the experiments in this study followed these culture activation steps.

2.2. Production of Base Formulation to Prepare Fermented Milks

Four base formulations were elaborated to produce the fermented milk with different amounts of GBP. The formulations' bases were composed of 10.0 g/100 g RSMP and 7.0 g/100 g sugar in relation to the water weight associated with different amounts of GBP: (i) control sample—without addition of GBP; (ii) addition of 3.0 g/100 g of GBP; (iii) addition of 6.0 g/100 g of GBP and (iv) addition of 9.0 g/100 g of GBP. According to the manufacturer (La Pianezza®, Industrial District Bandeirants, Brazil), 100 g of GBP is composed of 20.00 g of carbohydrates, 1.17 g of proteins, 7.83 g of fiber, 1.17 mg of iron, 20.16 mg of magnesium, 0.50 mg of manganese, 235.00 mg of potassium, and it is free of total fats. The samples were homogenized with a sterilized mixer, distributed in glass jars, and immediately autoclaved at 121 °C for 15 min.

2.3. Production of Fermented Milks and Determination of Kinetic Parameters of the Fermentation

The autoclaved base formulation samples were cooled and inoculated with 10% of the activated culture of *L. paracasei* subsp. *paracasei* LBC 81. The inoculated milk was incubated at 37 °C for 14 h.

After that, the kinetic parameters, pH and titratable acidity, were evaluated. pH was evaluated by a potentiometer (Digimed, modelo DM21, São Paulo, Brasil), and measures were made every two hours, until pH 4.6 or an equivalent value was reached. The titratable acidity was determined according to the methodology described by [13]; the results were expressed in g/100 g of lactic acid.

2.4. Chemical Composition

The chemical composition of the fermented milks enriched with GBP was determined by the evaluation of the moisture content [13]; the protein content was determined by the Kjeldahl method and ashes [14]; the crude fiber was evaluated using the Fiber Digester model MS444/CI (Marconi, Piracicaba, Brazil); and the total carbohydrate content present in the products was as the remainder—the values found for moisture, protein content, lipid content and ash content were subtracted from 100. The lipid content was measured using the fat extractor, Model ANKOM XT15 Extractor (Ankom Technology, New York, NY, USA) [15].

2.5. Sensory Evaluation

The sensory test for the fermented milk samples was performed with 113 panelists (age ranging from 18 to 58 years, 51% females and 49% males). The samples were randomized and monadically presented. The panelists evaluated five attributes: appearance, flavor, aroma, texture and overall acceptance, using a 9-point hedonic scale. The Free and Informed Consent Form was presented to the participants of the study and approved by the Research Ethics Committee (Parecer: 2.000.289) of the University of Brasilia.

2.6. Syneresis Measure in the Fermented Milks

The fermented milk syneresis was determined by the methodology described by Fiszman et al. [16] with adaptations. Flasks containing 10 mL of the fermented milk samples were rested at 4 °C, and at intervals of 3, 6, 9, 12, 18, 24 and 48 h, the serum released was collected with the aid of a pipette (20–200 µL). The syneresis was calculated as the ratio of the serum volume to the initial volume of the fermented milk samples and was expressed in mL/100 mL.

2.7. Characterization of the Fermented Milks during the Storage Period

The viability of the probiotics and the technological properties of the fermented milks enriched with GBP were evaluated in the beginning of the storage period and each 7 days until 28 days of storage was complete. The fermented milks were stored at 4 °C in a climatic chamber (Model MA 415, Marconi, Piracicaba, Brazil).

2.7.1. Determination of Viability

The viability of the probiotic culture was determined by the *Spread plate* technique on MRS agar medium. The fermented milk samples were subjected to several serial dilutions in 0.85 g/100 g saline solution. The selected dilutions were plated on MRS agar and immediately incubated at 37 °C for 48 h. After the incubation period, the number of Colony Forming Units (CFU) was determined. The final result was expressed as log CFU/mL.

2.7.2. Technological Properties of Fermented Milks

For the technological evaluation of the fermented milks during the refrigerated storage, the pH, the titratable acidity and the color were evaluated. The pH and the titratable acidity were determined as described in Section 2.3.

The evaluation of the color of the fermented milks was made by using the ColorQuest XE Spectrophotometer (HunterLab, Reston, VA, USA), obtaining the values of the coordinates L, a and b of the Hunter system. From the values of the coordinates, L, a and b, the parameters related the hue angle (*h*, Equation (1)), the chroma (*C*, Equation (2)) and the color difference (Δ*E*, Equation (3)) were obtained [17–19].

$$h = \text{arctang}(b/a) \tag{1}$$

$$C = \sqrt{(a^2 + b^2)} \tag{2}$$

$$\Delta E = \sqrt{(L - L_0)^2 + (a - a_0)^2 + (b - b_0)^2} \tag{3}$$

In which

L—measurable in terms of white to black intensity;
a—measurable in terms of red and green intensity;
b—measurable in terms of yellow and blue intensity;
L_0, a_0 and b_0—coordinates obtained at the beginning of the storage period of each of the fermented milks.

2.8. Statistical Analysis

Initially, we performed an analysis of variance with 5% probability and later we performed Tukey's test or a regression analysis. Post-hoc Tukey's test and contrasts were used for the comparison of the variables related to the chemical composition and sensorial quality of fermented milks, respectively. For the viability of probiotics in fermented milks with different concentrations of GBP during refrigerated storage post-hoc analysis was done with Tukey's test and Bonferroni's correction. For the results related to the kinetic parameters during the fermentation process, syneresis and technological properties during the refrigerated storage, regression analysis was used. The analysis of variance and Tukey's tests were performed in SPSS v. 19.0 (IBM Corporation, New York, NY, USA). SigmaPlot software v.10 (Systat Software Inc., Erkrath, Germany) was used. In each experiment, three replicates were adopted, except for the sensory analysis which was evaluated with 113 individuals.

3. Results and Discussion

3.1. Kinetic Parameters of Acidification

The pH and titratable acidity profile of the formulations of milks fermented by *L. paracasei* LBC 81 can be observed in Figure 1 and Table 1.

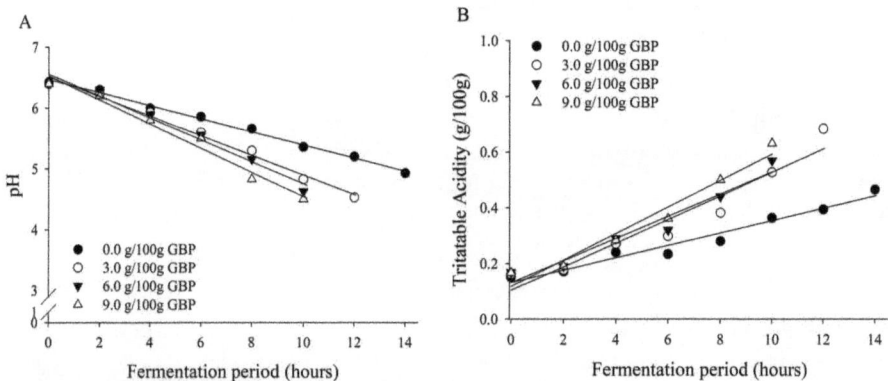

Figure 1. Regression curves of pH (**A**) and titratable acidity, expressed in g/100 g of lactic acid (**B**) of fermented milk by *L. paracasei* subsp *paracasei* LBC 81 with different concentrations (g/100 g) of green banana pulp (GBP) as a function of the fermentation period.

Table 1. Regression equations of pH and titratable acidity (g/100 g of lactic acid) of fermented milks by *L. paracasei* subsp. *paracasei* LBC 81 with different concentrations (g/100 g) of green banana pulp (GBP) as a function of the fermentation period.

Variable	GBP (g/100 g)	Adjusted Equation	R^2	SEE
pH	0.0	$\hat{y} = 6.47 - 0.11 ** X$	0.99	0.04
	3.0	$\hat{y} = 6.51 - 0.16 ** X$	0.99	0.08
	6.0	$\hat{y} = 6.56 - 0.18 ** X$	0.97	0.13
	9.0	$\hat{y} = 6.53 - 0.20 ** X$	0.98	0.13
Titratable Acidity (g/100 g)	0.0	$\hat{y} = 0.13 + 0.02 ** X$	0.96	0.02
	3.0	$\hat{y} = 0.10 + 0.04 ** X$	0.92	0.06
	6.0	$\hat{y} = 0.13 + 0.04 ** X$	0.95	0.04
	9.0	$\hat{y} = 0.11 + 0.05 ** X$	0.96	0.04

SEE = Standard error of estimate; ** Significant ($p < 0.01$); $n = 3$ sample replicates.

It was verified that as the concentration of GBP increased in the formulations, the decrease in the pH was faster and hence, there was a faster increase in titratable acidity. In regard to the pH variable (Figure 1A), estimated values equivalent to 5.37 and 4.53 after 10 h of fermentation were obtained for the control treatment control (0.0 g/100 g) and the treatment with 9.0 g/100 g of GBP, respectively. In relation to the titratable acidity (Figure 1B), the estimated values for the control treatment (0.0 g/100 g) and with 9.0 g/100 g of GBP were equivalent to 0.33 and 0.61 g/100 g of lactic acid, respectively.

Results referring to the fermentation kinetics demonstrated that GBP is an excellent substrate for the growth of *L. paracasei* LBC 81. GBP presents a great source of resistant starch (RS), phenolic acids, minerals and vitamins of importance to the human health [12] and, probably to the growth of *L. paracasei* LBC 81. Although the milk enriched with GBP was subjected to the autoclaving process, which reduces the presence of some thermosensitive nutrients, the amount of nutrients that remained was enough to accelerate the acidification of the product by the microorganism fermentation. Probably, the incorporation of GBP into the fermented milk allowed the prevalence of the homofermentative metabolism of the *L. paracasei* subsp *paracasei* LBC 81 culture. The addition of GBP stimulated the growth of *Lactobacillus acidophilus* after one day of fermentation in research carried out by Costa et al. [10].

L. paracasei strains present an optional heterofermentative metabolism, which makes them undesirable in some situations for use as starter cultures, being more used in the elaboration of dairy products as an adjunct culture. In anaerobic and nutrient-restricted conditions, the homofermentative pathway may undergo changes due to the activity of the NAD-dependent pyruvate decarboxylase enzyme, generating acetate and CO_2 from pyruvate, and thereby displacing the production of lactic acid [20].

Probiotic bacteria, when utilized as starter culture, are responsible for the slower acidification of a product, by a duration of almost 38 h [21]. Therefore, the elaboration of probiotic yoghurt has been one alternative used. The symbiotic association of the yogurt cultures (*Lactobacillus delbrueckii* and *Streptococcus thermophilus*) with probiotic strains stimulates the growth of other probiotic cultures. However, the elaboration of fermented milk using only one probiotic culture as a starter has been possible because this incorporates foods rich in nutrients which benefits the growth of the microorganism. The fermentation of the milk by probiotic strains (*L. rhamnosus* IMC 501® e *L. paracasei* IMC 502®) presented a higher decrease in pH when the milk was supplemented with wheat and oat bran [22].

3.2. Chemical Composition

There were significant differences ($p < 0.05$) only in the variables moisture and crude fiber (Table 2).

Table 2. Chemical composition of fermented milks by *L. paracasei* subsp *paracasei* LBC 81 with different concentrations (g/100 g) of green banana pulp (GBP).

Variable	Concentration of GBP (g/100 g)			
	0.0	3.0	6.0	9.0
Moisture (g/100 g)	85.90 ± 0.40 [a]	85.67 ± 0.41 [a]	84.52 ± 1.39 [a,b]	83.20 ± 0.74 [b]
Proteins (g/100 g)	2.71 ± 0.14	2.84 ± 0.13	2.85 ± 0.76	3.34 ± 0.63
Lipids (g/100 g)	0.34 ± 0.10	0.37 ± 0.12	0.38 ± 0.12	0.21 ± 0.07
Ash (g/100 g)	0.88 ± 0.11	0.81 ± 0.10	0.85 ± 0.04	0.81 ± 0.10
Crude fiber (g/100 g)	0.00 ± 0.00 [b]	0.40 ± 0.12 [a]	0.43 ± 0.00 [a]	0.48 ± 0.08 [a]
Carbohydrates (g/100 g)	10.14 ± 0.57	9.92 ± 0.44	10.97 ± 1.61	11.96 ± 0.39

For moisture and crude fiber, means followed by the same lower-case letter [a–b] on the lines did not differ statistically with Tukey's test ($p > 0.05$); $n = 3$ sample replicates.

The moisture obtained in the fermented milk enriched with 9.0 g/100 g of GBP was significantly lower ($p < 0.05$) than that obtained in the product with 3.0 g/100 g of GBP and the product without GBP. This result was expected, because when the total amount of GBP is higher, the percentage of dry matter increases and consequently, the amount of moisture reduces.

GBP samples presented more crude fiber ($p < 0.05$) than the control (0.0 g/100 g) sample due to the amount of fiber content present in green banana pulp [12,23]. The control sample (0.0 g/100 g) does not include any ingredient that contains fiber.

Dietary fiber has been widely associated with positive health outcomes (satiety, glycemic index regulation, intestinal regulation, cancer prevention and others) with the fiber content of food products being a potential basis for health claims in several countries [24]. Therefore, our product could have positive effects on human health, not only due to its probiotic effect, but also due to the effect of fiber on human organisms. In addition to the fiber content, GBP can also contribute to human health (as glycemic and cholesterol control, intestinal regulation, chronic disease prevention, and satiety) due to the presence of resistant starch and phenolic compounds [25,26]. Since we did not evaluate these compounds, further studies are necessary to evaluate the presence of these compounds and the effect of GBP fermented milk in human health.

It is important to highlight that the addition of GBP on these concentrations (3.0–9.0 g/100 g) did not significantly affect the composition of total protein content, lipids and carbohydrates. Therefore, there is probably no interference on total energetic value from the final formulation.

3.3. Sensory Properties

In all evaluated attributes, a significant difference ($p < 0.05$) was observed (Table 3).

Table 3. Sensory analysis of fermented milks by *L. paracasei* subsp *paracasei* LBC 81 with 0.0, 3.0, 6.0 and 9 g/100 g of green banana pulp (GBP).

Sensory Attribute	Concentration of GBP (g/100 g)			
	0.0	3.0	6.0	9.0
Appearance	5.13 ± 2.23 [d]	7.56 ± 1.46 [b]	8.12 ± 1.16 [a]	5.68 ± 1.94 [c]
Flavor	5.16 ± 2.32 [b]	6.25 ± 1.76 [a]	6.32 ± 1.89 [a]	4.83 ± 2.35 [b]
Aroma	6.48 ± 1.79 [b,c]	6.90 ± 1.45 [a,b]	7.00 ± 1.56 [a]	6.15 ± 2.00 [c]
Texture	4.98 ± 2.12 [c]	6.28 ± 1.90 [b]	7.05 ± 1.85 [a]	4.94 ± 2.23 [c]
Overall acceptability	5.30 ± 1.94 [b]	6.63 ± 1.48 [a]	6.78 ± 1.73 [a]	5.02 ± 2.10 [b]

For each sensory attribute, means followed by the same lower-case letters [a–d] on the lines do not differ significantly in post-hoc analysis via contrasts ($p > 0.05$); $n = 113$ panelists.

The fermented milk enriched with 6.0 g/100 g of GBP presented the highest mean acceptance regarding appearance and texture ($p < 0.05$). There was no significant difference ($p > 0.05$) when comparing fermented milk with 6.0 g/100 g of GBP with fermented milk with 3.0 g/100 g of GBP for flavor, aroma and overall acceptability. However, there was a significant difference ($p < 0.05$) when fermented milk without GBP (0.0 g/100 g) was compared with fermented milks with 3.0 and 6.0 g/100 g of GBP for flavor and overall acceptability.

It is important to highlight that 70.0% or more of the panelists expressed mean values ranging from 6–9 (on 9-point hedonic scale) for fermented milk with 6.0 g/100 g of GBP for all evaluated attributes. A sample is considered as having good acceptance when 70% or more of the individuals express mean values on the 9-point hedonic scale of higher than 5 [27]. Similarly, a study that evaluated the acceptance of yoghurt with GBP showed better acceptance for all evaluated attributes with the incorporation of GBP at a concentration of 5.0 g/100 g in yoghurt [11]. In relation to fermented milk with 3.0 g/100 g, the percentage of panelists expressing mean values of 6–9 on the 9-point hedonic scale was also 70.0% or more, except for texture. The difference in the texture is related to the addition of GBP which, among other functions, is employed to change the consistency of liquid products [24].

It is noted that the formulation with 9.0 g/100 g of GBP was less accepted regarding all attributes evaluated, compared to other formulations with GBP. Considering that the chemical composition of formulations with 6.0 and 9.0 g/100 g of GBP did not differ statistically, the use of the formulation with better acceptance (6.0 g/100 g of GBP) would probably not negatively affect the nutritional impact of this product. The concentration of 9.0 g/100 g of GBP negatively affected the acceptance of the product probably due to the acidification of the product caused by the increase in the concentration of GBP (Figure 1 and Table 1). Thus, the rejection observed related to the attributes, flavor and overall quality, can be associated with the higher acidity of the 9.0 g/100 g GBP product, since flavor impacts directly on the overall quality of the product. Moreover, the reduction in humidity and the increase in the solid content could be affected the texture of the 9.0 g/100 g GBP product.

3.4. Syneresis in the Fermented Milks

Regarding syneresis in the fermented milks for up to 48 h at 4 °C (Figure 2 and Table 4), it was observed that the fermented milk without GBP presented lower syneresis compared with fermented milks enriched with GBP.

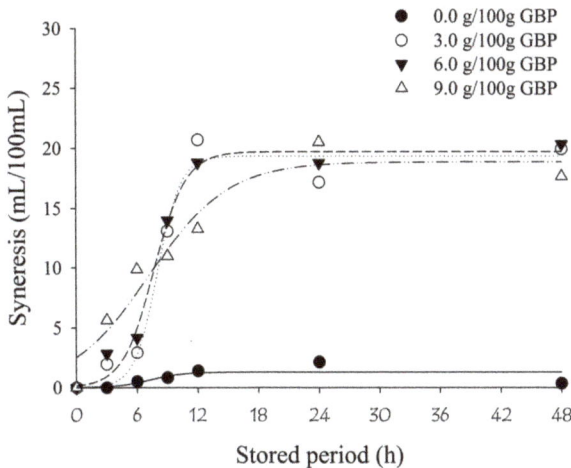

Figure 2. Regression curves of syneresis (g/100 g) of milk fermented by *L. paracasei* subsp *paracasei* LBC 81 with different concentrations of green banana pulp (GBP) over 48 h at 4 °C.

Table 4. Syneresis regression equations of fermented milks by *L. paracasei* subsp *paracasei* LBC 81 with different concentrations of green banana pulp (GBP) over 48 h at 4 °C.

GBP (g/100 g)	Adjusted Equation	R^2	SEE
0.0	$\hat{y} = \dfrac{1.29}{1 + e^{-\left(\frac{X-7.28}{1.63}\right)}}$	0.55	0.64
3.0	$\hat{y} = \dfrac{19.35}{1 + e^{-\left(\frac{X-8.04}{1.14}\right)}}$	0.98	1.74
6.0	$\hat{y} = \dfrac{19.71}{1 + e^{-\left(\frac{X-7.70}{1.57}\right)}}$	0.99	1.21
9.0	$\hat{y} = \dfrac{18.87}{1 + e^{-\left(\frac{X-7.24}{3.91}\right)}}$	0.94	2.12

SEE = Standard error of estimate; $n = 3$ sample replicates.

When the samples containing GBP were analyzed, faster syneresis was observed until 6 h of storage in the fermented milk with 9.0 g/100 g of GBP. In contrast, it was verified that there was a tendency toward higher syneresis in fermented milks containing 3.0 and 6.0 g/100 g of GBP until 24 h of storage. It should be highlighted that during the evaluation of the syneresis in the fermented milk with 9.0 g/100 g of GBP, a physical retention of the serum by the gel was observed, and it was not possible to collect it through the top of the bottles used to pack the product.

Due to its high content of starch, green banana pulp, [28], was probably responsible for enhancing the syneresis of the fermented milks [29]. Syneresis occurred due to the high tendency for hydrogen bonds to form between adjacent molecules of starch, when refrigerated. This process is known as retrogradation and results in the appearance of gel [30]. Over time, this formed gel has the tendency to release water, known as starch syneresis.

It is important to highlight that in dairy products, such as yoghurts and fermented milks, regardless of the presence of starch, syneresis can be observed during refrigerated storage due to the acidity and changes in protein binding [24]. Therefore, the addition of GBP that contains native and resistant starch accentuates the syneresis of our product.

3.5. Viability of L. paracasei LBC 81 during Storage

The mean values for the viability of *L. paracasei* LBC 81 in fermented milks made with different amounts of GBP for 28 days of storage at 4 °C are presented in Table 5.

Table 5. Evaluation of *Lactobacillus paracasei* subsp *paracasei* LBC81 in fermented milks enriched with different concentrations of green banana pulp (GBP) during a storage period of 28 days at 4 °C.

Stored Period (Days)	GBP Concentration (g/100 g)			
	0.0	3.0	6.0	9.0
0	8.89 ± 0.17 [a,A]	9.05 ± 0.15 [a,A]	8.98 ± 0.36 [a,B]	8.91 ± 0.27 [a,C]
7	8.36 ± 0.19 [c,B]	9.01 ± 0.30 [b,A]	9.83 ± 0.14 [a,A]	9.56 ± 0.19 [a,A,B]
14	8.90 ± 0.21 [b,A]	8.95 ± 0.20 [b,A]	9.47 ± 0.18 [a,A]	9.32 ± 0.12 [a,b,B,C]
21	8.95 ± 0.17 [c,A]	9.16 ± 0.54 [b,c,A]	9.60 ± 0.27 [a,b,A]	9.83 ± 0.30 [a,A]
28	8.66 ± 0.12 [b,A,B]	8.91 ± 0.70 [b,A]	9.43 ± 0.14 [a,A,B]	9.57± 0.32 [a,A,B]

Means followed by the same lower-case letters on the lines [(a–c)] did not differ significantly in post-hoc analyses by Tukey's tests ($p > 0.05$). Means followed by the same capital letters [(A–C)] in a column did not differ significantly by in post-hoc analyses by Bonferroni's corrections ($p > 0.05$).

Significant variation ($p < 0.05$) in the viability of *L. paracasei* LBC 81 was observed based on the interaction between the GBP concentration and storage period. During the storage period, only fermented milk enriched with 3.0 g/100 g of GBP showed no significant variation ($p > 0.05$) in the population size of *L. paracasei* LBC81. It should be noted that fermented milks with 6.0 and 9.0 g/100 g of GBP had higher counts of 9.0 log CFU/g after 28 days of storage at 4 °C.

Variations in the population size of the microorganisms, similar to that observed for *L. paracasei* LBC81 in fermented milks, are expected since microorganisms present in food stored under refrigeration undergo several physiological changes, which may lead to a decrease or increase in the microbial population. In addition, the decrease or increase in the population of *L. paracasei* LBC81 did not reach a logarithmic cycle. Although this variation was significant, it should be noted that all formulations developed were within the established standard for probiotic foods (10^6 to 10^9 CFU/g) [31].

When analyzing the effect of the addition of GBP on the viability of *L. paracasei* LBC 81 in each storage period, a significant variation ($p < 0.05$) was observed. In general, there was an increase in the population of *L. paracasei* LBC81, associated with the elevation in GBP concentration. Green banana is rich in various nutrients, and the availability of these nutrients in fermented milk may have favored the growth of *L. paracasei* LBC81 during the storage period. Stability or population increase of probiotic strains during the storage period is desirable when associated with the ingestion of a larger number of probiotic strains. On the other hand, it becomes undesirable because it is associated with post-acidification, which can make the product very acidic and of low acceptance by the consumer.

The results obtained are similar to those observed in fermented milks elaborated with fiber from oranges or quinoa [8,32]. However, previous studies have shown that supplementation does not always maintain the stability of a probiotic culture throughout the storage period. Supplementation of yogurt with fruit flours, such as banana, apple and grape, was not sufficient to maintain stability for 28 days of storage at 4 °C [9]. However, the reduction in viability was less than one log cycle, without compromising the functionality of the product.

3.6. Technological Properties

The technological properties of the fermented milk elaborated with different concentrations of GBP over 28 days of storage at 4 °C are presented in Figure 3 and Table 6.

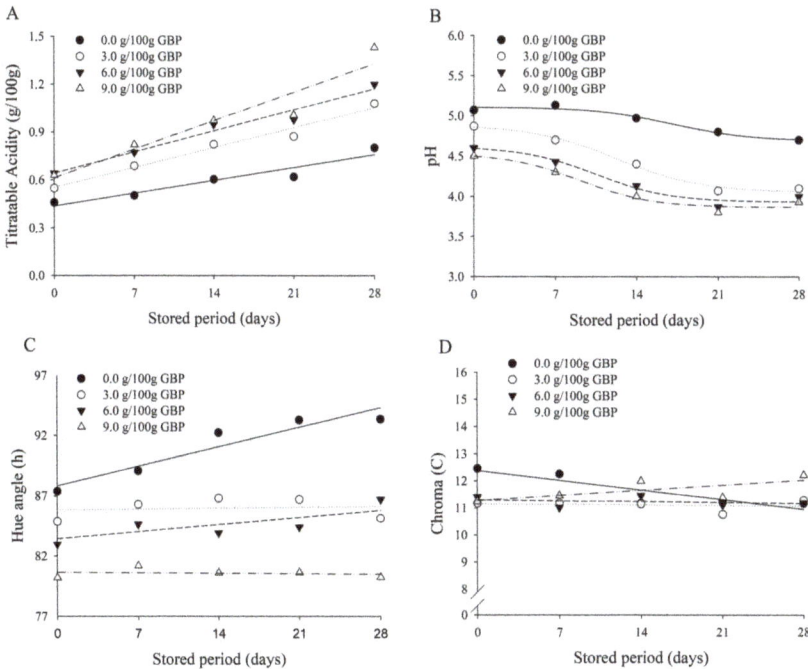

Figure 3. *Cont.*

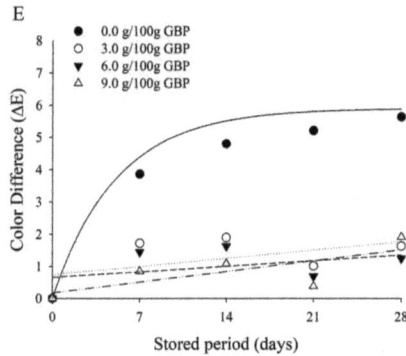

Figure 3. Regression curves of the titratable acidity expressed in g/100 g of lactic acid (**A**); pH (**B**); hue angle (**C**); Chroma (**D**) and Color Difference (ΔE) (**E**) of fermented milks by *L. paracasei* subsp *paracasei* LBC 81 with different concentrations (g/100 g) of green banana pulp (GBP) as a function of the fermentation period.

Table 6. Regression equations of titratable acidity expressed in g/100 g of lactic acid (A), pH (B), hue angle (C), Chroma (D) and Color Difference (ΔE) of fermented milks by *L. paracasei* subsp *paracasei* LBC 81 with different concentrations of GBP over 28 days at 4 °C.

Variable	GBP (g/100 g)	Adjusted Equation	R^2	SEE
Titratable Acidity (g/100 g)	0.0	$\hat{y} = 0.44 + 0.01 * X$	0.91	0.05
	3.0	$\hat{y} = 0.55 + 0.02 ** X$	0.97	0.04
	6.0	$\hat{y} = 0.64 + 0.02 ** X$	0.97	0.05
	9.0	$\hat{y} = 0.61 + 0.03 * X$	0.91	0.11
pH	0.0	$\hat{y} = 4.69 + \dfrac{0.41}{1 + e^{-\left(\frac{X-17.12}{3.36}\right)}}$	0.97	0.06
	3.0	$\hat{y} = 4.05 + \dfrac{0.83}{1 + e^{-\left(\frac{X-12.23}{3.63}\right)}}$	0.99	0.08
	6.0	$\hat{y} = 3.93 + \dfrac{0.69}{1 + e^{-\left(\frac{X-10.48}{-3.17}\right)}}$	0.97	0.12
	9.0	$\hat{y} = 3.87 + \dfrac{0.66}{1 + e^{-\left(\frac{X-9.11}{-3.87}\right)}}$	0.97	0.10
Hue angle	0.0	$\hat{y} = 87.83 + 0.23 * X$	0.89	0.99
	3.0	$\hat{y} = 85.79 + 0.01^{\text{ns}} X$	0.02	1.02
	6.0	$\hat{y} = 83.08 + 0.10^{\text{ns}} X$	0.68	0.89
	9.0	$\hat{y} = 80.67 - 0.01^{\text{ns}} X$	0.04	0.45
Chroma	0.0	$\hat{y} = 12.37 - 0.05 * X$	0.78	0.34
	3.0	$\hat{y} = 11.16 - 0.01^{\text{ns}} X$	0.04	0.23
	6.0	$\hat{y} = 11.30 - 0.01^{\text{ns}} X$	0.08	0.21
	9.0	$\hat{y} = 11.28 + 0.03^{\text{ns}} X$	0.48	0.35
Color Difference	0.0	$\hat{y} = 5.90\left(1 - e^{(-0.20X)}\right)$	0.91	0.88
	3.0	$\hat{y} = 0.74 + 0.04^{\text{ns}} X$	0.28	0.77
	6.0	$\hat{y} = 0.66 + 0.3^{\text{ns}} X$	0.18	0.70
	9.0	$\hat{y} = 0.17 + 0.05^{\text{ns}} X$	0.53	0.57

SEE = Standard error of estimate; ^{ns} Not significant; ** Significant ($p < 0.01$); * Significant ($p < 0.05$); $n = 3$ sample replicates.

In relation to the titratable acidity (Figure 2A), it was observed that there was a significant increase as a result of the interaction between the concentrations of GBP and the storage period.

It should be noted that fermented milk containing GBP had higher initial titratable acidity than fermented milk without GBP, and there was a trend for this difference to increase throughout the storage period. At the beginning of the storage period, the estimated difference in titratable acidity between the fermented milk without GBP and that with 9.0 g/100 g of GBP was 0.17 g/100 g of lactic acid. However, after 28 days of storage, the estimated difference was 0.73 g/100 g of lactic acid. Such a trend may be associated with the greater viability of *L. paracasei* LBC 81 in fermented milks containing GBP, as observed in Table 5.

Regarding the pH data (Figure 3B), a consistency was observed with the titratable acidity data, since there was a reduction in pH as the storage period increased, with an increase in the difference between values observed in the fermented milks without GBP and those with GBP. The differences between pH values in fermented milks without GBP and with 9.0 g/100 g of GBP were 0.64 and 0.83 at the beginning of the storage period and after 28 days, respectively.

The stability of the pH and acidity of fermented dairy products during refrigerated storage is desirable with respect to the acceptability and viability of the probiotic culture. In the present study, we verified that an increase in the concentration of GBP in fermented milk caused a greater decrease in pH, and consequently elevated the acidity of the product. Similarly, a decrease in pH was also observed in probiotic yogurt supplemented with lemon and orange fibers after 30 days of storage at 4 °C, where the pH of yogurts supplemented with lemon and orange fiber were 3.97 and 3.92, respectively [32].

The post-acidity in the different formulations of the fermented milks enriched with GBP over the storage period of 28 days at 4 °C is not desirable. The yoghurts and fermented milks present a shelf life of 28 to 30 days. This established shelf life is associated with the pH and acidity of the product. These parameters, after a prolonged storage period, make the products less acceptable for consumers. In our study, we observed that the product with higher acidity was less accepted by consumers. In addition to compromising product acceptance, the marked decrease in pH may affect the viability of probiotic strains. It is important to highlight that even with the decrease in pH and the increase in the titratable acidity of the fermented milks enriched with GBP, the viability of *L. paracasei* LBC 81 was not compromised over 28 days of storage at 4 °C (Table 5).

As for the coloration of fermented milks during storage, there was a significant variation in the variables, hue angle (*h*), chroma (*C*) and color difference (Δ*E*), due to the interaction between the concentration of GBP and the storage period. At the beginning of the storage period, the hue angle (Figure 3C) of the fermented milk without GBP was higher than in the fermented milks containing GBP. As the storage period increased, there was only a significant ($p < 0.05$) increase in the hue angle in fermented milk that did not contain GBP. Similar results were observed for the chroma (Figure 3D) and for the color difference (Figure 3E). In terms of chroma, there was a significant decrease ($p < 0.05$) only in the product without GBP over 28 days of storage. In the same sense, an expressive variation was observed only in the product elaborated without GBP, with an estimated value of 5.88, after 28 days of storage. On the other hand, the color differences in the fermented milks with GBP remained below 2.00 during storage at 4 °C.

In general, foods are susceptible to oxidation reactions when submitted to some storage conditions. Those foods rich in antioxidant substances are protected by the damage caused from the oxygen reactions, and therefore, present less alteration to flavor and color. Possibly, substances present in banana, such as antioxidants and phenolic compounds [33], acted as protective agents in the fermented milks against the action of reactive oxygen species. In this sense, these substances influenced the stability of the hue angle, chroma and color difference of fermented milk over 28 days of storage at 4 °C.

Although antioxidants and phenolic compounds are sensitive to high temperatures, it is possible that, after autoclaving, reduced concentrations of these substances were sufficient to ensure the color stability of the fermented milks. This stability of the color on the fermented milks with GBP can also justify the stability of the probiotic strain *L. paracasei* LBC 81 over the 28 days of storage at 4 °C. In the presence of antioxidant substances and phenolic compounds, *L. paracasei* LBC 81 would be least exposed to attack by reactive oxygen species. The oxygen reactive species attack proteins, nucleic acids and lipids and are considered one of the most important causes of injury and cellular death [34].

Thus, it is possible that the stability of the viability of *L. paracasei* LBC 81 is also associated with the protection of antioxidant substances and phenolic compounds.

4. Conclusions

The addition of GBP accelerated the growth and stabilized the viability of *L. paracasei* LBC 81 during a period of refrigerated storage. In addition to this benefit, the tonality, chroma and color difference of the fermented milks were less affected as the amount of GBP increased. The sensorial analysis of fermented milk enriched with 6.0% of GBP had better acceptance when compared to fermented milk without GBP and with the other formulations. One of the disadvantages of the incorporation of GBP into fermented milk was in relation to the increase in syneresis and the occurrence of post-acidification during the storage period. However, these technological variables can be improved with the use of stabilizers and with greater control of the fermentation process in further studies. It is also important to highlight that the use of green banana pulp can contribute to the nutritional quality of the fermented milk due to its phenolic compounds, resistant starch, fibers and other components. Therefore, our product could impact consumer health due to its probiotic and prebiotic effects. However, further studies should be conducted to evaluate the impact of this product on consumers' health.

Acknowledgments: All authors would like to acknowledge the financial support of Coordination for the Improvement of Higher Level Personnel (CAPES).

Author Contributions: E.d.S.L. and E.R.d.A. conceived and designed the experiments; C.d.O.V., P.A.A. and E.d.S.L. performed the experiments; E.d.S.L., E.R.d.A., E.R.N. and S.H. analyzed the data; V.C.G. contributed reagents/materials/analysis tools; E.d.S.L., E.R.d.A., R.P.Z. and C.d.O.V. wrote the paper.

Conflicts of Interest: The authors declare no conflict of interest.

References

1. Food and Agriculture Organization (FAO); World Health Organization (WHO). *Guidelines for the Evaluation of Probiotics in Food: Report of a Joint FAO/WHO Working Group. London Ontario;* FAO: Rome, Italy, 2002.
2. Fontana, L.; Bermudez-Brito, M.; Plaza-Diaz, J.; Muñoz-Quezada, S.; Gil, A. Sources, isolation, characterisation and evaluation of probiotics. *Br. J. Nutr.* **2013**, *109*, S35–S50. [CrossRef] [PubMed]
3. Vasiljevic, T.; Shah, N.P. Probiotics—From Metchnikoff to bioactives. *Int. Dairy J.* **2008**, *18*, 714–728. [CrossRef]
4. Mani-López, E.; Palou, E.; López-Malo, A.; Remeuf, F.; Corrieu, G.; Reinheimer, J.A.; Benedet, H.D. Probiotic viability and storage stability of yogurts and fermented milks prepared with several mixtures of lactic acid bacteria. *J. Dairy Sci.* **2014**, *97*, 2578–2590. [CrossRef] [PubMed]
5. Maganha, L.C.; Rosim, R.E.; Corassin, C.H.; Cruz, A.G.; Faria, J.A.F.; Oliveira, C.A.F. Viability of probiotic bacteria in fermented skim milk produced with different levels of milk powder and sugar. *Int. J. Dairy Technol.* **2014**, *67*, 89–94. [CrossRef]
6. Kailasapathy, K.; Harmstorf, I.; Phillips, M. Survival of *Lactobacillus acidophilus* and *Bifidobacterium animalis* ssp. *lactis* in stirred fruit yogurts. *Food Sci. Technol.-LEB* **2008**, *41*, 1317–1322. [CrossRef]
7. Montanuci, F.D.; Pimentel, T.C.; Garcia, S.; Prudencio, S.H. Effect of starter culture and inulin addition on microbial viability, texture, and chemical characteristics of whole or skim milk Kefir. *Food Sci. Technol.-Braz.* **2012**, *32*, 580–865. [CrossRef]
8. Casarotti, S.N.; Carneiro, B.M.; Penna, A.L.B. Evaluation of the effect of supplementing fermented milk with quinoa flour on probiotic activity. *J. Dairy Sci.* **2014**, *97*, 6027–6035. [CrossRef] [PubMed]
9. Casarotti, S.N.; Penna, A.L.B. Acidification profile, probiotic in vitro gastrointestinal tolerance and viability in fermented milk with fruit flours. *Int. Dairy J.* **2015**, *41*, 1–6. [CrossRef]
10. Costa, E.L.; Alencar, N.M.M.; Rullo, G.S.R.; Taralo, R.L. Green banana pulp on probiotic yoghurt. *Food Sci. Technol.-Braz.* **2017**, 1–6.
11. Silveira, A.C.R.; Silva, M.A.P.; Moura, L.C.; Souza, D.G.; Plácido, G.R.; Caliari, M. Parâmetros físico-químicos e sensoriais de iogurtes com biomassa da banana verde. *Glob. Sci. Technol.* **2017**, *10*, 29–42.
12. Da Mota, R.V.; Lajolo, F.M.; Cordenunsi, B.R.; Ciacco, C. Composition and functional properties of banana flour from different varieties. *Starch Stärke* **2000**, *52*, 63–68. [CrossRef]

13. Instituto Adolfo Lutz (IAL). *Métodos Físico-Químicos Para Análise de Alimentos*; IAL: São Paulo, Brazil, 2008; p. 1020.

14. AOAC International. *Official Methods of Analysis of AOAC International*, 18th ed.; AOAC International: Gaithersburg, MD, USA, 2005.

15. American Oil Chemists' Society (AOCS). *Official Methods and Recommended Pratices of the American Oil Chemist's Society*, 5th ed.; Firestone, D., Ed.; AOCS Press: Champaign, IL, USA, 1997.

16. Fiszman, S.M.; Salvador, A. Effect of gelatine on the texture of yoghurt and of acid-heat-induced milk gels. *Eur. Food Res. Technol.* **1999**, *208*, 100–105. [CrossRef]

17. Francis, F.J. The origin of tan^{-1} a/b. *J. Food Sci.* **1975**, *40*, 412. [CrossRef]

18. Little, A.C. A research note off on a tangent. *J. Food Sci.* **1975**, *40*, 410–411. [CrossRef]

19. Mclellan, M.R.; Lind, L.R.; Kime, R.W. Hue angle determinations and statistical analysis for multiquadrant Hunter L,a,b data. *J. Food Qual.* **1995**, *18*, 235–240. [CrossRef]

20. Kandler, O. Carbohydrate metabolism in lactic acid bacteria. *Antonie van Leeuwenhoek* **1983**, *49*, 209–224. [CrossRef] [PubMed]

21. Saxelin, M.; Grenov, B.; Svensson, U.; Fondén, R.; Reniero, R.; Mattila-Sandholm, T. The technology of probiotics. *Trends Food Sci. Technol.* **1999**, *10*, 387–392. [CrossRef]

22. Coman, M.M.; Verdenelli, M.C.; Cecchini, C.; Silvi, S.; Vasile, A.; Bahrim, G.E.; Orpianesi, C.; Cresci, A. Effect of buckwheat flour and oat bran on growth and cell viability of the probiotic strains *Lactobacillus rhamnosus* IMC 501®, *Lactobacillus paracasei* IMC 502® and their combination SYNBIO®, in synbiotic fermented milk. *Int. J. Food Microbiol.* **2013**, *167*, 261–268. [CrossRef] [PubMed]

23. Juarez-Garcia, E.; Agama-Acevedo, E.; Sayago-Ayerdi, S.G.; Rodriguez-Ambriz, S.L.; Bello-Pérez, L.A. Composition, digestibility and application in breadmaking of banana flour. *Plant Food Hum. Nutr.* **2006**, *61*, 131–137. [CrossRef] [PubMed]

24. Liao, H.J.; Hung, C.C. Chemical composition and in vitro starch digestibility of green banana (cv. Giant Cavendish) flour and its derived autoclaved/debranched powder. *LWT* **2015**, *64*, 639–644. [CrossRef]

25. De Souza, N.C.O.; De Oliveira, L.L.; De Alencar, E.L.; Moreira, G.P.; Leandro, E.S.; Ginani, V.C.; Zandonadi, R.P. Textural, physical and sensory impacts of the use of green banana puree to replace fat in reduced sugar pound cakes. *LWT* **2018**, *89*, 617–623. [CrossRef]

26. Brownlee, I.A.; Chater, P.I.; Pearson, J.P.; Wilcox, M.D. Dietary fibre and weight loss: Where are we now? *Food Hydrocoll.* **2017**, *68*, 186–191. [CrossRef]

27. Foley, M.; Beckley, J.; Ashman, H.; Moskowitz, H.R. The mind-set of teens towards food communications revealed by conjoint measurement and multi-food databases. *Appetite* **2009**, *52*, 554–560. [CrossRef] [PubMed]

28. Cereda, M.P. *Propriedades Gerais do Amido*; Fundação Cargill: São Paulo, Brazil, 2001.

29. Tovar, J.; Melito, C.; Herrera, E.; Rascón, A.; Pérez, E. Resistant starch formation does not parallel syneresis tendency in different starch gels. *Food Chem.* **2002**, *76*, 455–459. [CrossRef]

30. Hoover, R. Composition, molecular structure, and physicochemical properties of tuber and root starches: A review. *Carbohydr. Polym.* **2001**, *45*, 253–267. [CrossRef]

31. Nazzaro, F.; Fratianni, F.; Nicolaus, B.; Poli, A.; Orlando, P. The prebiotic source influences the growth, biochemical features and survival under simulated gastrointestinal conditions of the probiotic *Lactobacillus acidophilus*. *Anaerobe* **2012**, *18*, 280–285. [CrossRef] [PubMed]

32. Sendra, E.; Fayos, P.; Lario, Y.; Fernández-López, J.; Sayas-Barberá, E.; Pérez-Alvarez, J.A. Incorporation of citrus fibers in fermented milk containing probiotic bacteria. *Food Microbiol.* **2008**, *25*, 13–21. [CrossRef] [PubMed]

33. Aquino, C.F.; Salomão, L.C.C.; Ribeiro, S.M.R.; de Siqueira, D.L.; Cecon, P.R. Carbohydrates, phenolic compounds and antioxidant activity in pulp and peel of 15 banana cultivars. *Rev. Bras. Frutic.* **2016**, *38*. [CrossRef]

34. Van de Guchte, M.; Serror, P.; Chervaux, C.; Smokvina, T.; Ehrlich, S.D.; Maguin, E. Stress responses in lactic acid bacteria. *Antonie van Leeuwenhoek* **2002**, *82*, 187–216. [CrossRef] [PubMed]

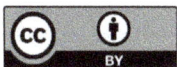

nutrients

MDPI

Article

Daily Intake of Milk Powder and Risk of Celiac Disease in Early Childhood: A Nested Case-Control Study

Elin M. Hård af Segerstad [1], Hye-Seung Lee [2], Carin Andrén Aronsson [1], Jimin Yang [2],
Ulla Uusitalo [2], Ingegerd Sjöholm [3], Marilyn Rayner [3], Kalle Kurppa [4], Suvi M. Virtanen [5],
Jill M. Norris [6], Daniel Agardh [1,*] and on behalf of the TEDDY Study Group

[1] The Diabetes and Celiac Disease Unit, Department of Clinical Sciences, Lund University, 202 05 Malmö,
    Sweden; elin.malmberg_hard_af_segerstad@med.lu.se (E.M.H.A.S.);
    carin.andren_aronsson@med.lu.se (C.A.A.)
[2] Health Informatics Institute, Morsani College of Medicine, University of South Florida, 33620 FL Tampa,
    USA; hye-seung.lee@epi.usf.edu (H.-S.L.); jimin.yang@epi.usf.edu (J.Y.); ulla.uusitalo@epi.usf.edu (U.U.)
[3] Department of Food Technology, Engineering and Nutrition, Chemical Center, Lund University,
    221 00 Lund, Sweden; ingegerd.sjoholm@food.lth.se (I.S.); marilyn.rayner@food.lth.se (M.R.)
[4] Tampere Center for Child Health Research, University of Tampere and Tampere University Hospital,
    33521 Tampere, Finland; kalle.kurppa@uta.fi
[5] Unit of Nutrition, National Institute for Health and Welfare, 00271 Helsinki, Finland; Faculty of Social
    Sciences, University of Tampere, Tampere Center for Child Health Research, University of Tampere and
    Tampere University Hospital and the Science Center of Pirkanmaa Hospital District Tampere,
    33521 Tampere, Finland; suvi.virtanen@thi.fi
[6] Department of Epidemiology, Colorado School of Public Health, University of Colorado Anschutz Medical
    Campus, 80045 CO Aurora, USA; jill.norris@ucdenver.edu
*   Correspondence: daniel.agardh@med.lu.se; Tel.: +1-464-039-1113

Received: 13 March 2018; Accepted: 26 April 2018; Published: 28 April 2018

Abstract: Milk powder and gluten are common components in Swedish infants' diets. Whereas
large intakes of gluten early in life increases the risk of celiac disease in genetically at-risk Swedish
children, no study has yet evaluated if intake of milk powder by 2 years of age is associated with celiac
disease. A 1-to-3 nested case-control study, comprised of 207 celiac disease children and 621 controls
matched for sex, birth year, and HLA genotype, was performed on a birth cohort of HLA-DR3-DQ2
and/or DR4-DQ8-positive children. Subjects were screened annually for celiac disease using tissue
transglutaminase autoantibodies (tTGA). Three-day food records estimated the mean intake of milk
powder at ages 6 months, 9 months, 12 months, 18 months, and 24 months. Conditional logistic
regression calculated odds ratios (OR) at last intake prior to seroconversion of tTGA positivity, and
for each time-point respectively and adjusted for having a first-degree relative with celiac disease and
gluten intake. Intake of milk powder prior to seroconversion of tTGA positivity was not associated
with celiac disease (OR = 1.00; 95% CI = 0.99, 1.03; p = 0.763). In conclusion, intake of milk powder in
early childhood is not associated with celiac disease in genetically susceptible children.

Keywords: infant feeding; Sweden; HLA; milk powder; formula; gluten; commercial infant foods

---

1. Introduction

Celiac disease is a common chronic small bowel disease caused by intolerance to gluten found
in foods containing wheat, rye or barley [1]. It has been debated whether the global differences in
prevalence are due to variations in infant feeding practices [2]. One affecting factor could be variations
in gluten intake during the first years of life [3]. The effects of dairy product intake on the risk of celiac

disease is less studied. Although the vast majority of patients with celiac disease have antibodies directed against tissue transglutaminase (tTGA) [4], a proportion also have detectable antibodies against milk protein [5]. Although a recent study did not find avoidance of cow´s milk-based products to protect from celiac disease compared with extensively hydrolyzed formula [5], it is not entirely clear whether other components in milk products may trigger celiac disease.

Commercial instant porridges and cereal milk drinks based on milk powder and gluten containing cereals are common infant food products in some parts of the world [6]. In milk powder production, advanced glycation end products (AGEs) are formed through Maillard reactions [7]. AGEs have pro-inflammatory effects and may induce increased oxidative stress in adults [8]. Notably, levels of AGEs increase during storage of commercial instant porridge and cereal milk drinks in room temperatures [9]. It could therefore be hypothesized that a high intake of commercial instant porridge and cereal milk drinks containing high concentrations of AGEs cause an initial inflammation that results in an increased gut permeability to gluten antigens that eventually leads to celiac disease in genetic at risk individuals.

The aim of this study was to investigate if intake of milk powder is associated with celiac disease in children. We prospectively collected food data from a birth cohort of genetically predisposed children that later developed celiac disease and compared it to matched controls in a nested case-control study.

2. Subjects and Methods

2.1. Study Population

The Environmental Determinants of Diabetes in the Young (TEDDY) study is an observational study conducted at 6 clinical centers in Finland, Germany, Sweden and the United States, investigating the environmental factors associated with type 1 diabetes and celiac disease [10]. Children carrying any of the HLA genotypes associated with type 1 diabetes and celiac disease were invited to participate in a 15-year follow-up [10], and among the enrolled participants 2525 were from the Swedish site. The TEDDY study is monitored by the National Institutes of Health and has been approved by ethics review boards at individual sites and informed consent from a parent or primary caretaker were obtained prior to screening.

2.2. Screening for Celiac Disease

Annual screening for celiac disease begins at 2 years of age by measurement of IgA and IgG autoantibodies against tTGA using radioligand binding assays as previously described [1]. Children positive for tTGA have their blood samples analyzed to determine the closest time point of tTGA seroconversion. Children positive for tTGA in two consecutive samples were evaluated for celiac disease at their health care provider. Diagnosis of celiac disease was established if a child had a biopsy showing Marsh score of 2 or higher and responded to a gluten-free diet with a significant decrease in tTGA levels.

As of July 31 in 2016, 2,077 Swedish TEDDY children had been screened for tTGA of whom 504 (24%) were tTGA positive at median 30 months of age (first quartile (Q1): 21, third quartile (Q3): 53) and 85 of those (17%) children seroconverted to tTGA prior to or at 24 months of age. Among the 238 tTGA positive children that were finally investigated with an intestinal biopsy, 207 of the 2077 (10%) children were diagnosed with celiac disease at median 45 months of age (Q1: 33, Q3: 70) (Figure 1).

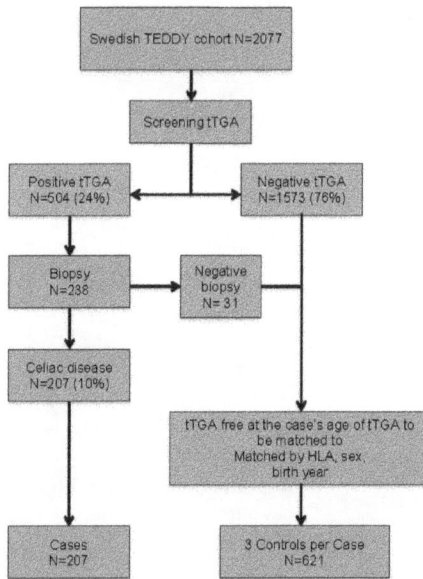

Figure 1. Flowchart of the study population.

2.3. Study Design

A nested case-control design included the 207 cases with biopsy-proven celiac disease and 3 controls randomly selected from the cohort for each case after matching on gender, the number of HLA DQ2 alleles and birth year (i.e., 1–3 nested case-control design) (Table 1). All controls were free of biopsy-proven celiac disease within 3 months of the matched case's age of biopsy, as well as tTGA negative within 3 months of the matched case's age of seroconversion. In this nested case-control study, 39 cases were selected as controls until seroconversion of tTGA.

Table 1. Characteristics of the identified cases with celiac disease in the Swedish TEDDY birth cohort used as matching factors in a nested 1-3 case-control study.

Matching Variable	Cases N = 207 (%)
Sex	
- Female	131 (63.3)
- Male	76 (36.7)
Birth year	
- 2004	11 (5.3)
- 2005	39 (18.8)
- 2006	28 (13.5)
- 2007	41 (19.8)
- 2008	37 (17.9)
- 2009	46 (22.2)
- 2010	5 (2.4)
HLA-genotype	
- DQ2/DQ8	64 (30.9)
- DQ8/DQ8	35 (16.9)
- DQ2/DQ2	100 (48.3)
- Other	8 (3.9)

2.4. Dietary Assessment

A study nurse collected a 24-h dietary recall at the first visit between 3 and 4.5 months of age. Three-day food records, including two weekdays and one weekend day, were then collected at follow-up visits at 6 months, 9 months, 12 months, 18 months, and 24 months of age, respectively. Normal food habits were encouraged during the time of the food record collection. Parents were provided with a manual including written instructions, as well as photos of portion sizes and drawings of foods of different sizes and as reference. When the child started daycare, a set of separate food record sheets and manual were provided for the daycare personnel. At the study visits, the study nurse performed a face-to-face interview, probing for missing or unclear information and revising the food record accordingly. A trained study dietitian or nutritionist entered the dietary information in a food database. The TEDDY database for Sweden was based on the Swedish National Food Composition Database, with information about nutrient content for foods and standard recipes for several composite dishes [11]. Products and brands different from standard food items in ingredients or nutritional values as well as unique recipes recorded by families were added to the database. For commercial baby foods, recipes were created based on the ingredient list together with information on the nutritional value, and added as a new food item if it changed in nutritional value or content. The study personnel entering the food data reached consensus estimates for the weight of foods when there was no information in the national food database or from the producer.

Intake of milk powder was either obtained directly from the database (including infant cereal milk drink and instant porridge), as an estimate for average content in a food type (including infant formula and chocolate) or an estimate based on brand name (including yoghurts). Based on the structure of the database, the content of milk powder could not be estimated for some specific products (such as ice cream, powder-based sauces, and certain prepared foods). From the dietary records, gluten intake was also assessed as it was considered a confounding factor. Total intake of wheat, rye and barley could be obtained from the database, and the amount of ingested gluten was calculated by multiplying the analyzed content of protein in each of these grains with 0.8 for wheat, 0.65 for rye, and 0.5 for barley [12].

Body weight was measured at every clinic visit at 3 months, 6 months, 9 months, 12 months, 18 months, and 24 months (Figure 2a). Scales were of different brands over the study period of which Tanita (Tanita Corp, Tokyo, Japan) was most commonly applied. Tanita scale was the most common and that scales were calibrated regularly. Energy intake for breastfed subjects was estimated using the energy requirement based on the child's age and weight at the time for the food record, then subtracting the energy intake from other reported food (Figure 2b) [13].

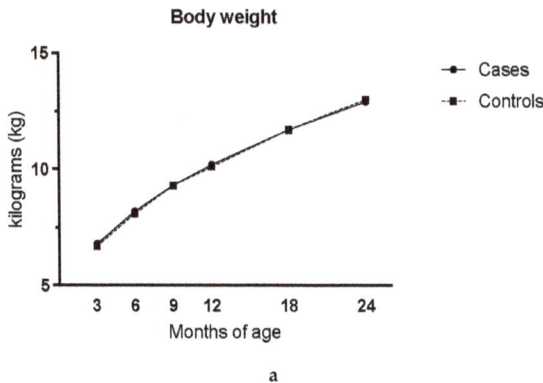

Body weight

a

Figure 2. *Cont.*

b

c

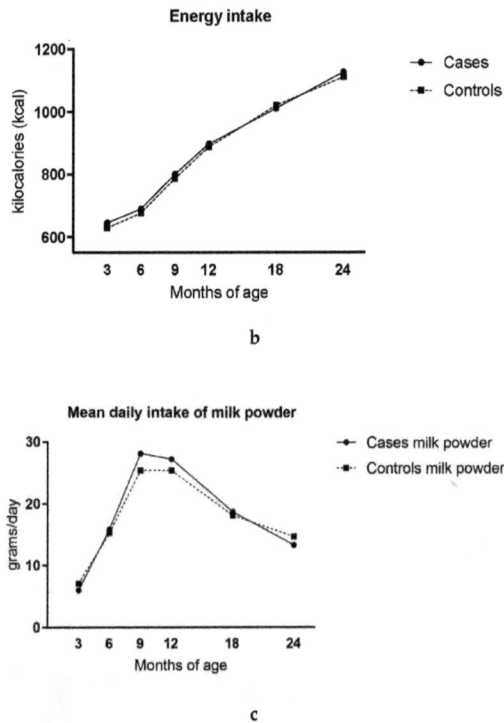

Figure 2. Body weight at clinic visit (**a**) and assessed daily mean intake of energy (kcal) (**b**), mean daily intake of milk powder (gram per day) from 3-day food records in cases with celiac disease and matched, healthy controls (1:3) (**c**). For breastfed subjects, energy intake was estimated using assessed energy requirement and subtracting energy intake from other reported food. Controls were matched to cases by gender, HLA genotype and birth year.

2.5. Statistical Analysis

Daily intake of milk powder in grams per day was assessed as the mean intake from the three-day diet records. Intake data were available until 24 months of age, but age of tTGA seroconversion for cases ranged from 10 to 120 months. Only available intakes reported prior to the case's tTGA seroconversion were included in analysis in order to compare between a case and matched control, using conditional logistic regression. Daily intake was also analyzed in grams per kilogram body weight (g/kg/day) in order to standardize intake between subjects. Intake reported at the visit prior to the case's tTGA seroconversion was as "last intake," and the sum of all intakes assessed as "total intake." Intake at a given age (3 months, 6 months, 9 months, 12 months, 18 months, or 24 months) was compared if it was available or appropriate for the case's age of seroconversion. We first adjusted for having a first-degree relative with celiac disease as a confounder. Milk powder intake was then analyzed with and without adjustment for gluten intake in order to separate the effect on risk of celiac disease between the two dietary exposures. Odds ratios were reported with 95% confidence intervals (CI), along with two-sided p-value. Statistical significance was determined when p-value <0.05. All statistical analyses were performed using SAS version 9.4 (SAS Institute Inc., Cary, NC, USA).

3. Results

Energy intake and body weight increased as expected with age for both cases and controls (Figure 2a,b). The mean daily intake of milk powder increased in both cases and controls by 12 months of age and more significantly between 6 months and 9 months of age, respectively (Figure 2c). At 6 months, the intake of milk powder was 15.9 g and 15.3 g per day for cases and controls respectively. At 9 months it had increased to 28.1 grams and 25.4 grams per day for cases and controls and at 24 months it had decreased to 13.3 grams and 14.7 grams per day for cases and controls.

Neither energy intake nor body weight were associated with celiac disease. Intake of milk powder in grams per day prior to seroconversion of tTGA positivity did not increase the risk of celiac disease, either for last intake, nor total intake or for intake at any given age. This was also true for the relative intake in grams per kg body weight (Table 2). In the unadjusted model, there was a small increased risk for celiac disease for the milk powder intake at 9 months of age in grams per day (OR = 1.01, 95%CI = 1.0–1.02; p = 0.037), as well as in grams per kilogram bodyweight per day (OR = 1.1, 95%CI = 1.0–1.2; p = 0.044).

Table 2. Comparison of mean daily intake of milk powder (grams per day and grams per kilo bodyweight) in cases with celiac disease and matched, healthy controls (1:3), and risk of celiac disease analyzed with conditional logistic regression expressed as odds ratio (OR) after adjusting for having a first-degree relative with celiac disease and for gluten intake at the given time point. Controls were matched to cases by gender, HLA genotype and birth year.

Time point	Number of cases analyzed	Number of cases missing intake	Milk powder intake (g/day)		Milk powder intake (g/kg/day)	
			OR (CI 95%)	p-value	OR (CI 95%)	p-value
Last intake [1]	207	0	1.0 (0.99–1.01)	0.937	0.99 (0.87–1.13)	0.861
Total intake [2]	207	0	1.0 (1.0–1.00)	0.662	1.0 (0.98–1.03)	0.763
Intake at						
3 months	207	0	0.99 (0.97–1.01)	0.159	0.92 (0.83–1.02)	0.125
6 months	202	5	1.0 (0.99–1.02)	0.643	1.02 (0.91–1.13)	0.788
9 months	198	9	1.01 (1.0–1.02)	0.069	1.09 (0.99–1.19)	0.072
12 months	192	9	1.01 (1.0–1.02)	0.181	1.08 (0.96–1.21)	0.184
18 months	146	21	1.0 (0.98–1.02)	0.983	1.01 (0.84–1.21)	0.923
24 months	103	19	0.99 (0.97–1.01)	0.202	0.88 (0.69–1.12)	0.301

[1] Last reported intake at the visit prior to seroconversion of tTGA; [2] Sum of all reported intakes prior to seroconversion of tTGA

Having a first-degree relative with celiac disease (OR = 2.53, 95%CI 1.37, 4.67, p = 0.003) and reported gluten intake when assessed in grams per day (OR = 1.09, 95%CI 1.03–1.16; p = 0.004) as well as in grams per kilograms per day (OR = 2.73, 95%CI 1.36–5.49; p = 0.005) were associated with celiac disease. When these confounders were included the adjusted model, the association between milk powder intake and celiac disease no longer remained significant.

4. Discussion

The present study showed that intake of milk powder does not increase the risk of celiac disease in genetically susceptible Swedish children. The peak intake of milk powder was observed at the age of 9 months after which it started to decrease, and may reflect a dietary intake pattern of formula, commercial porridge and milk cereal drink. The intake of milk powder observed was equivalent to the amount of commercial porridge and cereal milk drink consumed by Swedish infants as reported in a previous study [6].

The strength of the dietary assessment methods used in this study is that they allow for estimations of individual intake of foods. Repeated food records measure changes in dietary habits of infants and growing young children over time and is a suitable method when studying dietary intake and risk of disease [14]. Another advantage with the dietary data collected for this study is minimization of recall bias, which has been a limitation in previous studies using retrospective dietary assessment methods [15,16]. A prospective study design has the advantage of unawareness of the tTGA status at the time of the food data collection, which otherwise may influence parents to change their child's diet.

Analysis of relative dietary intake we also made, as recommended in nutrition research and disease [17]. The energy requirement of a child depends on age, weight, and growth [13]. A child larger in size may consume bigger portions than their smaller counterpart, resulting in a higher nutrient intake, but not necessarily higher intake in relation to body weight. We adjusted for the confounders of having a family member with celiac disease and for the gluten intake, respectively. The adjustments had a significant impact on the results, since we found an association with increased risk for celiac disease and intake of milk powder reported at the 9-month visit. We have previously published a study on the association between amount of gluten intake and celiac disease performed on the same cohort, which showed that the last intake of every gram gluten per day before seroconversion to tTGA positivity increased the risk of celiac disease by 28% [3].

The limitations of this study includes that milk powder intake was only studied in the first 2 years of life, whereas the majority of the celiac cases were diagnosed several years later. As 15.6% of the subjects also had missing food record data at 24 months, data collected at earlier timepoints was applied for the analyses, which may affect the reliability of the results. Additionally, we did not have access to complete information on content of milk powder for all food items; therefore, estimates had to be used. Although the excluded foods were considered less commonly used in the selected age groups, estimations on possible amounts of missing data were not performed. In this study, we analyzed two dietary exposures, and some common Swedish infant products contain both. Although the statistical analyses adjusted for the gluten intake, the study could be criticized for not quantifying the amount of gluten from products that also contained milk powder.

In conclusion, this nested case-control study on intake of milk powder during the first 2 years of life in genetically susceptible children showed that consumption of milk powder is not associated with celiac disease for Swedish children.

Author Contributions: The authors responsibilities were as follows – E.M.H., C.A.A., J.Y., U.U., I.S., M.R., K.K., S.M.V., J.M.N. and D.A.: designed the research project conception, developed the overall research plan, and oversaw the study; H.-S.L.: analyzed the data and performed the statistical analysis; E.H.M. and D.A.: wrote the manuscript and had primary responsibility for the final content; and all authors: approved the final version of the manuscript. None of the authors declared a conflict of interest. A list of members of the TEDDY study group is provided as followed.

Acknowledgments: This study was funded by U01 DK63829, U01 DK63861, U01 DK63821, U01 DK63865, 165 U01 DK63863, U01 DK63790, UC4 DK63829, UC4 DK63861, UC4 DK63821, UC4 166 DK63865, UC4 DK63863, UC4 DK63836, UC4 DK95300, and UC4 DK100238, and 167 Contract No. HHSN267200700014C from the National Institute of Diabetes and Digestive 168 and Kidney Diseases (NIDDK), National Institute of Allergy and Infectious Diseases 169 (NIAID), National Institute of Child Health and Human Development (NICHD), National 170 Institute of Environmental Health Sciences (NIEHS), Centers for Disease Control and 171 Prevention (CDC), and JDRF. This work supported in part by the NIH/NCATS Clinical and 172 Translational Science Awards to the University of Florida (UL1 TR000064) and the 173 University of Colorado (UL1 TR001082). National Institute of Health (NIH), Department of Health and Human Services (DHHS), the National Institute of Diabetes and Digestive and Kidney Diseases (NIDDK), National Institute of Allergy and Infectious Disease (NIAID), National Institute of Environmental Health Sciences (NIEHS), National Institute of Child Health and Human Development (NICHD), Centers for Disease Control and Prevention (CDC), JDRF.

Colorado Clinical Center: Marian Rewers, M.D., Ph.D., PI[1,4,5,6,10,11], Kimberly Bautista[12], Judith Baxter[9,10,12,15], Ruth Bedoy[2], Daniel Felipe-Morales, Kimberly Driscoll, Ph.D.[9], Brigitte I. Frohnert, M.D.[2,14], Marisa Gallant, M.D.[13], Patricia Gesualdo[2,6,12,14,15], Michelle Hoffman[12,13,14], Rachel Karban[12], Edwin Liu, M.D.[13], Jill Norris, Ph.D.[2,3,12], Adela Samper-Imaz, Andrea Steck, M.D.[3,14], Kathleen Waugh[6,7,12,15], Hali Wright[12]. University of Colorado, Anschutz Medical Campus, Barbara Davis Center for Childhood Diabetes.

Finland Clinical Center: Jorma Toppari, M.D., Ph.D., PI[¥,1,4,11,14], Olli G. Simell, M.D., Ph.D.[¥,1,4,11,13], Annika Adamsson, Ph.D.[*,12], Suvi Ahonen[*,±,§], Heikki Hyöty, M.D., Ph.D.[*,±,6], Jorma Ilonen, M.D., Ph.D.[¥,¶,3], Sanna Jokipuu[^], Tiina Kallio[^], Leena Karlsson[^], Miia Kähönen[µ,¤], Mikael Knip, M.D., Ph.D.[*,±,5], Lea Kovanen[*,±,§], Mirva Koreasalo[*,±,§,2], Kalle Kurppa, M.D., Ph.D.[*,±,13], Tiina Latva-aho[µ,¤], Maria Lönnrot, M.D., Ph.D.[*,±,6], Elina Mäntymäki[^], Katja Multasuo[µ,¤], Juha Mykkänen, Ph.D.[¥,3], Tiina Niininen±[*,12], Sari Niinistö[±,§,2], Mia Nyblom[*,±], Petra Rajala[^], Jenna Rautanen[±,§], Anne Riikonen[*,±,§], Mika Riikonen[^], Minna Romo[^], Juulia Rönkä[µ,¤], Jenni Rouhiainen[^], Tuula Simell, Ph.D., Ville Simell[¥,13], Maija Sjöberg[¥,12,14], Aino Stenius[µ,¤,12], Maria Leppänen[^], Sini Vainionpää[^], Eeva Varjonen[¥,12], Riitta Veijola, M.D., Ph.D.[µ,¤,14], Suvi M. Virtanen, M.D., Ph.D.[*,±,§,2], Mari Vähä-Mäkilä[^], Mari Åkerlund[*,±,§], Katri Lindfors, Ph.D.[*,13,¥] University of Turku, *University of Tampere, µUniversity of Oulu, ^Turku University Hospital, Hospital District of Southwest Finland, ±Tampere University Hospital, ¤Oulu University Hospital, §National Institute for Health and Welfare, Finland, ¶University of Kuopio.

Georgia/Florida Clinical Center: Jin-Xiong She, Ph.D., PI[1,3,4,11], Desmond Schatz, M.D.[*4,5,7,8], Diane Hopkins[12], Leigh Steed[12,13,14,1]5, Jamie Thomas[*6,12], Janey Adams[*12], Katherine Silvis[2], Michael Haller, M.D.[*14], Melissa Gardiner, Richard McIndoe, Ph.D., Ashok Sharma, Joshua Williams, Gabriela Young, Stephen W. Anderson, M.D.[^], Laura Jacobsen, M.D.[*14] Center for Biotechnology and Genomic Medicine, Augusta University. [*]University of Florida, [^]Pediatric Endocrine Associates, Atlanta.

Germany Clinical Center: Anette G. Ziegler, M.D., PI[1,3,4,11], Andreas Beyerlein, Ph.D.[2], Ezio Bonifacio Ph.D.[*5], Michael Hummel, M.D.[13], Sandra Hummel, Ph.D.[2], Kristina Foterek[¥2], Nicole Janz, Mathilde Kersting, Ph.D.[¥2], Annette Knopff[7], Sibylle Koletzko, M.D.[¶13], Claudia Peplow[12], Roswith Roth, Ph.D.[9], Marlon Scholz, Joanna Stock[9,12,14], Katharina Warncke, M.D.[14], Lorena Wendel, Christiane Winkler, Ph.D.[2,12,15]. Forschergruppe Diabetes e.V. and Institute of Diabetes Research, Helmholtz Zentrum München, and Klinikum rechts der Isar, Technische Universität München. [*]Center for Regenerative Therapies, TU Dresden, [¶]Dr. von Hauner Children's Hospital, Department of Gastroenterology, Ludwig Maximillians University Munich, [¥]Research Institute for Child Nutrition, Dortmund.

Sweden Clinical Center: Åke Lernmark, Ph.D., PI[1,3,4,5,6,8,10,11,15], Daniel Agardh, M.D., Ph.D.[13], Carin Andrén Aronsson[2,12,13], Maria Ask, Jenny Bremer, Ulla-Marie Carlsson, Corrado Cilio, Ph.D., M.D.[5], Emelie Ericson-Hallström, Lina Fransson, Thomas Gard, Joanna Gerardsson, Rasmus Bennet, Monica Hansen, Gertie Hansson, Susanne Hyberg, Fredrik Johansen, Berglind Jonsdottir, M.D., Helena Elding Larsson, M.D., Ph.D. [6,14], Marielle Lindström, Markus Lundgren, M.D.[14], Maria Månsson Martinez, Maria Markan, Jessica Melin[12], Zeliha Mestan, Karin Ottosson, Kobra Rahmati, Anita Ramelius, Falastin Salami, Sara Sibthorpe, Birgitta Sjöberg, Ulrica Swartling, Ph.D.[9,12], Evelyn Tekum Amboh, Carina Törn, Ph.D. [3,15], Anne Wallin, Åsa Wimar[12,14], Sofie Åberg. Lund University.

Washington Clinical Center: William A. Hagopian, M.D., Ph.D., PI[1,3,4, 5, 6,7,11,13, 14], Michael Killian[6,7,12,13], Claire Cowen Crouch[12,14,15], Jennifer Skidmore[2], Josephine Carson, Maria Dalzell, Kayleen Dunson, Rachel Hervey, Corbin Johnson, Rachel Lyons, Arlene Meyer, Denise Mulenga, Alexander Tarr, Morgan Uland, John Willis. Pacific Northwest Diabetes Research Institute.

Pennsylvania Satellite Center: Dorothy Becker, M.D., Margaret Franciscus, MaryEllen Dalmagro-Elias Smith[2], Ashi Daftary, M.D., Mary Beth Klein, Chrystal Yates. Children's Hospital of Pittsburgh of UPMC.

Data Coordinating Center: Jeffrey P. Krischer, Ph.D.,PI[1,4,5,10,11], Michael Abbondondolo, Sarah Austin-Gonzalez, Maryouri Avendano, Sandra Baethke, Rasheedah Brown[12,15], Brant Burkhardt, Ph.D.[5,6], Martha Butterworth[2], Joanna Clasen, David Cuthbertson, Christopher Eberhard, Steven Fiske[9], Dena Garcia, Jennifer Garmeson, Veena Gowda, Kathleen Heyman, Francisco Perez Laras, Hye-Seung Lee, Ph.D.[1,2,13,15], Shu Liu, Xiang Liu, Ph.D.[2,3,9,14], Kristian Lynch, Ph.D. [5,6,9,15], Jamie Malloy, Cristina McCarthy[12,15], Steven Meulemans, Hemang Parikh, Ph.D.[3], Chris Shaffer, Laura Smith, Ph.D.[9,12], Susan Smith[12,15], Noah Sulman, Ph.D., Roy Tamura, Ph.D.[1,2,13], Ulla Uusitalo, Ph.D.[2,15], Kendra Vehik, Ph.D.[4,5,6,14,15], Ponni Vijayakandipan, Keith Wood, Jimin Yang, Ph.D., R.D.[2,15]. Past staff: Lori Ballard, David Hadley, Ph.D., Wendy McLeod. University of South Florida.

Project scientist: Beena Akolkar, Ph.D.[1,3,4,5,6,7,10,11]. National Institutes of Diabetes and Digestive and Kidney Diseases.

Autoantibody Reference Laboratories: Liping Yu, M.D.[*5], Dongmei Miao, M.D.[^], Polly Bingley, M.D., FRCP[*5], Alistair Williams[*], Kyla Chandler[*], Saba Rokni[*], Claire Williams[*], Rebecca Wyatt[*], Gifty George[*], Sian Grace[*]. [^]Barbara Davis Center for Childhood Diabetes, University of Colorado Denver, [*]School of Clinical Sciences, University of Bristol UK.

HLA Reference Laboratory: Henry Erlich, Ph.D.[3], Steven J. Mack, Ph.D., Anna Lisa Fear. Center for Genetics, Children's Hospital Oakland Research Institute.

Repository: Sandra Ke, Niveen Mulholland, Ph.D. NIDDK Biosample Repository at Fisher BioServices.

Other contributors: Kasia Bourcier, Ph.D.[5], National Institutes of Allergy and Infectious Diseases. Thomas Briese, Ph.D.[6,15], Columbia University. Suzanne Bennett Johnson, Ph.D.[9,12], Florida State University. Eric Triplett, Ph.D.[6], University of Florida.

Committees: [1]Ancillary Studies, [2]Diet, [3]Genetics, [4]Human Subjects/Publicity/Publications, [5]Immune Markers, [6]Infectious Agents, [7]Laboratory Implementation, [8]Maternal Studies, [9]Psychosocial, [10]Quality Assurance, [11]Steering, [12]Study Coordinators, [13]Celiac Disease, [14]Clinical Implementation, [15]Quality Assurance Subcommittee on Data Quality.

Trial Identification Number: NCT00279318 (www.clinicaltrials.gov).

Conflicts of Interest: The authors declare no conflict of interest.

References

1. Liu, E.; Lee, H.S.; Aronsson, C.A.; Hagopian, W.A.; Koletzko, S.; Rewers, M.J.; Eisenbarth, G.S.; Bingley, P.J.; Bonifacio, E.; Simell, V.; et al. Risk of pediatric celiac disease according to HLA haplotype and country. *N. Engl. J. Med.* **2014**, *371*, 42–49. [CrossRef] [PubMed]
2. Ivarsson, A.; Myléus, A.; Norström, F.; van der Pals, M.; Rosén, A.; Högberg, L.; Danielsson, L.; Halvarsson, B.; Hammarroth, S.; Hernell, O.; et al. Prevalence of childhood celiac disease and changes in infant feeding. *Pediatrics* **2013**, *131*, e687–e694. [CrossRef] [PubMed]
3. Aronsson, C.A.; Lee, H.S.; Koletzko, S.; Uusitalo, U.; Yang, J.; Virtanen, S.M.; Liu, E.; Lernmark, A.; Norris, J.M.; Agardh, D.; et al. Effects of Gluten Intake on Risk of Celiac Disease: A Case-Control Study on a Swedish Birth Cohort. *Clin. Gastroenterol. Hepatol.* **2016**, *14*, 403–409. [CrossRef] [PubMed]
4. Dieterich, W.; Laag, E.; Schöpper, H.; Volta, U.; Ferguson, A.; Gillett, H.; Riecken, E.O.; Schuppan, D. Autoantibodies to tissue transglutaminase as predictors of celiac disease. *Gastroenterology* **1998**, *115*, 1317–1321. [CrossRef]
5. Hyytinen, M.; Savilahti, E.; Virtanen, S.M.; Härkönen, T.; Ilonen, J.; Luopajärvi, K.; Uibo, R.; Vaarala, O.; Åkerblom, H.K.; Knip, M.; et al. Avoidance of Cow's Milk-based Formula for At-risk Infants Does Not Reduce Development of Celiac Disease: A Randomized Controlled Trial. *Gastroenterology* **2017**, *153*, 961–970. [CrossRef] [PubMed]
6. Almquist-Tangen, G.; Dahlgren, J.; Roswall, J.; Bergman, S.; Alm, B. Milk cereal drink increases BMI risk at 12 and 18 months, but formula does not. *Acta Paediatr.* **2013**, *102*, 1174–1179. [CrossRef] [PubMed]
7. Kellow, N.J.; Savige, G.S. Dietary advanced glycation end-product restriction for the attenuation of insulin resistance, oxidative stress and endothelial dysfunction: A systematic review. *Eur. J. Clin. Nutr.* **2013**, *67*, 239–248. [CrossRef] [PubMed]
8. Van Puyvelde, K.; Mets, T.; Njemini, R.; Beyer, I.; Bautmans, I. Effect of advanced glycation end product intake on inflammation and aging: A systematic review. *Nutr. Rev.* **2014**, *72*, 638–650. [CrossRef] [PubMed]
9. Plaza, M.; Östman, E.; Tareke, E. Maillard Reaction Products in Powder Based for Infants and Toddlers. *Eur. J. Nutr. Food Saf.* **2016**, *6*, 65–74. [CrossRef]
10. Hagopian, W.A.; Erlich, H.; Lernmark, Å.; Rewers, M.; Ziegler, A.G.; Simell, O.; Akolkar, B.; Vogt, R., Jr.; Blair, A.; Llonen, J.; et al. The Environmental Determinants of Diabetes in the Young (TEDDY): Genetic criteria and international diabetes risk screening of 421 000 infants. *Pediatr. Diabetes* **2011**, *12*, 733–743. [CrossRef] [PubMed]
11. Livsmedelsverket. Swedish National Food Composition Database. 2016. Available online: http://www7.slv.se/SokNaringsinnehall (accessed on 8 December 2016).
12. Hoppe, C.; Trolle, E.; Gondolf, U.H.; Husby, S. Gluten intake in 6-36-month-old Danish infants and children based on a national survey. *J. Nutr. Sci.* **2013**, *2*, 1–7. [CrossRef] [PubMed]
13. Institute of Medicine. *Dietary Reference Intakes for Energy, Carbohydrate, Fiber, Fat, Fatty Acids, Cholesterol, Protein, and Amino Acids*; The National Academies Press: Washington, DC, USA, 2005.
14. Gibson, R.S. *Principles of Nutritional Assessment*, 2nd ed.; Oxford University Press: New York, NY, USA, 2005.
15. Ivarsson, A.; Hernell, O.; Stenlund, H.; Persson, L.Å. Breast-feeding protects against celiac disease. *Am. J. Clin. Nutr.* **2002**, *75*, 914–921. [CrossRef] [PubMed]
16. Akobeng, A.K.; Ramanan, A.V.; Buchan, I.; Heller, R.F. Effect of breast feeding on risk of coeliac disease: A systematic review and meta-analysis of observational studies. *Arch. Dis. Child.* **2006**, *91*, 39–43. [CrossRef] [PubMed]
17. Lachat, C.; Hawwash, D.; Ocké, M.C.; Berg, C.; Forsum, E.; Hörnell, A.; Larsson, C.I.; Sonestedt, E.; Wirfält, E.; Åkessonet, A.; et al. Strengthening the Reporting of Observational Studies in Epidemiology—nutritional epidemiology (STROBE-nut): An extension of the STROBE statement. *Nutr. Bull.* **2016**, *41*, 240–251. [CrossRef] [PubMed]

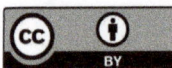

nutrients

MDPI

Article

Milk Fermented by Specific *Lactobacillus* Strains Regulates the Serum Levels of IL-6, TNF-*α* and IL-10 Cytokines in a LPS-Stimulated Murine Model

Aline Reyes-Díaz, Verónica Mata-Haro, Jesús Hernández, Aarón F. González-Córdova, Adrián Hernández-Mendoza, Ricardo Reyes-Díaz, María J. Torres-Llanez, Lilia M. Beltrán-Barrientos and Belinda Vallejo-Cordoba *

Centro de Investigación en Alimentación y Desarrollo, A.C. (CIAD), Carretera a La Victoria Km. 0.6, Apartado 1735, Hermosillo, Sonora 83304, Mexico; alredi22@hotmail.com (A.R.-D.); vmata@ciad.mx (V.M.-H.); jhdez@ciad.mx (J.H.); aaronglz@ciad.mx (A.F.G.-C.); ahernandez@ciad.mx (A.H.-M.); ricardo.reyes@ciad.mx (R.R.-D.); mtorres@ciad.mx (M.J.T.-L.); lilia.beltranb@gmail.com (L.M.B.-B.)
* Correspondence: vallejo@ciad.mx; Tel.: +52-662-289-2400

Received: 28 April 2018; Accepted: 23 May 2018; Published: 29 May 2018

Abstract: Studies report that metabolites, such as peptides, present in fermented milk with specific lactic acid bacteria, may regulate cytokine production and exert an anti-inflammatory effect. Hence, the cytokine regulatory effect of fermented milk by specific *Lactobacillus* strains was evaluated in a lipopolysaccharide (LPS)-stimulated murine model. From twelve strains, three (J20, J23 and J28) were selected for their high proteolytic and acidifying capacities in milk and used for the in vivo study. Three treatments (fermented milk, FM; pasteurized fermented milk, PFM; and its <10 kDa fractions, PFM10) were administrated daily for four weeks. After treatments, animals were induced to a systemic inflammation with LPS, and blood samples were collected 6 h post-LPS injection for cytokine analyses. Results showed that FM or PFM significantly ($p > 0.05$) reduced pro-inflammatory cytokine (IL-6 and TNF-α) concentrations and significantly increased anti-inflammatory (IL-10) cytokine concentrations in comparison to the control; also, pro-inflammatory cytokines were reduced for animals treated with PFM10 ($p < 0.05$). RP-HPLC-MS/MS analysis showed that water-soluble extracts (<10 kDa) from PFM with J28 presented 15 new peptides, which may be the metabolites involved in the cytokine regulatory effect of fermented milk.

Keywords: fermented milk; cytokine regulation; *Lactobacillus*; lipopolysaccharide

1. Introduction

The intake of dairy products fermented by *Lactobacillus* (L.) spp. have been associated with the ability to confer health benefits [1]. The modulation of the specific immune response through cytokine production regulation, which has shown to be strain dependent, is probably the most important health benefit [2,3]. The health-promoting effects may arise not only from bacteria themselves [4], but also from metabolites derived from milk fermentation, particularly bioactive peptides, that play a crucial role on these beneficial effects [5]. However, little attention has been paid to the modulation of cytokine production by bioactive peptides produced in milk fermented by lactic acid bacteria (LAB).

It has been reported that cell wall components of LAB or peptides liberated in milk may interact with specific receptors in the immune cells, which selectively influence the immune system through different mechanisms [6]. In fact, peptides derived from *L. helveticus*-fermented milk could enhance the systemic immune response following an *Escherichia* (E.) *coli* O157:H7 challenge [6]. Nevertheless, few reports have been published on the anti-inflammatory effects of fermented milk with other *Lactobacillus* strains. Indeed, most in vitro and in vivo related studies have been carried out with milk fermented with *L. helveticus* [7–9], and only one study was performed with *L. fermentum* [10].

Lipopolysaccharide (LPS) induces acute inflammation and endotoxic shock in experimental animals [3,11–13], and it is characterized by the production of cytokines and other mediators of inflammation. Therefore, LPS may be used to induce inflammation to evaluate the anti-inflammatory effect of fermented milk. During an infection by bacteria or viruses, among others, the host responds producing pro-inflammatory cytokines to contain infection. Pro-inflammatory cytokines such as interleukin-6 (IL-6) and tumor necrosis factor alpha (TNF-α) are responsible for early responses and amplify reactions, whereas anti-inflammatory cytokines such as IL-4 and IL-10 reduce inflammation and promote healing [14]. Pro-inflammatory cytokines contribute to defense mechanisms of the host and when secreted in excess, they may induce immunopathological disorders [15–18]. Therefore, it is necessary to find ways to downregulate its production or inhibit its effects in vivo. The aim of the present study was to evaluate the anti-inflammatory effects of milk fermented by specific *Lactobacillus* strains, on the serum cytokines levels in a LPS-stimulated murine model. Firstly, *Lactobacillus* strains were selected based on their technological properties such as proteolytic and acidifying activities. Then, selected strains were used to prepare fermented milk (FM), pasteurized fermented milk (PFM) and its fractions (<10 kDa) (PFM10), and the anti-inflammatory effects were tested in an in vivo study. In addition, peptides present in fractions (<10 kDa) were identified, since they may be associated to the potential anti-inflammatory effect.

2. Materials and Methods

2.1. Substrates and Chemicals

Lactobacilli MRS broth (De Man, Rogosa and Sharpe) was purchased from Difco (Sparks, MD, USA). Nonfat dry milk was obtained from Dairy America (Fresno, CA, USA). O-Phthaldialdehyde (OPA) was purchased from Fluka (Linz, Oberösterreich, Austria), and trichloroacetic acid (TCA), sodium dodecyl sulfate (SDS), 2-mercaptoethanol, acetonitrile, trifluoroacetic acid (TFA) and LPS from *E. coli* serotype O11:B4 were purchased from Sigma Chemical Co. (St. Louis, MO, USA).

2.2. Strains and Growth Conditions

Twelve *Lactobacillus* strains were obtained from the culture collection from the Dairy Laboratory at the Food Research and Development Center, A.C. (CIAD, A.C., Hermosillo, Sonora, Mexico). These wild strains were isolated from artisanal cheese and characterized [19]. *Lactobacillus* strains were cultured in 10 mL of sterile MRS Broth. Then, three consecutive subcultures were prepared (1%, v/v) and incubated for 24, 18 and 12 h, respectively, at 37 °C, in order to obtain fresh cultures. The initial average population (10^9 CFU/mL) of the inoculum was obtained in the 12-h fresh culture by the plate count method.

2.3. Preparation of Fermented Milk

Reconstituted nonfat dry milk (10%, w/v) was heated at 110 °C for 10 min, immediately cooled and stored overnight at 4 °C. To prepare starter cultures, a fresh culture of each strain was inoculated (1%, w/v) in sterile reconstituted nonfat milk, followed by incubation at 37 °C for 12 h. FM was produced by inoculation of sterile reconstituted commercial nonfat dry milk (10%, w/v) with starter cultures (3%, v/v), followed by incubation at 37 °C for 48 h. The final average population in each FM was 109 CFU/mL. PFM was prepared by heating fermented milk at 75 °C for 20 min and immediately cooling in an ice bath. PFM10 was prepared by centrifuging PFM in a Sorvall ST 16R centrifuge at 4696× g (Thermo Scientific, Osterode, Am Kalkberg, Germany) for 40 min at 4 °C; and supernatants were collected and ultra-filtered through 10 kDa cut-off membranes (Pall life Science, Port Washington, NY, USA) in a stirred ultrafiltration cell (Millipore Amicon, Bedford, MA, USA). Permeates (<10 kDa) were collected, frozen at −80 °C and lyophilized in a FreeZone 6 freeze dryer (Labconco, Kansas, MO, USA). For the in vivo study, PFM10 was daily prepared by reconstitution to the original volume. Meanwhile, control acidified milk (AM) was prepared with sterile nonfat milk and acidified with lactic acid (Faga Lab, Cd. México, México) until a pH of 4.3 was reached. Peptide content in PFM and PFM10 was determined in the water-soluble fractions after protein precipitation with TCA (14%) by the bicinchoninic acid (BCA) method [20].

2.4. Proteolytic and Acidifying Activity

Proteolysis during milk fermentation at 24 and 48 h was quantified by using the OPA method [19]. For this purpose, 5 mL of 0.75 N TCA were added to 2.5 mL of fermented milk and vortexed for 1 min. Samples were kept at 4 °C for 30 min, then they were centrifuged (4696× g, 40 min, 4 °C). The supernatants were filtered using Whatman No. 2 paper. All filtrates were frozen at −20 °C until further analysis. A 30 µL sample aliquot containing TCA-soluble peptides were added to 600 µL of the freshly prepared OPA reagent. After 2 min at 20 °C, absorbance was immediately measured at 340 nm using a spectrophotometer Nanodrop 2000C (Thermo Scientific, Claire, WI, USA).

During fermentation, pH measurements were taken at 24 and 48 h, using a HI 2211 pH and ORP Benchtop Meter (Hanna Instruments, Woonocket, RI, USA). Additionally, titratable acidity was monitored [21]. Measurements were taken in duplicate.

2.5. Assay in a Murine Model

Male Wistar rats (5–6 weeks old, 110–160 g body weight (BW)) were obtained from Bioinvert & Aprexbio S.A. de C.V. (Ciudad de México, México). All rats were fed with a standard diet (Standard Rodent Laboratory-Chow 5001 Diet, Purina Feeds, Inc., St. Louis, MO, USA) and purified water *ad libitum*. Rats were housed in sanitized polycarbonate cages (60 × 40 × 30 cm) with sterile sawdust bedding that was replaced daily. Room temperature was kept at 22 ± 2 °C, with a relative humidity between 40 and 60%, and 12 h light/dark cycles.

Animals were adapted (first week) and randomly assigned in pairs to experimental groups (n = 6). The bioassay included the eleven groups: AM (control), FM/20, PFM/J20, PFM10/J20, FM/J23, PFM/J23, PFM10/J23, FM/J28, PFM/J28, and PFM10/J28. Also, a PBS (phosphate-buffered saline solution) group without LPS-induced inflammation was included for the evaluation of cytokine concentrations in a nonstimulated group. During four weeks, animals were daily fed with 1 mL of each treatment.

After four weeks, animals were subcutaneously injected with LPS (7.5 mg/kg BW, diluted in milliQ water) to induce a systemic inflammatory process. Finally, rats were sacrificed 6 h post-LPS stimulation. Blood samples were taken and centrifuged at 2348× g for 8 min; serum was collected and kept at −20 °C until cytokine analyses. This study was approved by the ethical committee of the Food Research and Development Center, A.C. (CE/007/2015) and was carried out following the recommendations of the Committee on Care and Use of Laboratory Animals of the Institute of Laboratory Animals Resources [22].

2.6. Cytokine Determinations

IL-10, IL-6 and TNF-α serum cytokine concentrations were determined by the ELISA method (Enzyme-Linked Immunosorbent Assay) using commercially available kits (Thermo Scientific, Rockford, IL, USA). These tests comprised recombinant cytokines from *E. coli* and antibodies against anti-inflammatory and pro-inflammatory cytokines (with 3, 5 and 15 pg/mL detection limits, respectively).

2.7. Isolation of Peptide Fractions by Reversed-Phase HPLC

Peptide profiles of PFM10 samples were obtained by reversed-phase high performance liquid chromatography (RP-HPLC) (1100 series; Agilent Technologies Japan Ltd., Tokyo, Japan) at 214 nm. Separation was carried out with an Extend-C18 (4.6 × 250 mm, 5-µm particle size, 180-A pore size) column from Agilent Technologies (Santa Clara, CA, USA) at room temperature (22 °C) with a solvent flow rate of 0.25 mL/min. Solvent A was a mixture of water-trifluoroacetic acid (1000:0.4, v/v) and solvent B contained acetonitrile-trifluoroacetic acid (1000:0.3, v/v). 20 µL of sample were injected. Peptides were eluted with a linear gradient of solvent B in solvent A from 0.1 to 99.9% for 40 min. The concentration of solvent B was linearly increased from 0.1 to 60 % in 30 min and from 60 to 99.9% between 30 and 35 min, then it was decreased from 99.9% to 0.1% between 35–40 min. Fractions from five chromatographic runs were collected, freeze dried and stored for further analysis.

2.8. Analysis of Peptides by Tandem Mass Spectrometry

Mass spectrometry (MS) analysis was performed using a 1100 Series LC/MSD Trap (Agilent Technologies Inc., Waldbronn, Karlsruhe, Germany) equipped with an electrospray ionization source (LC-ESI-MS). The nanocolumn was a C18-300 (150 mm × 0.75 µm, 3.5 µm; Agilent Technologies Inc.). The sample injection volume was 1 µL. Solvent A was a mixture of water-acetonitrile-formic acid (10:90:0.1, $v/v/v$) and solvent B contained water-acetonitrile-formic acid (97:3:0.1, $v/v/v$). The gradient was based on the increment of solvent B, which was initially set at 3% for 10 min and it took 23 more min to reach 65%. The 0.7 µL/min flow rate was directed into the mass spectrometer via an electrospray interface. Nitrogen (99.99%) was used as the nebulizing and drying gas and operated with an estimated helium pressure of 5×10^2 Pa. The needle voltage was set at 4 kV. Mass spectra were acquired over a range of 300 to 2500 mass/charge (m/z). The signal threshold to perform auto MS analyses was 30,000. The precursor ions were isolated within a range of 4.0 m/z and fragmented with a voltage ramp from 0.35 to 1.1 V. Peptide sequences were obtained from mass spectrometry data using the Mascot [23] server through the UniProtKB/Swiss-Prot database (http://www.matrixscience.com/help/seq_db_ setup_Sprot.html (accessed on 5 September 2016) sequences.

2.9. Statistical Analysis

Data normality was tested as a prerequisite before one way analysis of variance (ANOVA) was carried out in order to compare groups. Differences among means were assessed by Fisher's least significant difference for multiple comparison test and considered significant when $p \leq 0.05$. Data analyses were performed with NCSS 2007.

3. Results and Discussion

3.1. Strain Selection

3.1.1. Proteolytic Activity

Lactobacillus strains from two species (six *L. fermentum* and six *L. pentosus*) were evaluated [19]. Proteolytic activity assessed at 24 and 48 h of fermentation showed significant differences ($p < 0.05$), and it was time and strain dependent (Figure 1). Strains of *Lactobacillus fermentum* J20, J23 and J28 presented the highest proteolytic activity ($p < 0.05$). On the other hand, strains J10, J24, J26, J27, J31, J32, J34, J37 and J38 were considered as weakly proteolytic. The high proteolytic activity for species *L. fermentum* may be related to a large number of proteases and peptidases present [24].

It has been reported that metabolites such as peptides, released during fermentation, are important for the bioactive properties attributed to highly proteolytic lactic acid bacteria [8]. In fact, a study of the effect of *L. helveticus* and its nonproteolytic variant reported that mice administrated with milk fermented by the proteolytic variant (wild) of *L. helveticus* enhanced the immunomodulatory effect in comparison to those fed with milk fermented with the nonproteolytic variant [8]. Moreover, in another study the peptidic fractions from *Lactobacillus helveticus*-fermented milk offered protection against *Salmonella* infection, possibly by interfering in the virulence function [9]

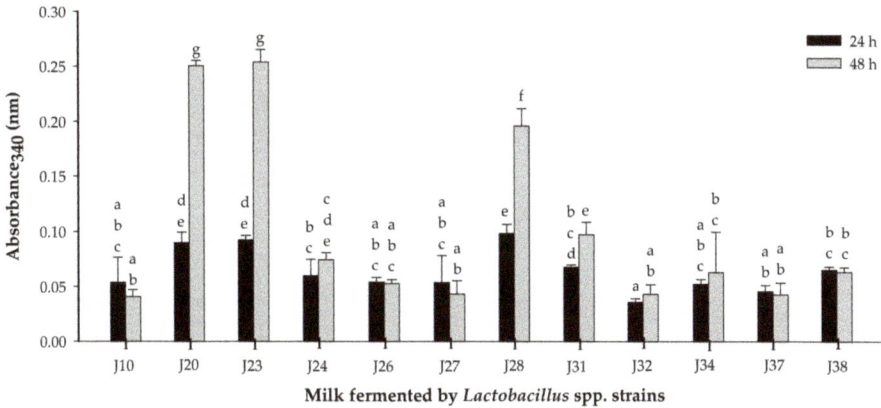

Figure 1. Proteolytic activity (o-phtaldialdehyde method) in milk fermented by different strains of *Lactobacillus* spp. at 24 or 48 h of fermentation (37 °C). Mean ± SD ($n = 3$). Different letters indicate significant differences ($p < 0.05$) among all fermented milks. Strains: J10, J20, J23, J28, J32 and J38 are *Lactobacillus fermentum*; J24, J26, J27, J31, J34 and J37 are *Lactobacillus pentosus*.

3.1.2. Acidifying Activity

The acidifying activity of *Lactobacillus* strains was evaluated by monitoring pH and titratable acidity at 24 and 48 h of fermentation (Figures 2 and 3). pH significantly decreased ($p < 0.05$) for milk fermented by *Lactobacillus* J20, J23 and J28 after 24 or 48 h. Similarly, titratable acidity was significantly ($p < 0.05$) different for these same strains of *Lactobacillus* J20, J23 and J28 after 24 and 48 h of fermentation. On the other hand, pH and titratable acidity did not significantly ($p > 0.05$) change for the rest of the strains. pH change and lactic acid production were strain dependent and may be explained in terms of differences in metabolic ability and growth requirements. While pH reduction depends on the amount of lactic acid and other organic acids released, which is directly linked to the culture metabolic capacity, titratable acidity depends only on the lactic acid produced [25].

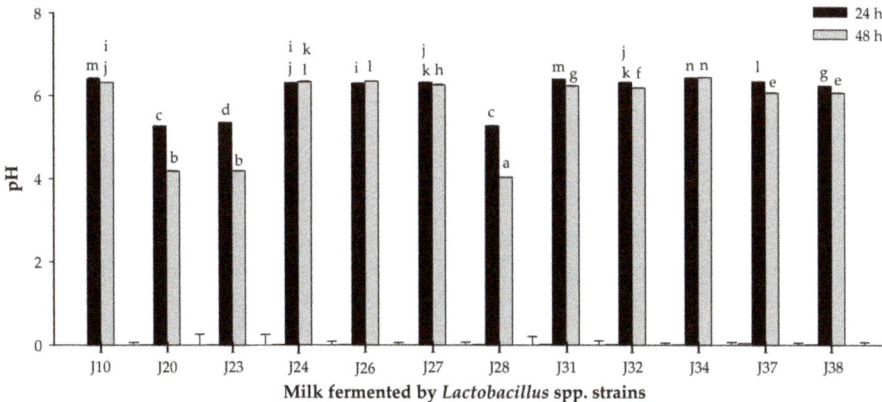

Figure 2. pH of milk fermented by *Lactobacillus* spp. strains at 24 or 48 h of fermentation. Mean ± SD ($n = 3$). Different letters indicate significant differences ($p < 0.05$) among all fermented milks. Strains: J10, J20, J23, J28, J32 and J38 are *Lactobacillus fermentum*; J24, J26, J27, J31, J34 and J37 are *Lactobacillus pentosus*.

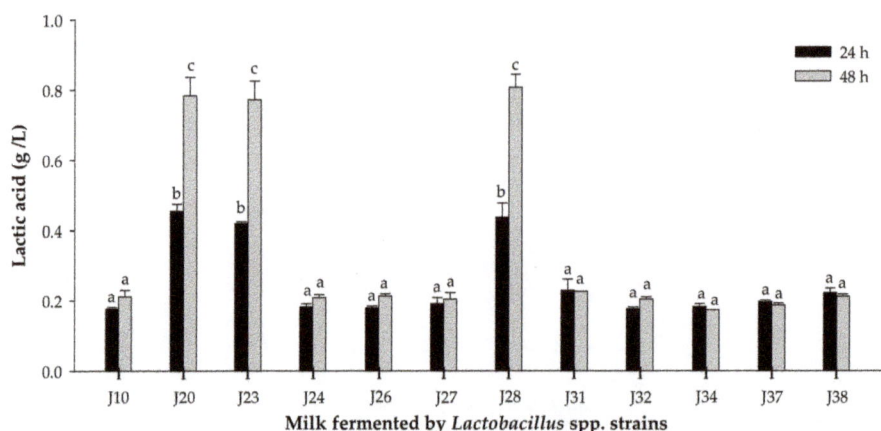

Figure 3. Lactic acid concentration in milk fermented by *Lactobacillus* spp. strains at 24 or 48 h of fermentation. Mean ± SD (*n* = 3). Different letters indicate significant differences (*p* < 0.05) among all fermented milks. Strains: J10, J20, J23, J28, J32 and J38 are *Lactobacillus fermentum*; J24, J26, J27, J31, J34 and J37 are *Lactobacillus pentosus*.

Since *Lactobacillus* J20, J23 and J28 showed the highest proteolytic and acidifying activities in milk, which are desirable technological properties; they were selected for further studies. Efficient proteolytic activity of some *Lactobacillus* sp. has been associated to the production of bioactive peptides with immunomodulatory activity derived from the hydrolysis of casein in milk. Additionally, acidification protects milk against spoilage by microorganisms and proliferation of pathogens, as well as contributes to the flavor and texture of fermented dairy products [25].

Bacterial growth for the selected strains of *L. fermentum* J20, J23 and J28 was monitored, and the point corresponding to the end of the exponential phase that reached 10^9 CFU/mL at 12 h was chosen as the initial average population for milk inoculum.

3.2. Cytokine Analysis in an LPS-Stimulated Murine Model

In this study, the effects of milk fermented by the three different selected strains of *L. fermentum* were evaluated, according to their capacity to modulate the production of IL-6, TNF-α and IL-10 cytokines in a LPS-stimulated murine model.

In a preliminary assay, it was found that 7.5 mg/kg of BW of LPS was an adequate dose to induce an increase on cytokine production in serum (data not shown). As expected, for all the cytokines tested, the LPS-stimulated control group (AM) presented significantly higher (*p* < 0.05) levels than the PBS group (without LPS stimulation) (Figures 4–6).

The IL-6 concentrations were determined in animals treated with LPS (Figure 4). Groups fed with FM/J23 or FM/J28 presented significantly lower (*p* < 0.05) IL-6 in serum, in contrast to the control group. However, FM/J20 did not show significant differences (*p* > 0.05) in IL-6 compared to the control group (AM). Furthermore, IL-6 concentrations in animals treated with PFM/J20, PFM/J23 or PFM/J28 were significantly (*p* < 0.05) lower than the control group (AM). Also, results showed that groups treated with PFM10/J28 significantly decreased (*p* < 0.05) concentrations of IL-6 in comparison to the control group. Nevertheless, PFM10/J20 and PFM/J23 were not significantly different (*p* > 0.05) from the control group.

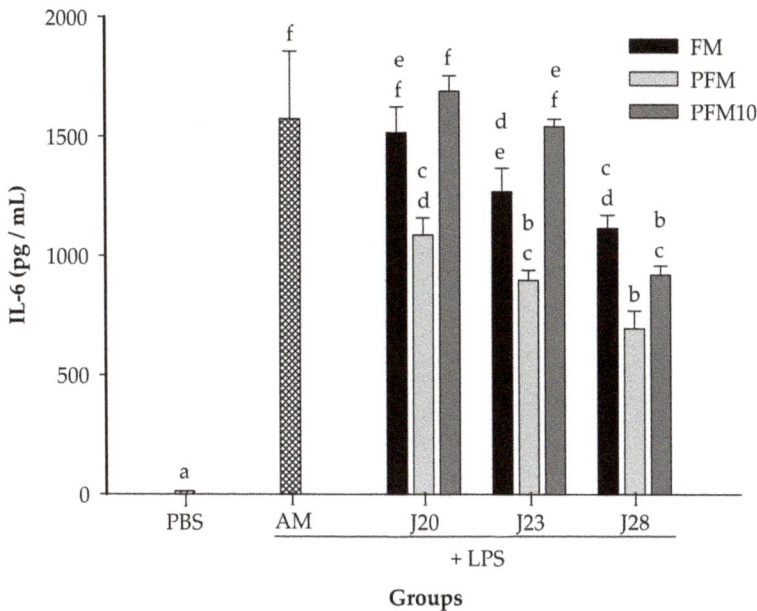

Figure 4. Serum concentrations of IL-6. Wistar rats were fed with fermented milk (FM), pasteurized fermented milk (PFM), fractions <10 kDa of PFM (PFM10) with *Lactobacillus* J20, J23 or J28; after 4 weeks, rats were injected with lipopolysaccharide, and sacrificed after 6 h post-injection. Control groups included: acidified milk (AM) injected with LPS; or phosphate buffer saline (PBS) without LPS. Bars represent means ± SE (*n* = 6). Different letters indicate significant differences (*p* < 0.05) among all groups.

In the case of TNF-α concentrations (Figure 5), animals treated with FM/J20 or FM/J28 showed a reduction (*p* < 0.05) of TNF-α compared to the control group. Nevertheless, FM/J23 was not significantly (*p* > 0.05) different from the control group. Also, all PFM/J20, PFM/J23 or PFM/J28 treatments significantly reduced (*p* < 0.05) TNF-α concentrations when compared to the control group. Moreover, results showed that groups treated with PFM10/J20, PFM/J23, and PFM/J28 significantly decreased (*p* < 0.05) concentrations of pro-inflammatory TNF-α cytokines, in comparison to the control group (AM) (Figure 5). It is noteworthy that FM/J28 was able to reduce TNF-α in all the treatments, whether in fermented milk, pasteurized fermented milk or its fractions.

Furthermore, the IL-10 concentrations were determined post-LPS treatments (Figure 6). Animals treated with FM/J20, FM/J23 or FM/J28 presented IL-10 concentrations that were significantly (*p* < 0.05) higher than the control group. Moreover, serum concentrations of this cytokine from PFM with J20, J23 or J28 groups were also significantly (*p* < 0.05) higher than those in the control group. Nevertheless, the IL-10 concentration for all administered groups with PFM10 did not increase in comparison to the control group (Figure 6). This may be due to the fact that the peptidic nitrogen content in PFM10/J28 was significantly (*p* < 0.05) lower than that in PFM (0.20 vs. 0.30%).

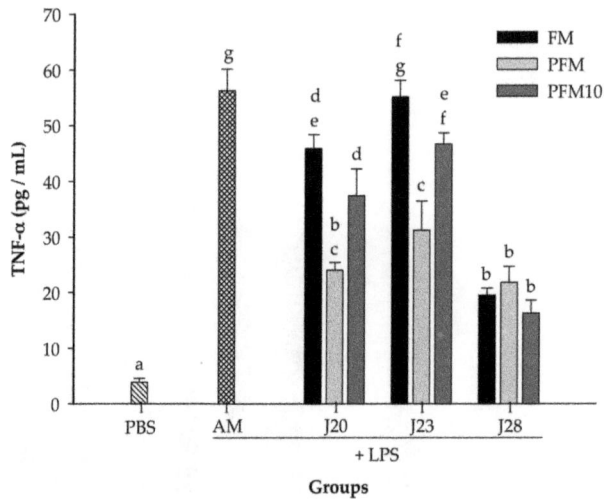

Figure 5. Serum concentrations of TNF-α. Groups were daily administrated for 4 weeks with fermented milk (FM), pasteurized fermented milk (PFM), fractions <10 kDa of PFM (PFM10) with *Lactobacillus* J20, J23 or J28; after 4 weeks, rats were injected with LPS, and sacrificed after 6 h post-injection. Control groups included: acidified milk (AM) injected with LPS; or phosphate buffer saline (PBS) without LPS. Bars represent means ± SE (n = 6). Different letters indicate significant differences (p < 0.05) among all groups.

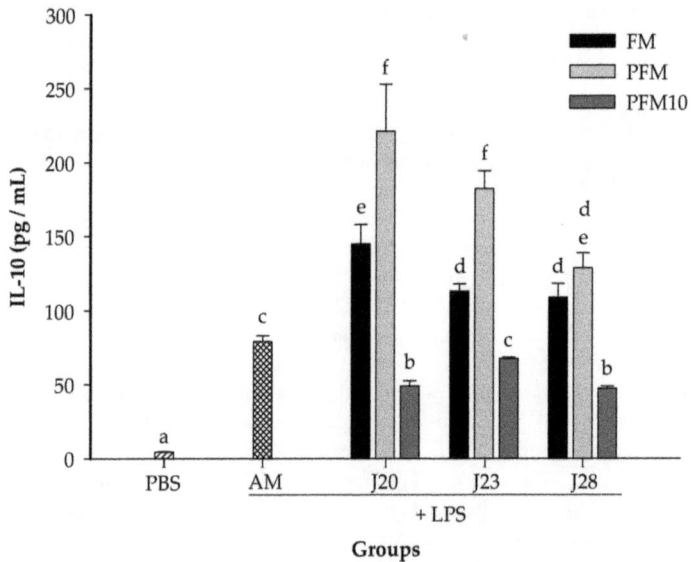

Figure 6. Serum concentration of IL-10. Groups were daily administrated for 4 weeks with fermented milk (FM), pasteurized fermented milk (PFM), fractions <10 kDa of PFM (PFM10) with *Lactobacillus* J20, J23 or J28; after 4 weeks, rats were injected with LPS, and sacrificed after 6 h post-injection. Control groups included: acidified milk (AM) injected with LPS; or phosphate buffer saline (PBS) without LPS. Bars represent means ± SE (n = 6). Different letters indicate significant differences (p < 0.05) among all groups.

3.3. Identification of Peptides in Milk Fermented by Lactobacillus Fermentum J28 with Potential Regulatory Effect on Cytokine Production

To the best of our knowledge, this is the first study that reports the anti-inflammatory effect of fermented milk with wild lactic acid bacteria different from *L. helveticus*. Indeed, the anti-inflammatory effect of FM with *L. helveticus* was reported in a murine model with LPS-induced inflammation and demonstrated that after three weeks of treatments, there was an inhibition of the production of the pro-inflammatory cytokine TNF-α, and an enhancement of the production of anti-inflammatory cytokine IL-10 [26].

The beneficial effects of fermented milk products may not only be attributed to bacteria themselves, but also to the metabolites produced during the fermentation [7]. The most important metabolites in fermented milks are peptides not present prior to fermentation; these bioactive peptides are potential modulators of various regulatory processes in the body [27]. In the present study, PFM treatment containing inactive bacteria presented a cytokine regulatory effect; therefore, this effect may not be attributable to live bacteria. It has been reported that nonviable bacteria may also exert beneficial effects [28]. In this sense, studies have reported that heat-treated whole nonviable bacterial cells, such as *L. casei Shirota* [29], *L. acidophilus* A2, *L. gasseri* A5, and *L. salivarius* A6 [30] presented anti-inflammatory effect. Thus, the anti-inflammatory effect of bacterial components present in PFM cannot be discarded.

Moreover, the regulatory effect of fermented milk was enhanced with heat treatment, which might be associated to structural protein changes. It has been reported that heat treatment changes the structural conformation of proteins and peptides in milk, promoting the formation of a large variety of bioactive peptides through digestion, since different protein bonds will be available for enzymes in the gastrointestinal tract [31]. Thus, peptides and proteins present in PFM may be more readily available for digestion in order to exert the regulatory effect. In fact, pro-inflammatory cytokine concentrations in PFM tended to be lower than in FM (Figures 4 and 5).

It is important to note that milk fermented by J28 (FM or PFM) was the most potent regulator for pro-inflammatory cytokines (IL-6 and TNF-α), while groups treated with FM/J20 or PFM/20 and PFM/23 were more potent inducers for the anti-inflammatory cytokine IL-10. Furthermore, it is worthwhile to highlight that although the proteolytic activity of J28 was significantly ($p < 0.05$) lower than that for J20 or J23 (Figure 1), treatments with J28, seem to have the greatest capacity to regulate pro-inflammatory cytokine production. Thus, it appears that what it is most important is the chemical structure of bioactive peptides.

It has been reported that peptides with the capacity to regulate the production of cytokines or the proliferation of immune cells consist of 2 to 32 AA, which may be contained in the fraction with a molecular weight of <10 kDa [32,33]. Hence, peptides present in PFM10 with J28 were identified.

A typical peptide profile produced by J28 showing five collected fractions (F1 to F5) is depicted in Figure 7. After fraction collection, peptides were identified by mass spectrometry. A typical mass spectrum of one of the peptides derived from β-casein is depicted in Figure 8. The proteolysis process gave rise to medium-sized peptides, ranging in length from 7 to 32 amino acids and a molecular weight mostly <3 kDa (Table 1).

Proteases and peptidases in J28 targeted mainly whey proteins, since twelve peptide sequences were derived from whey and only three from caseins. Peptides listed in Table 1 showed the action of mainly serine proteases, specifically trypsin, which cleaves the peptide chains mainly at the carboxyl side of the amino acids lysine (K) or arginine (R) [34].

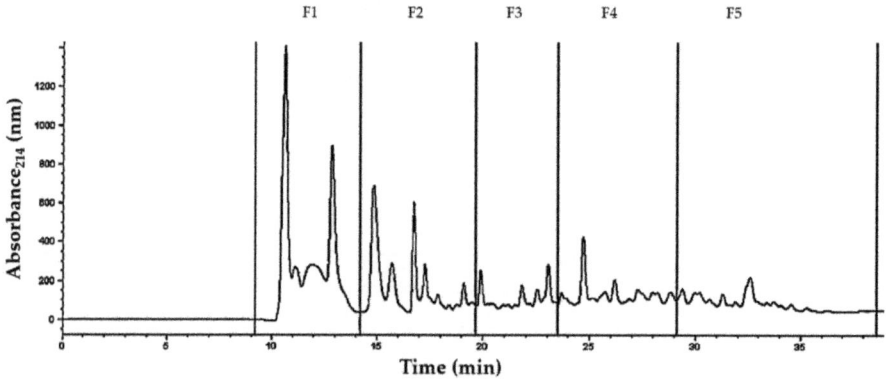

Figure 7. Peptide profiles in the water soluble fraction (<10 kDa) from pasteurized fermented milk (PFM10) with *Lactobacillus fermentum* J28, obtained by reversed-phase High Performance Liquid Chromatography at 214 nm. F1 to F5 correspond to collected fractions.

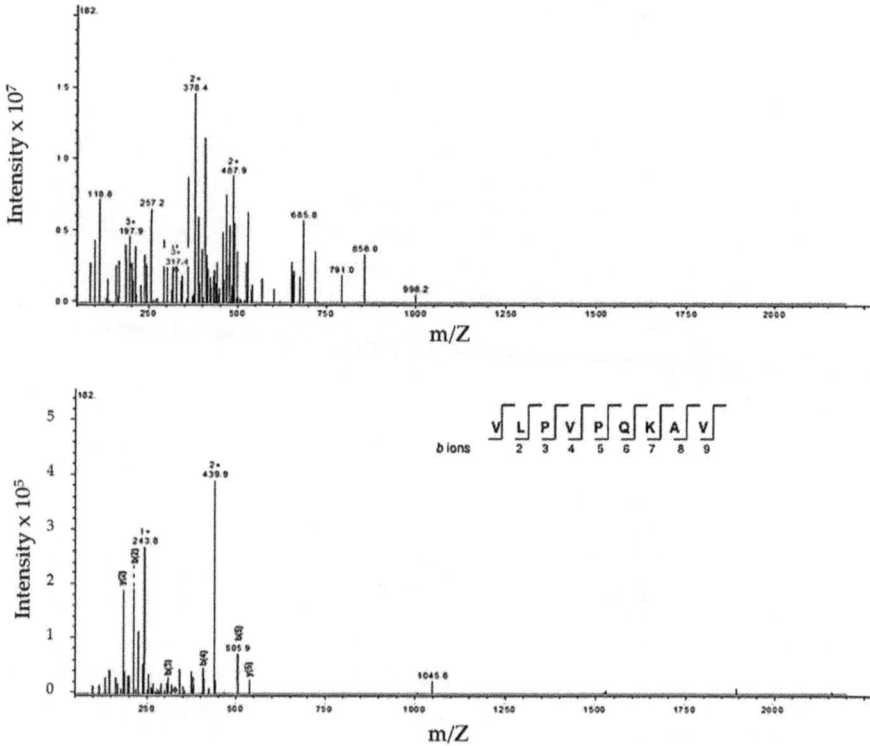

Figure 8. Typical mass spectrum corresponding to peptide sequence (VLPVPQKAV) collected from F4 obtained from milk fermented by *Lactobacillus fermentum* J28. (**A**) Triple-charged ion 317.4 m/z; (**B**) tandem mass spectrometry (MS/MS) spectrum for the specified ion in (**A**). After interpretation and comparison in the database, the fragment AA sequence matched β-CN (f185-193).

Table 1. Identification of peptides in the water soluble fraction (<10 kDa) obtained from milk fermented by *Lactobacillus fermentum* J28.

Sample [a]	Experimental Mass	Theoretical Mass	Molecular Ion (m/z) Selected for MS/MS [b] (Charge)	Protein Fragment	Sequence
F1	1622.75	1623.26	541.1 (+3)	α-La (f100–113)	LDDDLTDDIMCVKK
	2028.52	2028.09	2029.5 (+1)	β-Lg (f48–65)	LDAQSAPLRVYVEELKPT
F2	1877.74	1878.87	1878.7 (+1)	αs1-CN (50–66)	EKVNELSKDIGSESTED
	708.21	708.34	237.1 (+3)	α-La (f33–39)	DLKGYGG
F3	1029.86	1030.65	344.3 (+3)	β-Lg (f91–99)	KTKIPAVFK
	729.22	729.43	244.1 (+3)	Lactotransferrin (f67–73)	AIAEKKA
	3409.04	3409.73	1705.5 (+2)	Lactotransferrin (f73–104)	ADAVTLDGGMVFEAGRDPYKLRPVAAEIYGTK
	2036.38	2036.87	2037.4 (+1)	Lactotransferrin (f564–581)	NDTVWENTNGESTADWAK
	810.65	811.40	407.3 (+2)	Serotransferrin (f668–674)	AKKTYDS
	831.44	832.42	832.4 (+1)	Serotransferrin (f683–689)	AMTNLRQ
F4	967.94	968.47	484.9 (+2)	κ-CN (f55–62)	RYPSYGLN
	949.23	949.59	317.4 (+3)	β-CN (185–193)	VLPVPQKAV
	2236.12	2237.17	2237.1 (+1)	Lactotransferrin (f628–647)	QVLLHQQALFGKNGKNCPDK
F5	916.00	916.45	459.0 (+2)	β-Lg (f117–123)	KYLLFCM
	1133.62	1133.50	284.4 (+4)	Lactotransferrin (f523–533)	LCAGDDQGLDK

[a] F1 to F5 are collected fractions. [b] MS/MS: tandem mass spectrometry. Abbreviations used in table: α-La, alpha-lactalbumin; β-Lg, beta-lactoglobulin; αs1-CN, alpha-S1-casein; κ-CN, kappa-casein; β-CN, beta-casein.

A key point in the cytokine regulatory effect of bioactive peptides is the type of amino acid in the N-terminal and C-terminal positions [35]. Evidence suggests that the amino acid R in the extreme (N-terminal or C-terminal) of bioactive peptides is the dominant entity recognized by receptors on macrophages and lymphocytes, which may enhance their maturation and proliferation [36,37]. In this study, only one sequence with R (RYPSYGLN) derived from casein was present in milk fermented by J28. Portions of this sequence (YPSYGL and YPSYG) were reported to have angiotensin converting enzyme inhibitory activity (ACEI), in milk fermented by *Lactococcus lactis* NRRL B-50571 [38]. Also, sequence RYPSYG was reported to have ACEI in bovine casein hydrolysate prepared by neutral protease [39].

Similarly, a peptide (VLPVPQKAV) from β-casein was identified (Figure 8). It was reported that a portion of this peptide VLPVPQ presented ACEI activity [40]. Also, another peptide (VLPVPQK) derived from this same sequence inhibited lipoxygenase (enzyme associated to inflammatory process) activity in vitro. Thus, this peptide was linked to modulating inflammation [41]. Furthermore, the peptide VLPVPQK has also been reported to have anti-oxidative potential effect [42]. Additionally, it was reported that this peptide may be absorbed intact with PepT1-like transporters in a human intestinal cell model (Caco-2) [43]. Milk derived peptides have different biological effects, such as antihypertensive (ACEI), antioxidant and immunomodulatory [42,44]. Thus, one particular peptide sequence may have multiple bioactivities. These peptides, are inactive in the milk protein, and may be released and activated through milk fermentation by microorganisms and gastrointestinal digestion [45].

Likewise, the antihypertensive peptide VY [45] and the hypotriglyceridemic peptide VTL, which may be liberated during gastrointestinal digestion [46], are contained in the whey protein derived peptides, such as LDAQSAPLRVYVEELKPT and ADAVTLDGGMVFEAGRDPYKLRPVAAEIYGTK, respectively (Table 1). Additionally, the dipeptide YG contained in this sequence was reported to enhance the proliferation of peripheral blood lymphocytes and be used as an immunomodulatory peptide [47].

When LPS is released into the bloodstream causes inflammation via activation of monocytes and endothelial cells. It can lead to septic shock and even death. One strategy to prevent endotoxic shock is to neutralize the negatively charged phosphoryl groups present in lipid A, the most conserved part and major mediator of LPS activity bear by positively charged LPS-binding molecules, such as proteins or peptides [48]. In this sense, some examples of dairy peptides with proven LPS-binding ability that can reduce LPS activity have been reported [49,50]. Nevertheless, further studies are needed to evaluate the possible LPS-binding activity of peptides from milk fermented by J28.

The literature has reported the immunomodulatory effect of peptides mainly derived from caseins, and just few were related to the anti-inflammatory process [35]. Thus, these results open the possibility for finding new peptide sequences with anti-inflammatory activity.

In conclusion, FM by specific strains of *L. fermentum* are able to modulate the balance of LPS-induced pro- and anti-inflammatory serum cytokines. The cytokine regulatory effect was possibly due to components released in fermented milk, since pasteurized fermented milk and fractions <10 kDa also showed the effect. Thus, cytokine regulation may be associated to peptides present in fermented milk, nevertheless the effect of other milk components cannot be discarded. Furthermore, more studies are needed in order to elucidate the components responsible for the observed effect. Thus, fermented milk with these specific strains of *L. fermentum* show potential for the development of novel functional foods for the attenuation of systemic inflammatory disorders.

Author Contributions: The author's responsibilities were as follows: B.V.-C., A.F.G.-C., V.M.-H., J.H., A.H.-M. and A.R.-D. designed the study. A.R.-D. conducted the study and wrote the manuscript. B.V.-C. revised the manuscript and had primary responsibility for the final content of the manuscript. M.J.T.-L. identified peptide profiles. R.R.-D. and L.M.B.-B. edited the manuscript and performed statistical analysis. A.F.G.-C., A.H.-M., V.M.-H. and J.H. supplied valuable knowledge and scientific consultation throughout the study; and all authors read and approved the final manuscript.

Nutrients **2018**, *10*, 691

Acknowledgments: The authors express their gratitude to the Mexican Council of Science and Technology (CONACYT) for the doctoral scholarship granted to author Aline Reyes-Díaz. Also, authors would like to thank Rocio Hernández-Mendoza and Isidro Mendez Romero for their technical assistance.

Conflicts of Interest: The authors hereby declare no conflict of interests.

References

1. Shiby, V.K.; Mishra, H.N. Fermented Milks and Milk Products as Functional Foods—A Review. *Crit. Rev. Food Sci. Nutr.* **2013**, *53*, 482–496. [CrossRef] [PubMed]
2. Chiu, Y.H.; Lin, S.L.; Ou, C.C.; Lu, Y.C.; Huang, H.Y.; Lin, M.Y. Antiinflammatory effect of lactobacilli bacteria on HepG2 cells is through cross-regulation of TLR4 and NOD2 signalling. *J. Funct. Foods* **2013**, *5*, 820–828. [CrossRef]
3. Juarez, G.E.; Villena, J.; Salva, S.; Font de Valdez, G.; Rodriguez, A.V. *Lactobacillus reuteri* CRL1101 beneficially modulate lipopolysaccharide-mediated inflammatory response in a mouse model of endotoxic shock. *J. Funct. Foods* **2013**, *5*, 1761–1773. [CrossRef]
4. Maldonado Galdeano, C.; Novotny Núñez, I.; de Moreno de LeBlanc, A.; Carmuega, E.; Weill, R.; Perdigón, G. Impact of a probiotic fermented milk in the gut ecosystem and in the systemic immunity using a non-severe protein-energy-malnutrition model in mice. *BMC Gastroenterol.* **2011**, *11*, 64. [CrossRef] [PubMed]
5. Agyei, D.; Ongkudon, C.M.; Wei, C.Y.; Chan, A.S.; Danquah, M.K. Bioprocess challenges to the isolation and purification of bioactive peptides. *Food Bioprod. Process.* **2016**, *98*, 244–256. [CrossRef]
6. LeBlanc, J.; Fliss, I.; Matar, C. Induction of a humoral immune response following an *Escherichia coli* O157:H7 infection with an immunomodulatory peptidic fraction derived from *Lactobacillus helveticus*-fermented milk. *Clin. Diagn. Lab. Immunol.* **2004**, *11*, 1171–1181. [CrossRef] [PubMed]
7. Vinderola, G.; Matar, C.; Palacios, J.; Perdigón, G. Mucosal immunomodulation by the non-bacterial fraction of milk fermented by *Lactobacillus helveticus* R389. *Int. J. Food Microbiol.* **2007**, *115*, 180–186. [CrossRef] [PubMed]
8. Matar, C.; Valdez, J.C.; Medina, M.; Rachid, M.; Perdigon, G. Immunomodulating effects of milks fermented by *Lactobacillus helveticus* and its nonproteolytic variant. *J. Dairy Res.* **2001**, *68*, 601–609. [CrossRef] [PubMed]
9. Tellez, A.; Corredig, M.; Turner, P.; Morales, R.; Griffiths, M.W. A peptidic fraction from milk fermented with *L. helveticus* protects mice against *Salmonella* infection. *Int. Dairy J.* **2011**, *21*, 607–614. [CrossRef]
10. Sharma, R.; Kapila, R.; Kapasiya, M.; Saliganti, V.; Dass, G.; Kapila, S. Dietary supplementation of milk fermented with probiotic *Lactobacillus fermentum* enhances systemic immune response and antioxidant capacity in aging mice. *Nutr. Res.* **2014**, *34*, 968–981. [CrossRef] [PubMed]
11. Deng, B.; Wu, J.; Li, X.; Men, X.; Xu, Z. Probiotics and probiotic metabolic product improved intestinal function and ameliorated lps-induced injury in rats. *Curr. Microbiol.* **2017**, *74*, 1306–1315. [CrossRef] [PubMed]
12. Koscik, R.J.E.; Reid, G.; Kim, S.O.; Li, W.; Challis, J.R.G.; Bocking, A.D. Effect of *Lactobacillus rhamnosus* GR-1 Supernatant on cytokine and chemokine output from human amnion cells treated with lipoteichoic acid and lipopolysaccharide. *Reprod. Sci.* **2017**, *25*, 239–245. [CrossRef] [PubMed]
13. Shigemori, S.; Namai, F.; Yamamoto, Y.; Nigar, S.; Sato, T.; Ogita, T.; Shimosato, T. Genetically modified *Lactococcus lactis* producing a green fluorescent protein–bovine lactoferrin fusion protein suppresses proinflammatory cytokine expression in lipopolysaccharide-stimulated RAW 264.7 cells. *J. Dairy Sci.* **2017**, *100*, 7007–7015. [CrossRef] [PubMed]
14. Dinarello, C.A. Proinflammatory cytokines. *Chest* **2000**, *118*, 503–508. [CrossRef] [PubMed]
15. Miettinen, M.; Vuopio-Varkila, J.; Varkila, K. Production of human tumor necrosis factor alpha, interleukin-6, and interleukin-10 is induced by lactic acid bacteria. *Infect. Immun.* **1996**, *64*, 5403–5405. [PubMed]
16. Gabay, C. Interleukin-6 and chronic inflammation. *Arthritis Res. Ther.* **2006**, *8*, S3. [CrossRef] [PubMed]
17. Louis, H.; LeMoine, O.; Peny, M.O.; Quertinmont, E.; Fokan, D.; Goldman, M.; Devière, J. Production and role of interleukin-10 in concanavalin A induced hepatitis in mice. *Hepatology* **1997**, *25*, 1382–1389. [CrossRef] [PubMed]
18. Sang, H.; Wallis, G.L.; Stewart, C.A.; Kotake, Y. Expression of cytokines and activation of transcription factors in lipopolysaccharide-administered rats and their inhibition by phenyl N-tert-butylnitrone (PBN). *Arch. Biochem. Biophys.* **1999**, *363*, 341–348. [CrossRef] [PubMed]

19. Heredia, C.P.Y.; Méndez-Romero, J.I.; Hernández-Mendoza, A.; Acedo-Félix, E.; González-Córdova, A.F.; Vallejo-Cordoba, B. Antimicrobial activity and partial characterization of bacteriocin-like inhibitory substances produced by *Lactobacillus* spp. isolated from artisanal Mexican cheese. *J. Dairy Sci.* **2015**, *98*, 8285–8293. [CrossRef] [PubMed]

20. Smith, P.K.; Krohn, R.I.; Hermanson, G.T.; Mallia, A.K.; Gartner, F.H.; Provenzano, M.D.; Fujimoto, E.K.; Goeke, N.M.; Olson, B.J.; Klenk, D.C. Measurement of protein using bicinchoninic acid. *Anal. Biochem.* **1987**, *150*, 76–85. [CrossRef]

21. AOAC. *Official Methods of Analysis of AOAC*, 17th ed.; Association of Analytical Communities: Gaithersburg, MD, USA, 2000.

22. National Research Council (NRC). *Guide for the Care and Use of Laboratory Animals*, 8th ed.; The National Academies Press: Washington, DC, USA, 2011. [CrossRef]

23. Perkins, D.; Pappin, D.J.; Creasy, D.M.; Cottrell, J.S. Probability-based protein identification by searching sequence databases using mass spectrometry data. *Electrophoresis* **1999**, *20*, 3551–3567. [CrossRef]

24. Shihata, A.; Shah, N.P. Proteolytic profiles of yogurt and probiotic bacteria. *Int. Dairy J.* **2000**, *10*, 401–408. [CrossRef]

25. Widyastuti, Y.; Rohmatussolihat; Febrisiantosa, A. The role of lactic acid bacteria in milk fermentation. *Food Nutr. Sci.* **2014**, *5*, 435–442. [CrossRef]

26. Zhou, J.; Ma, L.; Xu, H.; Gao, Y.; Jin, Y.; Zhao, L.; David, X.A.L.; Zhan, D.; Zhang, S. Immunomodulating effects of casein-derived peptides QEPVL and QEPV on lymphocytes in vitro and in vivo. *Food Funct.* **2014**, *5*, 2061–2069.

27. Meisel, H.; Bockelmann, W. Bioactive peptides encrypted in milk proteins: Proteolytic activation and thropho-functional properties. *Antonie Leeuwenhoek* **1999**, *76*, 207–215. [CrossRef] [PubMed]

28. Taverniti, V.; Guglielmetti, S. The immunomodulatory properties of probiotics microorganisms beyond their viability (ghost probiotics: Proposal of paraprobiotic concept). *Genes Nutr.* **2011**, *6*, 261–274. [CrossRef] [PubMed]

29. Cross, M.L.; Ganner, A.; Teilab, D.; Fray, L.M. Patterns of cytokine induction by gram-positive and gram-negative probiotic bacteria. *FEMS Immunol. Med. Microbiol.* **2004**, *42*, 173–180. [CrossRef] [PubMed]

30. Chuang, L.; Wu, K.G.; Pai, C.; Hsieh, P.S.; Tsai, J.J.; Yen, J.H.; Lin, M.Y. Heat-killed cells of lactobacilli skew the immune response toward T helper polarization in mouse splenocytes and dentritic cell-treated T cells. *J. Agric. Food Chem.* **2007**, *55*, 11080–11086. [CrossRef] [PubMed]

31. Sánchez-Rivera, L.; Ménard, O.; Recio, I.; Dupont, D. Peptide mapping during dynamic gastric digestion of heated and unheated skimmed milk powder. *Food Res. Int.* **2015**, *77*, 132–139. [CrossRef]

32. Gill, H.S.; Doull, F.; Rutherfurd, K.J.; Cross, M.L. Immunoregulatory peptides in bovine milk. *Br. J. Nutr.* **2000**, *84* (Suppl. 1), S111–S117. [CrossRef] [PubMed]

33. Requena, P.; González, R.; López-Posadas, R.; Abadía-Molina, A.; Suárez, M.D.; Zarzuelo, A.; de Medina, F.S.; Martínez-Augustin, O. The intestinal antiinflammatory agent glycomacropeptide has immunomodulatory actions on rat splenocytes. *Biochem. Pharmacol.* **2010**, *79*, 1797–1804. [CrossRef] [PubMed]

34. Rodriguez, J.; Gupta, N.; Smith, R.D.; Pevzner, P.A. Does trypsin cut before proline? *J. Proteome Res.* **2008**, *7*, 300–305. [CrossRef] [PubMed]

35. Reyes-Díaz, A.; González-Córdova, A.F.; Hernández-Mendoza, A.; Reyes-Díaz, R.; Vallejo-Cordoba, B. Immunomodulation by hydrolysates and peptides derived from milk proteins. *Int. J. Dairy Technol.* **2018**, *71*, 1–9. [CrossRef]

36. Meisel, H.; FitzGerald, R.J. Biofunctional peptides from milk proteins: Mineral binding and cytomodulatory effects. *Curr. Pharm. Des.* **2003**, *9*, 1289–1295. [PubMed]

37. Haque, E.; Chand, R. Antihypertensive and antimicrobial bioactive peptides from milk proteins. *Eur. Food Res. Technol.* **2008**, *227*, 7–15. [CrossRef]

38. Rodríguez-Figueroa, J.C.; González-Córdova, A.F.; Torres-Yanez, M.J.; Garcia, H.S.; Vallejo-Cordoba, B. Novel angiotensin I-converting enzyme inhibitory peptides produced in fermented milk by specific wild *Lactococcus lactis* strains. *J. Dairy Sci.* **2010**, *95*, 5536–5543. [CrossRef] [PubMed]

39. Jiang, Z.; Tian, B.; Brodkorb, A.; Huo, G. Production, analysis and in vivo evaluation of novel angiotensin-I-converting enzyme inhibitory peptides from bovine casein. *Food Chem.* **2010**, *123*, 779–786. [CrossRef]

40. Hernández-Ledesma, B.; Amigo, L.; Ramos, M.; Recio, I. Angiotensin converting enzyme inhibitory activity in commercial fermented products. Formation of peptides under simulated gastrointestinal digestion. *J. Agric. Food Chem.* **2004**, *52*, 1504–1510. [CrossRef] [PubMed]

41. Rival, S.G.; Boeriu, C.G.; Wichers, H.J. Caseins and casein hydrolysates. 2. Antioxidative properties and relevance to lipoxygenase inhibition. *J. Agric. Food Chem.* **2001**, *49*, 295–302. [CrossRef] [PubMed]

42. Shanmugam, V.P.; Kapila, S.; Kemgang, T.S.; Kapila, R. Antioxidative peptide derived from enzymatic digestion of buffalo casein. *Int. Dairy J.* **2015**, *42*, 1–5. [CrossRef]

43. Vij, R.; Reddi, S.; Kapila, S.; Kapila, R. Transepithelial transport of milk derived bioactive peptide VLPVPQK. *Food Chem.* **2016**, *190*, 681–688. [CrossRef] [PubMed]

44. Qian, B.; Xing, M.; Cui, L.; Deng, Y.; Xu, Y.; Huang, M.; Zhang, S. Antioxidant, antihypertensive, and immunomodulatory activities of peptide fractions from fermented skim milk with *Lactobacillus delbrueckii* ssp. *bulgaricus* LB340. *J. Dairy Res.* **2011**, *78*, 72–79. [CrossRef] [PubMed]

45. Matsui, T.; Tamaya, K.; Seki, E.; Osajima, K.; Matsumo, K.; Kawasaki, T. Absorption of Val-Tyr with in vitro angiotensin i-converting enzyme inhibitory activity into the circulating blood system of mild hypertensive subjects. *Biol. Pharm. Bull.* **2002**, *25*, 1228–1230. [CrossRef] [PubMed]

46. Kagawa, K.; Matsutaka, H.; Fukuhama, C.; Watanabe, Y.; Fujino, H. Globin digest, acidic protease hydrolysate, inhibits dietary hypertriglyceridemia and Val-Val-Tyr-Pro, one of its constituents, possesses most superior effect. *Life Sci.* **1996**, *58*, 1745–1755. [CrossRef]

47. Kayser, H.; Meisel, H. Stimulation of human peripheral blood lymphocytes by bioactive peptides derived from bovine milk proteins. *FEBS Lett.* **1996**, *383*, 18–20. [CrossRef]

48. Van Amersfoort, E.S.; Van Berkel, T.J.C.; Kuiper, J. Receptors, mediators, and mechanisms involved in bacterial sepsis and septic shock. *Clin. Microbiol. Rev.* **2003**, *16*, 379–414. [CrossRef] [PubMed]

49. Cheng, X.; Gao, D.; Chen, B.; Mao, X. Endotoxin-binding peptides derived from casein glycomacropeptide inhibit lipopolysaccharide-stimulated inflammatory responses via blockade of NF-κβ activation in macrophages. *Nutrients* **2015**, *7*, 3119–3137. [CrossRef] [PubMed]

50. Iskandar, M.M.; Dauletbaev, N.; Kubow, S.; Mawji, N.; Lands, L.C. Whey protein hydrolysates decrease IL-8 secretion in lipopolysaccharide (LPS)-stimulated respiratory epithelial cells by affecting LPS binding to Toll-like receptor 4. *Br. J. Nutr.* **2013**, *110*, 58–68. [CrossRef] [PubMed]

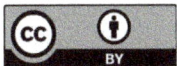

nutrients

MDPI

Article

Associations of Dairy Intake with Arterial Stiffness in Brazilian Adults: The Brazilian Longitudinal Study of Adult Health (ELSA-Brasil)

Amanda Gomes Ribeiro [1], José Geraldo Mill [1], Nágela Valadão Cade [1],
Gustavo Velasquez-Melendez [2], Sheila Maria Alvim Matos [3]
and Maria del Carmen Bisi Molina [1,*]

[1]   Centro de Ciências da Saúde, Universidade Federal do Espírito Santo, Vitória CEP 29042-755, Brazil;
       amandagribeiro@gmail.com (A.G.R.); josegmill@gmail.com (J.G.M.); nagelavc@terra.com.br (N.V.C.)
[2]   Escola de Enfermagem, Universidade Federal de Minas Gerais, Belo Horizonte CEP 30130-100, Brazil;
       jguveme@ufmg.br
[3]   Instituto de Saúde Coletiva, Universidade Federal da Bahia, Salvador CEP 40110-040, Brazil;
       sheilaalvim@gmail.com
*   Correspondence: mdcarmen2007@gmail.com; Tel.: +55-27-3335-7146

Received: 25 April 2018; Accepted: 29 May 2018; Published: 31 May 2018

Abstract: Recent studies have suggested the possible effect of dairy product intake on cardiovascular risk markers, including arterial stiffness. Our aim was to investigate whether dairy food intake is associated with arterial stiffness, which we assessed by carotid-femoral pulse wave velocity (cfPWV) and pulse pressure (PP) in a cross-sectional analysis of baseline data (2008–2010; n = 12,892) of the Brazilian Longitudinal Study of Adult Health (ELSA-Brasil). Dairy consumption was evaluated with a validated food-frequency questionnaire (FFQ) by computing servings per day for total and subgroups of dairy products. Dairy consumption was described in four categories ($\leq$1 serving/day to >4 servings/day). Covariance analysis (ANCOVA) was used to compare cfPWV across increasing intake of dairy food, adjusting for confounding factors, including non-dairy food groups. The intake of total dairy was inversely associated with cfPWV and PP (-0.13 m/s and -1.3 mmHg, from the lowest and to the highest category of dairy intake). Low-fat dairy, fermented dairy and cheese showed an inverse relationship with cfPWV and PP. These findings suggest a beneficial effect of dairy consumption to reduce arterial stiffness. However, further evidence from longitudinal studies or long-term intervention is needed to support reduction of cfPWV and PP mediating the beneficial effects of dairy products on cardiovascular health.

Keywords: dairy; cardiovascular health; pulse wave velocity; arterial stiffness

---

1. Introduction

Cardiovascular diseases (CVD) are the leading cause of death worldwide. There were 17.7 million deaths due to CVD in 2015, representing 31% of the total mortality rate recorded in that year. More than 75% of these deaths were recorded in low- and middle-income countries where CVDs most often affect individuals of working age and have a high economic and social impact [1]. According to estimates, 80% of the CVD burden is associated with modifiable behaviors, mainly eating behaviors, that affect risk factors such as arterial hypertension, diabetes mellitus (DM) and obesity [2].

Longitudinal studies suggested an inverse association between dairy product intake and risk of CVD, coronary disease and infarction [3,4]. These findings were consistent with observational studies that showed an inverse relation between milk intake and CVD risk factors such as hypertension [5,6]. The Dietary Approaches to Stop Hypertension (DASH) study was one of the first intervention studies supporting such an inverse relation and showed that diets rich in fruits, vegetables and low-fat dairy products (3 servings/day) were associated with lower systolic (SBP) and diastolic blood pressure (DBP) [7]. A meta-analysis of randomized clinical trials corroborated these findings and showed significant reductions in SBP (by 6.74 mmHg) and DBP (by 3.54 mmHg), values associated with the DASH diet [8].

Recent studies have also suggested the possible effect of dairy product intake on other cardiovascular risk markers, mainly arterial stiffness [9,10]. Stiffening of large arteries is characteristic of the aging process and may influence the development of chronic diseases such as isolated systolic hypertension. Conversely, arterial stiffness can also increase as a consequence of several factors, including type-II diabetes mellitus (DM), obesity and lifestyle characteristics such as smoking, physical activity and diet [11].

Carotid–femoral pulse wave velocity (cfPWV) is accepted as the 'gold standard' measurement of arterial stiffness, and it has been used to predict cardiovascular events [12]. There are a limited number of studies investigating the effect of diet on arterial stiffness. Epidemiological studies suggest that dairy may be inversely associated with cfPWV [9,13,14]. A cross-sectional and multi-center study showed a lower cfPWV of 0.10 m/s for every 100-g/day increase in low-fat dairy intake ($p = 0.011$) [13]. In the Maine-Syracuse Longitudinal Study, the frequency of the overall dairy consumption was also inversely associated with cfPWV [9]. The greater consumption of reduced-fat dairy was also correlated with lower cfPWV in a population with type 1 and type 2 diabetes [14].

There have been limited randomized controlled trials examining the effect of dairy on arterial stiffness. A systematic review concerning the effect of dietary interventions on arterial stiffness evidenced the limited, although consistent, beneficial effects of fermented dairy products [15]. More recently, a randomized, cross-over study found that the addition of non-fat dairy products reduced cfPWV and improved endothelial function [16]. On the other hand, in a cohort with diabetes, improving dietary quality by increasing consumption of fruits, vegetables and dairy did not reduce cfPWV, compared with a control group [17].

The aim of the current study was to assess the association between dairy product intake and arterial stiffness in the Brazilian Longitudinal Study of Adult Health (ELSA-Brasil) cohort. The assessment was done by taking into consideration the impact of CVD on the morbidity and mortality profile of middle-income countries such as Brazil; the relatively scarce data about diet and these diseases in such contexts; and evidence of the relation among dairy product intake, cardiovascular events and their risk factors.

2. Materials and Methods

The Brazilian Longitudinal Study of Adult Health (ELSA-Brasil), registered in clinicaltrials.gov as NCT02320461, is a multi-center cohort study designed to investigate the development of chronic diseases, primarily diabetes and cardiovascular diseases, and their risk factors over long-term follow-ups. ELSA-Brasil enrolled and assessed 15,105 civil servants (35–74 years) of five public universities and one research institution from six different cities (Salvador, Belo Horizonte, Rio de Janeiro, São Paulo, Vitoria, and Porto Alegre). Therefore, the sample came from the northeast (13.4% of participants), southeast (72.9% of participants), and southern (13.7% of participants) regions of Brazil. The study was approved by the National Research Ethics Commission (CONEP—976/2006) and by the research ethics committee of each institution. All participants signed an informed consent form.

The baseline procedures (2008–2010) included an interview for recruitment and signature of the informed consent. Clinic exams, blood and urine collection, and application of the questionnaires were done during a single visit to one of the six investigation centers (IC). All subjects were interviewed using a structured interviewer-administered questionnaire that included information on socio-demographic characteristics, lifestyle habits and detailed medical history; on the same day, the dietary intake of nutrients was collected with a validated semi-quantitative food frequency questionnaire (FFQ) [18].

The sample included volunteers and people who were actively recruited from lists of employees provided by the institutions. The exclusion criteria were as follows: Intention to leave the institution; being pregnant or having been pregnant less than four months before; having severe cognitive or communication difficulty and; if retired, living outside the metropolitan region. Sample size was calculated based on estimations of the incidences of type-2 DM and myocardial infarction in the Brazilian population and was compensated for sex differences and possible losses during follow-up. For a better distribution, recruitment goals were defined by sex (50% each), age (15% aged 35–44, 30% aged 45–54, 40% aged 55–64 and 15% aged 65–74 years) and occupational category (35% of support level, with incomplete elementary school; 35% with high school; and 30% with higher education/teaching level) [19].

For the present analysis, baseline data from ELSA-Brasil were used. We excluded participants with self-reported previous cardiovascular disease ($n = 1001$) and bariatric surgery ($n = 107$). Individuals who reported caloric intake <500 or >6000 kcal/day ($n = 408$), and individuals with an unvalidated cfPWV value ($n = 372$) were also excluded, which left 12,892 subjects with complete data for analysis.

2.1. Dietary Assessment and Dairy Measurement

Dietary intake was measured by an FFQ that was specific and validated in this population and included 114 food items relevant to the past 12 months [20]. For each food item ascertained, the FFQ included measures of portions and frequency of consumption, the latter of which with 8 response options: >3 times/day, 2–3 times/day, 1 time/day, 5–6 times/week, 2–4 times/week, 1 time/week, 1–3 times/month, and never/almost never.

Cow milk, cheese curds, yogurt, and cheeses were classified as "Milk and Cheese Group", and butter is described as a dairy product that should be consumed in moderation according to the Dietary Guidelines for the Brazilian Population [21]. In the ELSA FFQ, questions on dairy products included milk (skimmed milk, low-fat milk and whole milk), yogurt (regular, low-fat), cheese (regular, low-fat) and butter.

Servings of specific dairy foods were converted into daily servings, and total daily servings of dairy foods were calculated by summing all dairy foods. For each dairy food, a standard serving size was specified: 240 g for milk, 120 g for yogurt, 30 g for cheese and 5 g for butter.

We computed servings per day for total dairy intake (with butter) and the following dairy subgroups: Full-fat dairy without butter (whole milk, regular yogurt and cheese), low-fat dairy (skimmed milk, low-fat milk, low-fat yogurt and cheese), fermented dairy (total yogurt and cheese), milk, cheese, yogurt and butter.

2.2. Pulse Wave Velocity and Blood Pressure

Carotid-femoral pulse wave velocity (cfPWV), pulse pressure (PP) and systolic blood pressure (SBP) were used as dependent variables in the current study.

The cfPWV was measured using an automatic device (Complior, Artech Medical, France) with the subject in the supine position in accordance with the ELSA-Brasil protocols. The distance from the sternal furcula to the right femoral site where the pulse was recorded was measured with a metric tape, regardless of abdominal curvature. Pulse sensors were positioned in the right carotid and femoral arteries, and pulse waves were recorded and visualized on a computer screen. cfPWV was calculated by dividing the distance from the furcula to the femoral pulse by the difference between the delay between the rising phases of the carotid and femoral pulses, and it was expressed in m/s. A subject's cfPWV was the arithmetic average of readings obtained in ten consecutive cardiac cycles at a regular heart rate. Exams were recorded in each of the six investigation centers by trained and certificated researchers. Training and certification of each investigator was performed by a senior investigator. Validation of all exams obtained at the six investigations centers were performed in a central reading laboratory of cardiovascular physiology [22].

Systolic blood pressure (SBP) was measured using a validated oscillometric device (Omron HEM 705CPINT) after a 5-minute rest with the subject in a sitting position. Three measurements were taken at 1-minute intervals. The mean of the two latest BP measurements was considered as the casual BP. Pulse pressure was calculated as the arithmetic difference between SBP and DBP.

2.3. Covariates

Socio-demographic characteristics were included as covariables (potential confounders) of the study: Sex, age (continuous variable; years), race, per capita income (continuous variable); and lifestyle: Alcohol intake (g ethanol/day), physical activity (metabolic equivalent min/week) and smoking status (never smoked, ex-smoker, current smoker).

As adjustment for height when assessing cfPWV has been recommended [23], height, weight and waist circumference were used rather than BMI. Anthropometric measurements were obtained while participants were standing and dressed in a light uniform standardized for the study. We measured body weight to the nearest 0.1 kg with a calibrated scale (Toledo 2096PP) and height with a wall-mounted stadiometer (Seca-SE-216) to the nearest 0.1 cm. Waist circumference was measured using a non-stretchable tape around the midpoint between the lower border of ribs and the iliac crest.

Traditional cardiovascular risk factors with an effect on arterial stiffness were also included: Fasting glycaemia (mg/dL), total cholesterol (mg/dL) and mean blood pressure (MAP, mmHg), calculated as (PAS + (2 × PAD))/3. In addition, the use of antihypertensive, lipid-lowering and antidiabetic drugs (yes/no) were also included.

The following non-dairy food groups (g/day) were considered as possible confounders in our analyses: Fruit, vegetables, whole grains, fish, processed and unprocessed red and white meat.

2.4. Statistical Analyses

Data were analyzed with SPSS (Version 18, Chicago, IL, USA). Preliminary analyses were performed to assess correlations between dairy intake, cfPWV and other demographic, health status, and nutrition and lifestyle factors. Participant characteristics in the study were compared according to the dairy intake group ($\leq$1 serving/day, >1–2 servings/day, >2–4 servings/day and >4 servings/day). For continuous variables, analysis of variance (ANOVA) was used. For categorical variables, Chi-square tests were performed.

Covariance analysis (ANCOVA) was used to compare cfPWV across increasing intake of dairy food consumption ranging from $\leq$1 serving/day to >4 servings/day. Adjustments for multiple comparisons among dairy food intake groups were made and reported in terms of the Bonferroni adjustment. Linear trend was tested by modelling categorical dairy servings per day ($\leq$1 serving/day, >1–2 servings/day, >2–4 servings/day, >4 servings/day) as a continuous variable in the multivariable regression models.

We adjusted for covariates in 4 models as follows: Model 1: Demographic characteristics (age, sex, race, and income); Model 2: Model 1 + anthropometric variables (weight, height, and waist circumference) + lifestyle factors (smoking status, alcohol intake, and physical activity); Model 3: Model 2 + fasting glucose, total cholesterol, MAP (only for cfPWV) and use of drugs (antihypertensive, antidiabetic and lipid-lowering drugs); and Model 4: Model 3 + caloric intake (kcal/d) and non-dairy food groups (g/day; fruit, vegetables, whole grains, fish, and processed and unprocessed red and white meat).

These variables were selected if significantly associated in a simple correlation matrix with dairy food intake (the predictor) or cfPWV (the primary outcome variable), or if known to be related according to previously published studies.

3. Results

The median of total dairy product intake was 2.6 servings/day (interquartile range (IQR): 1.43–4.10), 1.00 serving/day of low-fat dairy (IQR: 0.13–2.20), and 1.07 serving/day of whole dairy

(IQR: 0.27–2.24). Cheese had the highest median intake in servings/day (1.00, IQR: 0.37–2.00), followed by milk (0.80, IQR: 0.07–1.25). The analysis in grams per day showed that the most consumed dairy product was milk (mean: 235.6 g/day), mainly whole milk (mean: 113.8 g/day), which was followed by cheese (mean: 43.3 g/day) and yogurt (mean: 37.4 g/day). In Table 1, we present the consumption of dairy subgroups according to categories of total dairy intake.

Table 1. Intake of dairy products according to categories of total dairy intake. ELSA-Brasil, 2008–2010 [1].

Dairy Products, Servings/Day	Categories of Dairy Consumption (Servings/Day)				
	≤1 (*n* = 2036)	>1–2 (*n* = 2862)	>2–4 (*n* = 4700)	>4 (*n* = 3294)	*p*
Dairy [2]	0.52	1.53	2.90	5.49	
Low-fat dairy [2]	0.10	0.60	1.27	2.80	
Skimmed milk, low-fat milk	0.06 ± 0.18	0.24 ± 0.40	0.52 ± 0.79	1.00 ± 1.34	<0.001
Low-fat yogurt	0.02 ± 0.09	0.08 ± 0.23	0.15 ± 0.35	0.21 ± 0.45	<0.001
Low-fat cheese	0.13 ± 0.19	0.36 ± 0.39	0.77 ± 0.75	1.79 ± 1.77	<0.001
Full-fat dairy [2]	0.23	0.93	1.40	2.80	
Whole milk	0.12 ± 0.23	0.30 ± 0.43	0.49 ± 0.79	0.82 ± 1.37	<0.001
Regular yogurt	0.04 ± 0.11	0.11 ± 0.23	0.20 ± 0.38	0.30 ± 0.54	<0.001
Regular cheese	0.14 ± 0.19	0.32 ± 0.37	0.56 ± 0.64	1.22 ± 1.42	<0.001
Fermented dairy [2]	0.23	0.90	1.67	3.20	
Yogurt (regular, low-fat)	0.06 ± 0.13	0.19 ± 0.29	0.35 ± 0.45	0.52 ± 0.61	<0.001
Cheese (regular, low-fat)	0.26 ± 0.26	0.68 ± 0.47	1.32 ± 0.84	3.00 ± 1.99	<0.001
Butter	0.04 ± 0.13	0.12 ± 0.28	0.26 ± 0.52	0.67 ± 1.08	<0.001

[1] ELSA-Brasil, Brazilian Longitudinal Study of Adult Health. Unless otherwise specified, all values are means ±SDs.
[2] Values are medians.

Table 2 summarizes the sociodemographic, health and diet data. The mean (±SD) age was 51.7 ± 8.9 years. Dairy product intake was higher in women, as well as among white people. Participants with higher dairy product intake reported lower alcohol intake and smoking habits as well as a higher physical activity level. Groups presenting higher dairy product intake also showed higher per capita family income and lower SBP, DBP, MAP, PP and glycaemia values.

Table 2. Baseline characteristics by categories of dairy consumption of Brazilian participants: ELSA-Brasil, 2008–2010 [1].

Characteristics of Participants	Categories of Dairy Consumption (Servings/Day)				*p*
	≤1 (*n* = 2036)	>1–2 (*n* = 2862)	>2–4 (*n* = 4700)	>4 (*n* = 3294)	
Age, years	51.2 ± 8.3	51.3 ± 8.9	51.7 ± 9.0	52.3 ± 9.2	<0.001
Sex, *n* (%)					
Men	1111 (54.6)	1356 (47.4)	1924 (40.9)	1339 (40.9)	
Women	925 (45.4)	1506 (52.6)	2776 (59.1)	2001 (59.1)	<0.001
Race, *n* (%)					
White	845 (41.5)	1368 (47.8)	2646 (56.3)	1963 (59.6)	
Other	1191 (58.5)	1494 (52.2)	2054 (43.7)	1331 (40.4)	<0.001
Educational level, *n* (%)					
Completed secondary school	872 (42.8)	1081 (37.8)	1516 (32.3)	923 (28.0)	
University degree	728 (35.8)	1399 (48.9)	2743 (58.4)	2133 (64.8)	<0.001
Weight, kg	73.1 ± 14.2	73.7 ± 14.6	72.6 ± 14.7	73.2 ± 15.1	0.019
BMI, kg/m²	26.8 ± 4.5	27.0 ± 4.6	26.7 ± 4.6	26.8 ± 4.6	0.111
Waist circumference, cm	91.1 ± 12.2	91.1 ± 12.3	90.1 ± 12.5	90.4 ± 12.7	0.001
Smoking status, *n* (%)					
Never smoker	1033 (50.7)	1642 (57.4)	2829 (60.2)	1980 (60.1)	
Ex-smoker	631 (31.0)	830 (29.0)	1361 (29.0)	943 (28.6)	
Current smoker	372 (18.3)	390 (13.6)	510 (10.8)	371 (11.3)	<0.001
Alcohol intake, g ethanol/day	71.8 ± 142.7	55.7 ± 118.3	47.0 ± 91.2	47.2 ± 90.0	<0.001
Physical activity, min/week	467.1 ± 884.2	557.5 ± 954.0	623.8 ± 1051.8	725.2 ± 1158.7	<0.001
cfPWV, m/s	9.51 ± 1.90	9.33 ± 1.81	9.22 ± 1.79	9.17 ± 1.74	<0.001
Systolic blood pressure, mm Hg	123.7 ± 18.7	122.0 ± 17.5	119.4 ± 16.5	119.2 ± 15.8	<0.001
Diastolic blood pressure, mm Hg	78.0 ± 11.3	77.0 ± 10.9	75.2 ± 10.3	75.1 ± 10.2	<0.001
Mean blood pressure, mm Hg	95.4 ± 12.9	94.0 ± 12.0	91.9 ± 11.4	91.8 ± 11.3	<0.001
Pulse pressure, mm Hg	45.8 ± 11.5	45.0 ± 10.7	44.2 ± 10.3	44.1 ± 9.9	<0.001
Fasting glucose, mg/dL	114.5 ± 35.6	111.3 ± 29.1	110.0 ± 27.8	109.6 ± 26.8	<0.001
Total cholesterol, mg/dL	218.0 ± 43.4	215.9 ± 41.7	214.8 ± 41.3	214.7 ± 41.0	0.019

Table 2. *Cont.*

Characteristics of Participants	Categories of Dairy Consumption (Servings/Day)				*p*
	≤1 (*n* = 2036)	>1–2 (*n* = 2862)	>2–4 (*n* = 4700)	>4 (*n* = 3294)	
Drugs, *n* (%)					
Antidiabetic drugs	170 (8.3)	217 (7.6)	334 (7.1)	231 (7.0)	0.247
Lipid-lowering drugs	208 (10.2)	318 (11.1)	572 (12.2)	403 (12.2)	0.066
Antihypertensive drugs	561 (27.6)	813 (28.4)	1235 (26.3)	842 (25.6)	0.055
Food groups, g/day					
Fruit	460.7 ± 405.3	504.3 ± 407.9	548.6 ± 401.8	616.9 ± 452.2	<0.001
Vegetables	191.1 ± 148.8	198.5 ± 136.7	217.5 ± 142.1	240.9 ± 159.4	<0.001
Unprocessed meat	153.7 ± 126.7	161.0 ± 112.4	165.6 ± 114.3	179.3 ± 124.5	<0.001
Processed meat	18.7 ± 23.2	20.1 ± 22.6	21.3 ± 23.0	27.1 ± 28.6	<0.001
Fish	46.8 ± 61.2	50.5 ± 61.3	50.2 ± 58.5	52.2 ± 59.9	0.016
Whole grains	30.4 ± 68.7	37.3 ± 71.1	44.6 ± 70.3	52.6 ± 77.0	<0.001

[1] Values are presented as the mean ±SD unless otherwise indicated.

The cfPWV, PP and SBP values decreased as the dairy product intake increased (from ≤1 serving/day to >4 servings/day). Table 3 shows the confidence interval (95%) associated with the mean of the outcomes of each intake group and summarizes the results of the statistical analyses applied to the adjusted models according to the sociodemographic, anthropometric, lifestyle, clinical and dietary variables. The lowest cfPWV values (mean = 9.17 m/s) in the model adjusted for demographic variables were recorded in the group presenting the highest dairy product intake (>4 servings/day). Such a trend remained in the models adjusted for anthropometric, lifestyle, clinical and dietary variables.

Table 3. Adjusted cfPWV, PP and SBP means [1] according to dairy servings per day among Brazilian adults: ELSA-Brasil, 2008–2010.

Outcome		Categories of Dairy Consumption (Servings/Day)								p^2
		≤1		>1–2		>2–4		>4		
		n = 2036		*n* = 2862		*n* = 4700		*n* = 3294		
		Mean	95% CI	Mean	95% CI	Mean	95% CI	Mean	95% CI	
cfPWV	Model 1	9.43	9.36–9.49	9.33	9.27–9.38	9.26	9.22–9.31	9.17	9.12–9.22	<0.001 [‡]
	Model 2	9.43	9.36–9.49	9.32	9.26–9.38	9.27	9.22–9.31	9.17	9.12–9.22	<0.001 [‡]
	Model 3	9.34	9.28–9.40	9.28	9.23–9.33	9.29	9.25–9.34	9.21	9.16–9.26	0.006 [†]
	Model 4	9.34	9.27–9.40	9.28	9.23–9.33	9.29	9.26–9.34	9.21	9.16–9.26	0.014 [‡]
PP	Model 1	45.3	44.9–45.7	44.9	44.6–45.3	44.4	44.2–44.7	44.1	43.8–44.5	<0.001 [‡]
	Model 2	45.3	44.8–45.7	44.9	44.6–45.3	44.4	44.2–44.7	44.2	43.9–44.5	<0.001 [‡]
	Model 3	45.1	44.7–45.5	44.9	44.5–45.2	44.4	44.2–44.7	44.3	44.0–44.6	0.003 [‡]
	Model 4	45.3	44.9–45.8	45.0	44.7–45.3	44.4	44.2–44.7	44.0	43.7–44.4	<0.001 [‡]
SBP	Model 1	122.4	121.7–123.0	121.6	121.1–122.2	119.9	119.5–120.4	119.6	119.1–120.1	<0.001 [‡]
	Model 2	122.2	121.6–122.9	121.5	121.0–122.1	120.0	119.6–120.4	119.7	119.2–120.2	<0.001 [‡]
	Model 3	122.0	121.3–122.6	121.4	120.9–121.9	120.0	119.6–120.5	119.9	119.4–120.5	<0.001 [‡]
	Model 4	122.4	121.8–123.1	121.7	121.2–122.2	120.1	119.7–120.5	119.3	118.8–119.9	<0.001 [‡]

[1] cfPWV, carotid-femoral pulse wave velocity; MAP, mean arterial pressure; PP, pulse pressure; and SBP, systolic blood pressure. Adjusted mean determined by ANCOVA for each of the following variables: Model 1: demographic characteristics (including age (continuous variable; years), sex, race, income (continuous variable. R$)); Model 2: model 1 + anthropometric measurements (weight (kg), height (m), waist circumference (cm)), lifestyle habits (smoking status, alcohol intake (grams of ethanol per day), physical activity (metabolic equivalent min/week)); Model 3: model 2 + fasting glucose (mg/dL), total cholesterol (mg/dL), MAP (mmHg), antidiabetic drugs (yes/no), lipid-lowering drugs (yes/no), antihypertensive drugs (yes/no); Model 4: extended set 2 + dietary (calorie intake (kcal/day) and non-dairy food groups (g/day)). [2] *p* for F-test. [‡] *p* <0.01 for statistically significant linear trend. Linear trend was tested by modelling dairy servings per day (≤1 serving/day, >1–2 servings/day, >2–4 servings/day and >4 servings/day) as a continuous variable in the multivariable regression models.

The cfPWV values in the lowest intake category (≤1 serving/day) were significantly higher than those in the highest intake category (*p* = 0.02). Comparisons between intake categories showed that participants who consumed more than 4 servings of dairy products/day presented lower PP and SBP values than those who consumed less than 1 serving/day or between 1 and 2 servings/day after the model was adjusted to avoid possible confounding factors (Figure 1).

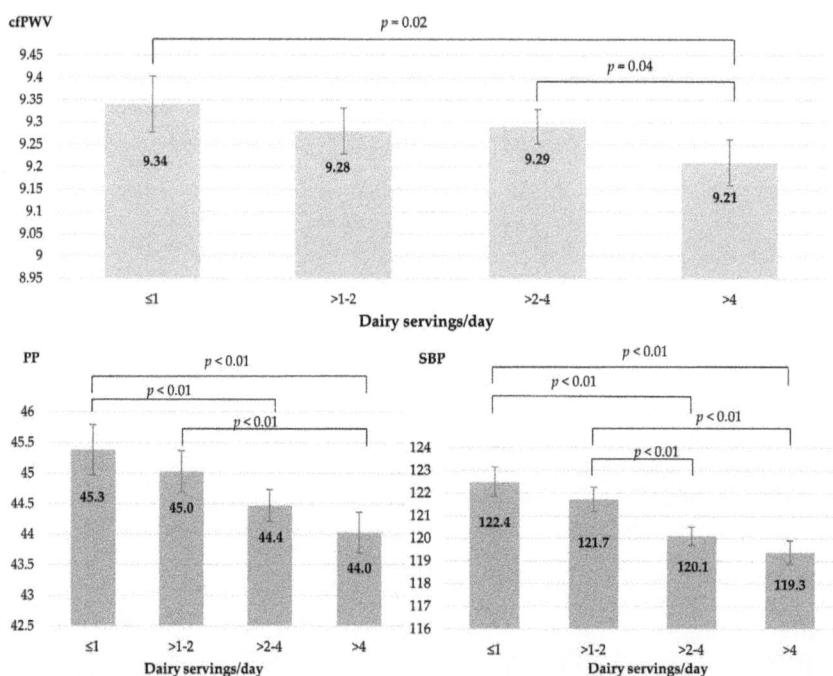

Figure 1. Mean values of carotid-femoral pulse wave velocity (cfPWV), pulse pressure (PP) and systolic blood pressure (SBP) in dairy intake groups after adjustment for variables in Model 4.

Table 4 shows differences in cfPWV, SBP and PP values according to the intake (servings/day) of different dairy subgroups. Low-fat dairy products, fermented dairy, and cheese showed a significant inverse association with cfPWV and PP. Whole and low-fat dairy products, fermented dairy, milk, and cheese showed a significant inverse association with SBP. Butter showed a significant inverse association only with cfPWV.

Table 4. Adjusted differences in cfPWV, PP and SBP associated with a 1 serving/day increase in the intake of dairy products: ELSA-Brasil, 2008–2010 [1].

Subgroups of Dairy, Servings/Day [1]	cfPWV (m/s)	PP (mmHg)	SBP (mmHg)
Low-fat dairy	−0.02 (−0.04, −0.01)	−0.3 (−0.35, −0.15)	−0.4 (−0.58, −0.26)
Full-fat dairy (without butter)	−0.00 (−0.02, 0.01)	−0.0 (−0.16, 0.06)	−0.2 (−0.40, −0.06)
Fermented dairy	−0.02 (−0.04, −0.01)	−0.3 (−0.43, −0.21)	−0.5 (−0.66, −0.33)
Milk	0.01 (−0.01, 0.03)	−0.0 (−0.19, 0.12)	−0.4 (−0.61, −0.12)
Cheese	−0.02 (−0.04, −0.01)	−0.4 (−0.47, −0.24)	−0.5 (−0.69, −0.33)
Yogurt	−0.02 (−0.07, 0.03)	−0.1 (−0.47, 0.24)	−0.5 (−1.05, 0.08)
Butter	−0.05 (−0.09, −0.02)	0.0 (−0.22, 0.25)	−0.1 (−0.51, 0.24)

[1] Values are presented as the mean (95% CI) adjusted by using multivariable linear regression for variables in model 4.

4. Discussion

The intake of dairy products in the current study was inversely associated with cfPWV, PP and SBP, adjusted by sociodemographic, anthropometric, lifestyle, clinical and other dietary factors. The cfPWV value was significantly lower in participants presenting a higher intake of dairy products than in those classified in the lowest intake category. These results were supported by SBP and PP findings (replacing haemodynamic indices used to assess arterial stiffness), which linearly decreased as the dairy product intake increased. Recent epidemiological findings suggested an inverse association between dairy product intake, particularly fermented dairy, and CVD [4]. One of the possible mechanisms of the beneficial effect of dairy products on cardiovascular health lies with the inverse relation between the consumption of these products and BP [24] and, possibly, between these products and arterial stiffness, which can be evaluated by measuring the PWV (as in the present study) or by the augmentation index (AI)) obtained in arterial tonometry [9,10,13].

Dairy intake was associated with lower BP and lower risk of developing hypertension in observational studies [24], but randomized controlled trials have shown mixed results [16,25]. Meta-analysis of seven mostly short-term randomized controlled studies with 711 adults found no significant effects of increased dairy food on the BP. However, most of the trials were small and of modest quality [25].

The current results corroborate with observational studies assessing the relation between dairy product intake and measures of arterial stiffness in populations in the United States and Wales. Crichton et al. [9] found lower cfPWV values in individuals consuming dairy products more than 5–6 times per week than in individuals presenting lower regular intake (1–4 times per week). In an analysis based on data from the Caerphilly Prospective Study, Livingstone et al. [10] observed that the AI was 1.8% lower in individuals in the highest dairy product intake quartile, after a 22.8-year follow-up, but no association was found for cfPWV. On other hand, Petersen et al. [14] found an inverse association between higher dairy intake and cfPWV, but not AI, in a cohort with diabetes. Previous research supports a dissociation between cfPWV and AI, and this phenomenon may be modulated by the presence of several factors, e.g., aging, use of medicaments and insulin resistance [26].

Intervention trials examining the effect of dairy on arterial stiffness are lacking. A randomized, cross-over study showed that an additional 4 servings of non-fat dairy per day reduced cfPWV compared with the no-dairy condition (4 servings of fruit juice). However, fruit juice may have a detrimental effect on arterial stiffness and the result could be a reflection of this [16]. In a cohort of individuals with type 1 and type 2 diabetes, AI and cfPWV were not improved with fruit and dairy increased in the intervention group after 12 months. However, the result may have been limited by the poor compliance of the participants with the intervention [17].

The mechanisms by which dairy products could reduce BP and arterial stiffness are not yet fully understood. However, it is hypothesized that bioactive peptides released during milk-protein digestion and milk-fermentation processes may be involved in this relation. Peptides deriving from casein were capable of reducing the action of the angiotensin converting enzyme (ACE) in experimental models, and it could reduce the circulating angiotensin II levels, thus preventing vasoconstriction and oxidative stress and increasing endothelium-dependent vasorelaxation [27,28]. Furthermore, there is evidence that certain milk peptides can inhibit the release of the vasoconstrictor endothelin-1 by endothelial cells, thus avoiding increased BP [29]. Randomized clinical trials reported the benefit of fermented dairy products rich in casein [30] and whey [31] on reducing BP and arterial stiffness.

A variety of other biologically active components, such as calcium, potassium and magnesium in dairy products, may also have an impact on BP and arterial stiffness [28]. Several possible mechanisms associated with the role played by calcium in cardiovascular health have been investigated. There is evidence that calcium can lower BP by regulating the renin-angiotensin system and by improving the sodium-potassium balance in humans [32]. A consistent set of results recorded in observational studies, clinical trials and meta-analyses indicated that high dietary potassium intake is associated with lower BP. Dietary potassium intake is important because it leads to vasodilation through sodium-potassium pump stimulation and through the opening of potassium channels. In addition to vasodilation, many other mechanisms by which potassium can influence BP, such as natriuresis, changes in intracellular sodium and tonicity, baroreceptor sensitivity modulation, and reduced sensitivity to norepinephrine and angiotensin II, have been investigated [33]. For magnesium, several mechanisms such as calcium channel blockade, competition with sodium for binding sites in vascular smooth muscle cells, increased prostaglandin E, endothelium-dependent vasodilatation and endothelial dysfunction improvement may also be involved in BP regulation. Magnesium is the most effective in reducing BP when it is used in combination with calcium and potassium [34].

In the present study, fermented dairy was inversely associated with cfPWV, PP and SBP values. However, the individual analysis applied to the dairy products showed that only for cheese this inverse association was found. Such a finding supports the result of a recent dose-response meta-analysis that assessed the relation between fermented dairy product intake and the risk of developing CVD. Cheese (10 g/day) was marginally inversely related to CVD (RR: 0.98; 95% CI: 0.95–1.00; 11 populations), whereas no significant association was found between yogurt and CVD [35].

Furthermore, we found an inverse association between the intake of low-fat dairy products and cfPWV, corroborating with observational [13] and interventional [16] studies. Recio-Rodriguez et al. found a decrease in cfPWV of 0.10 m/s estimated for every 100 g/day increase in low-fat dairy intake. However, the authors also found a cfPWV increase by 0.11 m/s estimated for each 100-g/day increase in the intake of whole dairy products. In the present study, there was no statistically significant association between the intake of whole dairy products (without butter) and cfPWV, and there was a smaller but significant association with SBP, comparing with low-fat dairy products. One hypothesis for the different results presented between full-fat and low-fat dairy in BP could be the bioavailability of minerals. It is possible that when consumed with fatty acids, released from the diet during digestion in the small intestine, the divalent cations of calcium and magnesium form insoluble soaps not absorbed by enterocytes [36].

In sensitivity analyses, we investigated whether intake of cheese was driving the associations with cfPWV for low-fat dairy intake by excluding this item from this variable. As a result, the association was not found for the subgroup with skimmed milk, low-fat milk and, low-fat yogurt, but the significant association remained for low-fat cheese alone ($B = -0.04$, $p < 0.001$). The same result was not found for full-fat cheese.

Interestingly, butter was inversely associated with cfPWV, a finding not detected for the other haemodynamic indexes. Previous analysis in the ELSA-Brasil population showed a graded inverse association between full-fat dairy and butter consumption and metabolic syndrome, and the results suggested that saturated fatty acids (SFAs) found in dairy products could be responsible for this association [37]. Saturated fat consumption has been classically related to elevated LDL (plasma cholesterol) and to increased cardiovascular risk. However, prospective cohort studies and clinical trials investigating the association between milk fat and CVD did not find clear evidence on the intake of whole dairy products and CVD [38,39]. According to a recent meta-analysis, the intake of high-fat dairy products (around 200 g/day) did not show an association with CVD (RR: 0.93; 95% CI: 0.84–1.03) [35]. A prospective study investigating the association between the intake of different dietary sources and the incidence of cardiovascular events in the Multi-Ethnic Study of Atherosclerosis (MESA) population found that a higher intake of saturated fat from dairy products was associated with a lower incidence of CVD. Replacement of 2% of the energy of the saturated fat derived from meat by the energy of the saturated fat derived from milk was associated with 25% less risk of developing CVD [40]. Moreover, in two prospective cohorts, higher plasma dairy fatty acid concentrations were associated with lower incident diabetes [41]. However, in the present study inverse association was only found between cfPWV and butter, but not for whole fat dairy (milk, cheese, and yogurt). It is possible that butter consumption has been acting as a marker for an unknown confounding variable.

The differences in cfPWV and SBP associated with increased dairy product intake were relatively small in the current study, 0.13 m/s for cfPWV and 3.1 mmHg for SBP between the lowest and the highest intake category. Even though they are small, these differences may be clinically relevant. Meta-analysis of the predictive cfPWV value in cardiovascular and death events estimated a cfPWV increase of 1 m/s represents a 14%, 15% and 15% increase in the risk (adjusted for age and sex) of cardiovascular events, death by CVD, and all-cause mortality, respectively [42]. According to Selmer et al. [43], the reduction of 4 mmHg in SBP would be equivalent to a 15.7% lower risk of death by stroke and to a 9.9% lower risk of myocardial infarction. Therefore, our study supports the view that reduction of cfPWV and BP can mediate the beneficial effects of dairy food on cardiovascular outcomes.

Our study has strengths and limitations. It is the first study to examine the relationship between dairy food intake and arterial stiffness, as measured by cfPWV, in Latin America. Moreover, this relationship was examined in a large sample (12,892 individuals from both sexes) with a wide age range and controlled for relevant demographic, health and dietary variables. However, the cross-sectional and observational nature of the study has limitations to be considered, since the findings may result from residual confusion despite the extensive adjustment for other food variables and confounding factors. The cross-sectional nature of the study, with a single measure of cfPWV and BP, does not allow conclusions regarding causality.

In addition, although FFQs have been widely adopted in epidemiological studies, the method also presents limitations, mainly because it produces a retrospective and subjective diet evaluation. FFQ depends on participant memory, and it may lead to reports of insufficient or excessive food intake. Another limitation was the absence of any objective biomarker of dairy intake, e.g., levels of pentadecanoic and margaric acid levels.

5. Conclusions

Higher dairy food intake was associated with lower cfPWV and accompanying lower PP and SBP values. However, dairy food intake was associated with many confounders that are generally associated with better health, such as less smoking status, higher physical activity and fruit and vegetable intake, and higher socioeconomic status. Therefore, additional evidence from longitudinal and randomized studies are necessary to conclude if reduction of arterial stiffness and BP effectively mediate the beneficial effects of dairy products on cardiovascular health, thus preventing development of CVD.

Author Contributions: A.G.R., M.C.B.M. and N.V.C. conceived and designed the study. A.G.R. performed the data analysis. A.G.R., M.C.B.M., G.V.-M., J.G.M. and S.M.A.M. reviewed the data quality, interpreted the data and drafted the manuscript. A.G.R. and M.C.B.M. wrote the majority of the paper, with all authors reviewing and approving the manuscript.

Funding: The ELSA-Brasil Study was supported by the Brazilian Ministry of Health (Science and Technology Department) and the Brazilian Ministry of Science, Technology and Innovation (Financiadora de Estudos e Projetos-FINEP and Conselho Nacional de Desenvolvimento Científico e Tecnológico-CNPq), grants 01 06 0010.00 RS, 01 06 0212.00 BA, 01 06 0300.00 ES, 01 06 0278.00 MG, 01 06 0115.00SP, 01 06 0071.00 RJ.

Acknowledgments: The authors thank the staff and participants of ELSA-Brasil for their important contributions and the Research Support Foundation of Espírito Santo (FAPES).

Conflicts of Interest: The authors declare no conflict of interest.

References

1. Pan American Health Organization (PAHO/WHO). Deaths Due to Noncommunicable Diseases in Countries of the Americas. Available online: http://www.paho.org/hq/index.php?option=com_content&view=article&id=10169&Itemid=41167&lang=en (accessed on 9 August 2017).
2. GBD 2016 Risk Factors Collaborators. Global, regional, and national comparative risk assessment of 84 behavioural, environmental and occupational, and metabolic risks or clusters of risks, 1990–2016: A systematic analysis for the Global Burden of Disease Study 2016. *Lancet* **2017**, *390*, 1345–1422. [CrossRef]
3. Alexander, D.D.; Bylsma, L.C.; Vargas, A.J.; Cohen, S.S.; Doucette, A.; Mohamed, M.; Irvin, S.R.; Miller, P.E.; Watson, H.; Fryzek, J.P. Dairy consumption and CVD: A systematic review and meta-analysis. *Br. J. Nutr.* **2016**, *115*, 737–750. [CrossRef] [PubMed]
4. Qin, L.-Q.; Xu, J.-Y.; Han, S.-F.; Zhang, Z.-L.; Zhao, Y.-Y.; Szeto, I.M. Dairy consumption and risk of cardiovascular disease: An updated meta-analysis of prospective cohort studies. *Asia Pac. J. Clin. Nutr.* **2015**, *24*, 90–100. [PubMed]

5. Wang, H.; Fox, C.S.; Troy, L.M.; Mckeown, N.M.; Jacques, P.F. Longitudinal association of dairy consumption with the changes in blood pressure and the risk of incident hypertension: The Framingham Heart Study. *Br. J. Nutr.* **2015**, *114*, 1887–1899. [CrossRef] [PubMed]

6. Zong, G.; Sun, Q.; Yu, D.; Zhu, J.; Sun, L.; Ye, X.; Li, H.; Jin, Q.; Zheng, H.; Hu, F.B.; et al. Dairy consumption, type 2 diabetes, and changes in cardiometabolic traits: A prospective cohort study of middle-aged and older Chinese in Beijing and Shanghai. *Diabetes Care* **2014**, *37*, 56–63. [CrossRef] [PubMed]

7. Azadbakht, L.; Mirmiran, P.; Esmaillzadeh, A.; Azizi, T.; Azizi, F. Beneficial effects of a Dietary Approaches to Stop Hypertension eating plan on features of the metabolic syndrome. *Diabetes Care* **2005**, *28*, 2823–2831. [CrossRef] [PubMed]

8. Saneei, P.; Salehi-Abargouei, A.; Esmaillzadeh, A.; Azadbakht, L. Influence of Dietary Approaches to Stop Hypertension (DASH) diet on blood pressure: A systematic review and meta-analysis on randomized controlled trials. *Nutr. Metab. Cardiovasc. Dis. NMCD* **2014**, *24*, 1253–1261. [CrossRef] [PubMed]

9. Crichton, G.E.; Elias, M.F.; Dore, G.A.; Abhayaratna, W.P.; Robbins, M.A. Relations between dairy food intake and arterial stiffness: Pulse wave velocity and pulse pressure. *Hypertension* **2012**, *59*, 1044–1051. [CrossRef] [PubMed]

10. Livingstone, K.M.; Lovegrove, J.A.; Cockcroft, J.R.; Elwood, P.C.; Pickering, J.E.; Givens, D.I. Does dairy food intake predict arterial stiffness and blood pressure in men?: Evidence from the Caerphilly Prospective Study. *Hypertension* **2013**, *61*, 42–47. [CrossRef] [PubMed]

11. Wu, C.-F. Therapeutic modification of arterial stiffness: An update and comprehensive review. *World J. Cardiol.* **2015**, *7*, 742. [CrossRef] [PubMed]

12. Mikael, L.R.; de Paiva, A.M.G.; Gomes, M.M.; Sousa, A.L.L.; Jardim, P.C.B.V.; de Vitorino, P.V.O.; Euzébio, M.B.; de Sousa, W.M.; Barroso, W.K.S. Vascular Aging and Arterial Stiffness. *Arq. Bras. Cardiol.* **2017**. [CrossRef] [PubMed]

13. Recio-Rodriguez, J.I.; Gomez-Marcos, M.A.; Patino-Alonso, M.-C.; Sanchez, A.; Agudo-Conde, C.; Maderuelo-Fernandez, J.A.; Garcia-Ortiz, L. Association between fat amount of dairy products with pulse wave velocity and carotid intima-media thickness in adults. *Nutr. J.* **2014**, *13*. [CrossRef] [PubMed]

14. Petersen, K.S.; Keogh, J.B.; Meikle, P.J.; Garg, M.L.; Clifton, P.M. Dietary predictors of arterial stiffness in a cohort with type 1 and type 2 diabetes. *Atherosclerosis* **2015**, *238*, 175–181. [CrossRef] [PubMed]

15. Pase, M.P.; Grima, N.A.; Sarris, J. The effects of dietary and nutrient interventions on arterial stiffness: A systematic review. *Am. J. Clin. Nutr.* **2011**, *93*, 446–454. [CrossRef] [PubMed]

16. Machin, D.R.; Park, W.; Alkatan, M.; Mouton, M.; Tanaka, H. Effects of non-fat dairy products added to the routine diet on vascular function: A randomized controlled crossover trial. *Nutr. Metab. Cardiovasc. Dis. NMCD* **2015**, *25*, 364–369. [CrossRef] [PubMed]

17. Petersen, K.; Clifton, P.; Lister, N.; Keogh, J. Effect of Improving Dietary Quality on Arterial Stiffness in Subjects with Type 1 and Type 2 Diabetes: A 12 Months Randomised Controlled Trial. *Nutrients* **2016**, *8*, 382. [CrossRef] [PubMed]

18. Molina, M.C.B.; Benseñor, I.M.; de Cardoso, L.O.; Velasquez-Melendez, G.; Drehmer, M.; Pereira, T.S.S.; de Faria, C.P.; Melere, C.; Manato, L.; Gomes, A.L.C.; et al. Reprodutibilidade e validade relativa do Questionário de Frequência Alimentar do ELSA-Brasil. *Cadernos de Saúde Pública* **2013**, *29*, 379–389. [CrossRef]

19. Aquino, E.M.; Araujo, M.J.; Almeida, M.D.C.C.; Conceicao, P.; Andrade, C.R.D.; Cade, N.V.; Carvalho, M.S.; Figueiredo, R.C.D.; da Fonseca, M.D.J.M.; Giatti, L.; et al. *Revista de Saúde Pública*, 2013; *47*, 10–18. [CrossRef]

20. Sichieri, R.; Everhart, J.E. Validity of a Brazilian food frequency questionnaire against dietary recalls and estimated energy intake. *Nutr. Res.* **1998**, *18*, 1649–1659. [CrossRef]

21. Ministério da Saúde. *Guia Alimentar Para a População Brasileira*, 2nd ed.; Ministério da Saúde: Brasília, Brazil, 2014; ISBN 978-85-334-2176-9.

22. Mill, J.G.; Pinto, K.; Griep, R.H.; Goulart, A.; Foppa, M.; Lotufo, P.A.; Maestri, M.K.; Ribeiro, A.L.; Andreao, R.V.; Dantas, E.M.; et al. Afericoes e exames clinicos realizados nos participantes do ELSA-Brasil. *Revista de Saúde Pública* **2013**, *47*, 54–62. [CrossRef] [PubMed]

23. Smulyan, H.; Marchais, S.J.; Pannier, B.; Guerin, A.P.; Safar, M.E.; London, G.M. Influence of body height on pulsatile arterial hemodynamic data. *J. Am. Coll. Cardiol.* **1998**, *31*, 1103–1109. [CrossRef]

24. Soedamah-Muthu, S.S.; Verberne, L.D.M.; Ding, E.L.; Engberink, M.F.; Geleijnse, J.M. Dairy consumption and incidence of hypertension: A dose-response meta-analysis of prospective cohort studies. *Hypertension* **2012**, *60*, 1131–1137. [CrossRef] [PubMed]

25. Benatar, J.R.; Sidhu, K.; Stewart, R.A.H. Effects of high and low fat dairy food on cardio-metabolic risk factors: A meta-analysis of randomized studies. *PLoS ONE* **2013**, *8*, e76480. [CrossRef] [PubMed]

26. Protogerou, A.; Safar, M. Dissociation between Central Augmentation Index and Carotid–Femoral Pulse-Wave Velocity: When and Why? *Am. J. Hypertens.* **2007**, *20*, 648–649. [CrossRef] [PubMed]

27. Fekete, Á.A.; Givens, D.I.; Lovegrove, J.A. The impact of milk proteins and peptides on blood pressure and vascular function: A review of evidence from human intervention studies. *Nutr. Res. Rev.* **2013**, *26*, 177–190. [CrossRef] [PubMed]

28. Lovegrove, J.A.; Hobbs, D.A. New perspectives on dairy and cardiovascular health. *Proc. Nutr. Soc.* **2016**, *75*, 247–258. [CrossRef] [PubMed]

29. Maes, W.; Van Camp, J.; Vermeirssen, V.; Hemeryck, M.; Ketelslegers, J.M.; Schrezenmeir, J.; Van Oostveldt, P.; Huyghebaert, A. Influence of the lactokinin Ala-Leu-Pro-Met-His-Ile-Arg (ALPMHIR) on the release of endothelin-1 by endothelial cells. *Regul. Pept.* **2004**, *118*, 105–109. [CrossRef] [PubMed]

30. Jauhiainen, T.; Rönnback, M.; Vapaatalo, H.; Wuolle, K.; Kautiainen, H.; Groop, P.; Korpela, R. Long-term intervention with Lactobacillus helveticus fermented milk reduces augmentation index in hypertensive subjects. *Eur. J. Clin. Nutr.* **2010**, *64*, 424–431. [CrossRef] [PubMed]

31. Pal, S.; Ellis, V. The chronic effects of whey proteins on blood pressure, vascular function, and inflammatory markers in overweight individuals. *Obes. Silver Spring* **2010**, *18*, 1354–1359. [CrossRef] [PubMed]

32. Rautiainen, S.; Wang, L.; Manson, J.E.; Sesso, H.D. The Role of Calcium in the Prevention of Cardiovascular Disease—A Review of Observational Studies and Randomized Clinical Trials. *Curr. Atheroscler. Rep.* **2013**, *15*. [CrossRef] [PubMed]

33. Houston, M.C. The Importance of Potassium in Managing Hypertension. *Curr. Hypertens. Rep.* **2011**, *13*, 309–317. [CrossRef] [PubMed]

34. Houston, M. The Role of Magnesium in Hypertension and Cardiovascular Disease: Magnesium, Hypertension, and Cardiovascular Disease. *J. Clin. Hypertens.* **2011**, *13*, 843–847. [CrossRef] [PubMed]

35. Guo, J.; Astrup, A.; Lovegrove, J.A.; Gijsbers, L.; Givens, D.I.; Soedamah-Muthu, S.S. Milk and dairy consumption and risk of cardiovascular diseases and all-cause mortality: Dose–response meta-analysis of prospective cohort studies. *Eur. J. Epidemiol.* **2017**, *32*, 269–287. [CrossRef] [PubMed]

36. Corte-Real, J.; Bohn, T. Interaction of divalent minerals with liposoluble nutrients and phytochemicals during digestion and influences on their bioavailability—A review. *Food Chem.* **2018**, *252*, 285–293. [CrossRef] [PubMed]

37. Drehmer, M.; Pereira, M.A.; Schmidt, M.I.; Alvim, S.; Lotufo, P.A.; Luft, V.C.; Duncan, B.B. Total and Full-Fat, but Not Low-Fat, Dairy Product Intakes are Inversely Associated with Metabolic Syndrome in Adults. *J. Nutr.* **2016**, *146*, 81–89. [CrossRef] [PubMed]

38. Elwood, P.C.; Pickering, J.E.; Givens, D.I.; Gallacher, J.E. The consumption of milk and dairy foods and the incidence of vascular disease and diabetes: An overview of the evidence. *Lipids* **2010**, *45*, 925–939. [CrossRef] [PubMed]

39. German, J.B.; Gibson, R.A.; Krauss, R.M.; Nestel, P.; Lamarche, B.; van Staveren, W.A.; Steijns, J.M.; de Groot, L.C.P.G.M.; Lock, A.L.; Destaillats, F. A reappraisal of the impact of dairy foods and milk fat on cardiovascular disease risk. *Eur. J. Nutr.* **2009**, *48*, 191–203. [CrossRef] [PubMed]

40. De Oliveira Otto, M.C.; Mozaffarian, D.; Kromhout, D.; Bertoni, A.G.; Sibley, C.T.; Jacobs, D.R.; Nettleton, J.A. Dietary intake of saturated fat by food source and incident cardiovascular disease: The Multi-Ethnic Study of Atherosclerosis. *Am. J. Clin. Nutr.* **2012**, *96*, 397–404. [CrossRef] [PubMed]

41. Yakoob, M.Y.; Shi, P.; Willett, W.C.; Rexrode, K.M.; Campos, H.; Orav, E.J.; Hu, F.B.; Mozaffarian, D. Circulating Biomarkers of Dairy Fat and Risk of Incident Diabetes Mellitus Among Men and Women in the United States in Two Large Prospective Cohorts. *Circulation* **2016**, *133*, 1645–1654. [CrossRef] [PubMed]

42. Vlachopoulos, C.; Aznaouridis, K.; Stefanadis, C. Prediction of cardiovascular events and all-cause mortality with arterial stiffness: A systematic review and meta-analysis. *J. Am. Coll. Cardiol.* **2010**, *55*, 1318–1327. [CrossRef] [PubMed]

43. Selmer, R.; Kristiansen, I.; Haglerod, A.; Graff-Iversen, S.; Larsen, H.; Meyer, H.; Bonaa, K.; Thelle, D. Cost and health consequences of reducing the population intake of salt. *J. Epidemiol. Community Health* **2000**, *54*, 697–702. [CrossRef] [PubMed]

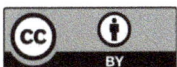

nutrients

MDPI

Article

The Consumption of Dairy and Its Association with Nutritional Status in the South East Asian Nutrition Surveys (SEANUTS)

Khanh Le Nguyen Bao [1], Sandjaja Sandjaja [2], Bee Koon Poh [3], Nipa Rojroongwasinkul [4], Chinh Nguyen Huu [1], Edith Sumedi [2], Jamil Nor Aini [3], Sayamon Senaprom [4], Paul Deurenberg [5], Marjolijn Bragt [6], Ilse Khouw [6,*] and on behalf of the SEANUTS Study Group [†]

[1] National Institute of Nutrition, 48B Tang Bat Ho Street, Hanoi 10000, Vietnam; bkhanhnin@gmail.com (K.L.N.B.); nguyenhuuchinhvdd@gmail.com (C.N.H.)
[2] Persatuan Ahli Gizi Indonesia, Jalan Hang Jebat III/F3, Kebayoran Baru, Jakarta 12120, Indonesia; san_gizi@yahoo.com (S.S.); edith.sumedi@yahoo.com (E.S.)
[3] Universiti Kebangsaan Malaysia, Jalan Raja Muda Abdul Aziz, 50300 Kuala Lumpur, Malaysia; pbkoon@ukm.edu.my (B.K.P.); ainijamil@ukm.edu.my (J.N.A.)
[4] Institute of Nutrition Mahidol University, Phuttamonthon 4, Nakhon Pathom 73170, Thailand; nipa.roj@mahidol.ac.th (N.R.); sayamon.sen@mahidol.ac.th (S.S.)
[5] Nutrition Consultant, 055 Laurel Street, 3319 Ramon, Isabela, the Philippines; paul.deurenberg@gmail.com
[6] FrieslandCampina, Stationsplein 4, 3818 LE Amersfoort, the Netherlands; marjolijn.bragt@frieslandcampina.com
[*] Correspondence: ilse.tan-khouw@frieslandcampina.com; Tel.: +65-6578-5921
[†] The SEANUTS Study Group comprises the following. Vietnam: Khanh Le Nguyen Bao, Chinh Nguyen Huu, Hop Le Thi, Truong Nguyen Hong, Van Anh Nguyen Do, Do Tran Thanh, Nga Tran Thuy, Nhung Bui Thi, Dzung Nguyen Dinh, Tuoc Bui Van, Khang Nguyen Van, Dzung Nguyen Viet, Luan Nguyen Viet, Ha Nguyen Thu Ha, Xuyen Hoang Thi, Long Nguyen Van, Hai Tran Thi, Long Pham Si, Huong Nguyen Thi, Ngan Nguyen Thi, Thao Le Thanh, Kieu Dau Thi, Thang Dinh Tat, Mai Nguyen Thi Tuyet. Indonesia: Sandjaja Sandjaja, Basuki Budiman, Moesijanti Soekatri, Heryudarini Harahap, Fitrah Ernawati, Yekti Widodo, Edith Sumedi, Nurmeida S. Syarief, Rustan Effendi, Gustina Sofia, Minarto, Hidayat Syarief. Malaysia: Poh Bee Koon, Norimah A Karim, Ruzita A Talib, Siti Balkis Budin, Alvin Ng Lai Oon, Siti Haslinda Mohd Din, Wong Jyh Eiin, Mohd Ismail Noor, Rahman Jamal, Nor Azmi Kamaruddin, Nik Shanita Safii, Chin Yit Siew, Wee Bee Suan, Nor Aini Jamil A. Wahab. Thailand: Nipa Rojroongwasinkul, Atitada Boonpraderm, Pattanee Winichagoon, Petcharat Kunaphan, Uruwan Yamborisut, Wanphen Wimonpeerapattana, Sayamon Senaprom, Kallaya Kijboonchoo, Wiyada Thasanasuwan, Weerachat Srichan, Kusol Soonthorndhada, Sasiumphai Purttiponthanee. FrieslandCampina: Ilse Khouw, Panam Parikh, Swee Ai Ng, Anne Schaafsma, Marjolijn Bragt.

Received: 28 April 2018; Accepted: 5 June 2018; Published: 13 June 2018

Abstract: Despite a major decrease in undernutrition worldwide over the last 25 years, underweight and stunting in children still persist as public health issues especially in Africa and Asia. Adequate nutrition is one of the key factors for healthy growth and development of children. In This study, the associations between dairy consumption and nutritional status in the South East Asian Nutrition Survey (SEANUTS) were investigated. National representative data of 12,376 children in Indonesia, Malaysia, Thailand, and Vietnam aged between 1 and 12 years were pooled, representing nearly 88 million children in This age category. It was found that the prevalence of stunting and underweight was lower in children who consumed dairy on a daily basis (10.0% and 12.0%, respectively) compared to children who did not use dairy (21.4% and 18.0%, respectively) ($p < 0.05$). The prevalence of vitamin A deficiency and vitamin D insufficiency was lower in the group of dairy users (3.9% and 39.4%, respectively) compared to non-dairy consumers (7.5% and 53.8%, respectively) ($p < 0.05$). This study suggests that dairy as part of a daily diet plays an important role in growth and supports a healthy vitamin A and vitamin D status.

Keywords: dairy; SEANUTS; stunting; underweight; vitamin A; vitamin D; haemoglobin

1. Introduction

Although the proportion of under nutrition in the Southeast Asian region decreased tremendously from 31% in 1990 to 10% in 2015, 16% of the children under 5 years of age are still moderately to severely underweight [1]. Moreover, it is projected that more than 25% or 165 million children under 5 years of age are stunted, of which 90% reside in Africa and Asia [2].

In line with these numbers, the South East Asian Nutrition Surveys (SEANUTS) also showed that under nutrition is still a major issue in the four countries of Indonesia, Malaysia, Thailand, and Vietnam, yet at different degrees [3–6]. Overall, the prevalence of stunting in children 0.5–12 years of age in these four countries was around 15%, with rural Indonesia having the highest prevalence (38.8%) and urban Thailand the lowest prevalence (4.2%). The prevalence of underweight varied between 6.4% for urban Thai children and 28.9% for rural Indonesian children. Moreover, SEANUTS also found a high prevalence of vitamin D insufficiency in all of the four countries, varying from 20% in Thailand up to 44% in Malaysia [7].

Nutrition is an important factor for healthy growth and development in children. Dietary guidelines recommend a well-balanced diet including all major food groups for sufficient intake of necessary macro- and micronutrients [8]. However, SEANUTS showed that a large proportion of children did not meet their daily recommended intake (RDI) of many nutrients including calcium, iron, vitamin C, and vitamin D [3–6]. It was also found that with the exception of meat/poultry, Malaysian children did not meet the recommendations of daily intake for each food group [9].

Dairy products contribute to a healthy diet by providing energy, protein, and micronutrients such as calcium, magnesium, and vitamins B1, B2, and B12 [10]. Dairy protein is considered to be of high quality as it provides all the essential amino acids, with high bioavailability [11]. In many recommendation and guidelines, dairy is often advised as part of a healthy diet [12]. Analyses of SEANUTS data of Vietnam and Indonesia showed that children consuming dairy products were better in achieving RDI levels for protein, calcium, iron, zinc, vitamins A, B1, B2, B3, C, and D, compared to children who did not consume dairy [13,14].

A few studies have linked dairy consumption with nutritional status [12,15], but many of them were relatively small or conducted in selected groups. The objective of This SEANUTS analysis was to determine whether children who consumed dairy products as part of their daily diet had a better nutritional status as measured by anthropometric indices and blood status for iron, vitamin A and D compared to children who did not.

2. Materials and Methods

SEANUTS is a nationally-representative multi-centre survey in Indonesia, Malaysia, Thailand, and Vietnam, conducted between 2010 and 2011, to assess the nutritional status and lifestyle factors of over 16,500 children aged 0.5–12 years old. A multi-stage cluster sampling, stratified for geographical location, gender and age was carried out. The survey was conducted according to the guidelines laid down in the Declaration of Helsinki and in each country the survey and its procedures were approved by local ethical committees. The survey is registered in the Netherlands Trial Register as NTR2462. Details of SEANUTS methodology are described elsewhere [3–6,16]. In the current study only data of children older than 1 year were used.

Nutrient intake and dairy consumption were calculated from 24 h recall questionnaires (Indonesia, Thailand, and Vietnam) and/or from semi-quantitative food frequency questionnaires (FFQ, Indonesia, Malaysia, Thailand) using the local food composition tables.

Even though different local dietary guidelines advice children to consume 2–3 servings of dairy per day (500–750 g dairy), many children in South East Asia do not meet This recommendation. Therefore, we decided to use lower criteria. A child was defined as 'dairy user' if he/she consumed a minimum of either 15 g milk powder (equals about 100 mL milk when dissolved in water), 100 g UHT/flavoured/cultured milk or drink yoghurt, 50 g yoghurt, 10 g condensed milk or ice cream, or 5 g cheese on a daily basis. Each of these amounts was also considered to reflect one dairy consumption. If the consumption of each individual dairy product was below these criteria but the sum of all dairy products exceeded 100 g, the child was classified as 'dairy user' as well. If different dairy products were consumed in the above mentioned minimum amounts, consumption would be categorized as ≥2 consumptions per day.

Information on the level of education of the child's mother and family income was collected from the parents or primary caregivers using a structured questionnaire. Income was categorized into country specific quintiles, while education was classified into three groups as primary school or lower, secondary education or tertiary education.

Weight was measured using calibrated digital scales accurate to 0.1 kg. Height was measured using wall-mounted stadiometers accurate to 0.1 cm. Body mass index (BMI, kg/m^2) was calculated as weight divided by height squared. Weight for age Z-scores (WAZ), BMI for age Z-scores (BAZ) and height for age Z-scores (HAZ) were calculated based on WHO references [17,18]. Children with HAZ, WAZ and BAZ lower than −2 SD of the reference value were classified as stunted, underweight and thin, respectively. The cut-off values for overweight and obesity among children <5 years were +2 SD and +3 SD, whereas they were +1 SD and +2 SD, respectively, for children aged ≥5 years.

Blood from a subsample of subjects was analysed for haemoglobin (Hb), ferritin, vitamin A (serum retinol), and vitamin D (25-hydroxyvitamin D (25(OH)D)). Details of the methodologies used are described in Schaafsma et al. [16]. Anaemia was defined as Hb concentrations <110 g/L for subjects <5 years, <115 g/L for subjects aged 5–11.9 years, and <120 g/L for subjects aged ≥12 years [19]. Iron deficiency was defined as serum ferritin concentrations <12 µg/L for children aged <5 years and <15 µg/L for children aged ≥5 years [20]. Serum retinol concentration <0.70 µmol/L was used as an indicator for vitamin A deficiency [21], whereas circulating 25(OH)D concentration <50 nmol/L was used as an indication for vitamin D insufficiency [22].

Data were weighted using age, gender and residence weight factors to extrapolate to the total population per country. The weight factors were based on data from the relevant national Statistical Offices. In the pooled analyses, the population size of each country was taken into account to avoid bias due to the effect of larger population number.

Data were analysed using SPSS version 20.0 (IBM Cooperation 2011, Armonk, NY, USA) with complex sample techniques. Differences between groups were tested using analysis of (co)variance after correction for possible confounders. Differences in categorical variables across groups were tested using logistic regression with correction for confounding variables (age, residence, mother's educational level, and income level). Values are expressed as mean and SE and level of significance is set at $p < 0.05$.

3. Results

The total sample size in the present analyses was 12,376, representing nearly 88 million children. Table 1 shows the anthropometric characteristics of the children and their blood profiles.

Overall, 68% of the children consumed dairy (Table 2) according to the criteria as defined in the Materials and Methods, although it varied per country. Most of the children in Thailand (98%) consumed dairy on a daily basis, followed by Malaysia (69%), Indonesia (52%), and Vietnam (47%), respectively. For the types of dairy product, amongst the four countries, UHT/flavoured milk was the most consumed (32%), followed by powder milk (22%), but the consumptions varied across countries. In Malaysia, mostly powder milk was consumed (41%). In Thailand and Vietnam, the children drank mainly UHT/flavoured milk (84% and 34%, respectively). In Indonesia mainly condensed milk was consumed (27%). Yoghurt and cheese were dairy formats less consumed by the children (data not shown).

Table 1. Characteristics of the children (1–12 years old) per country and in the four countries combined.

	Indonesia		Malaysia		Thailand		Vietnam		All Four Countries	
Sample size	3163		3472		2943		2798		12,376	
Population	53,184,526		5,740,266		9,662,074		19,402,735		87,989,601	
	Mean	SE	Mean	SE	Mean	SE	Mean	SE	Mean	SE
Age (years)	6.6	0.1	7.1	0.1	7.2	0.1	7.4	0.1	7.1	0.0
Weight (kg)	19.4	0.2	25.5	0.4	24.3	0.3	22.1	0.2	22.9	0.1
Height (cm)	110.5	0.4	118.2	0.6	118.2	0.5	118.0	0.3	116.2	0.2
BMI (kg/m^2)	15.4	0.1	17.0	0.1	16.4	0.1	15.4	0.0	16.1	0.0
HAZ	−1.44	0.03	−0.55	0.03	−0.52	0.02	−0.88	0.02	−0.84	0.01
WAZ	−1.23	0.04	−0.33	0.03	−0.39	0.03	−0.81	0.03	−0.70	0.02
BAZ	−0.47	0.03	0.14	0.03	−0.10	0.03	−0.54	0.03	−0.23	0.02
Hb (g/L)	122	0	131	0	125	1	127	1	126	0
Ferritin (µg/L)	46.8	1.0	48.5	1.5	59.4	1.9	49.1	2.3	51.0	0.9
Retinol (µmol/L)	1.47	0.02	1.06	0.01	1.23	0.02	1.05	0.03	1.18	0.01
25-hydroxyvitamin D (nmol/L)	53.1	0.9	52.7	1.0	59.5	1.1	55.9	1.7	55.7	0.7

BMI: body mass index; HAZ: height for age Z-score; WAZ: weight for age Z-score; BAZ: body mass index for age Z-score, Hb: Haemoglobin. Recommended values for Hb are >110 g/L for subjects <5 years, >115 g/L for subjects aged 5–11.9 years and >120 g/L for subjects aged ≥12 years. Recommended iron values are >12 µg/L for children aged <5 years and >15 µg/L for children aged ≥5 years. Recommended values for retinol is >70 µmol/L and for vitamin D >50 nmol/L.

Table 2. Percentage of children consuming different dairy products and percentage of dairy users per country and for the four countries combined.

	Indonesia	Malaysia	Thailand	Vietnam	All Four Countries
UHT/flavoured milk (>100 g)	5	3	84	34	32
Milk powder (>15 g)	19	41	14	11	22
Condensed milk (>10 g)	27	15	0	4	12
Dairy user *	52	69	98	47	68

* Dairy user is defined as a minimum average consumption of either 15 g powder milk, 100 g UHT/flavoured milk, 50 g yoghurt, 10 g condensed milk or ice cream, or 5 g cheese on a daily basis. In case the consumption of each individual dairy product was below these criteria but the sum of all dairy products exceeded 100 g, the child was classified as 'dairy user' as well.

There were less dairy users in the older children (from approx. 6 years onwards), except for Thailand where almost 100% of the children were dairy consumers irrespective of their age. Dairy consumption did not differ between boys and girls, but in Indonesia and Vietnam more urban children (62% and 72%, respectively) consumed dairy compared to rural children (44% and 34%, respectively, $p < 0.05$). The consumption was also dependent on maternal education level and socio-economic status except for Thailand. Significant more children consumed dairy when their mothers were higher educated and when their families were in the higher income quintiles (data not shown).

Some 42.6% of the children were categorized in the <1 dairy consumption per day group, while 39.3% and 18.1% had 1 and ≥2 dairy consumptions per day, respectively. Mean dairy intake in the group of 1 dairy consumption per day was 281 ± 6 g/day and in the group of ≥2 dairy consumptions per day 521 ± 6 g/day. Children in the groups of 1 or ≥2 dairy consumptions per day had higher total dietary intakes compared to children consuming <1 dairy consumption per day when compared to the different local recommended dietary allowances of each country (Table 3).

In Table 4 the mean (SE) of anthropometric variables in the three dairy user groups and the prevalence for malnutrition is shown. Weight, height, WAZ, and HAZ were significantly higher in children in the groups of 1 or ≥2 dairy consumptions per day compared to children who consumed <1 dairy consumption per day. Consequently, the prevalence for underweight and stunting was lower in the children drinking more than 1 or ≥2 dairy consumptions per day. For height, HAZ, WAZ, and stunting, there were also significant differences between 1 and ≥2 dairy consumptions per day.

However, BMI, BAZ, or the prevalence for thinness, overweight, and obesity did not differ between the three groups.

Table 3. Total dietary intake as percent of local RDA for the three different dairy user groups.

Dairy Per Day	<1 Dairy Consumption		1 Dairy Consumption		≥2 Dairy Consumptions	
	Mean	SE	Mean	SE	Mean	SE
Energy	74 [a]	1	90 [b]	1	97 [c]	1
Protein	119 [a]	1	158 [b]	1	179 [c]	1
Calcium	55 [a]	1	96 [b]	1	83 [c]	1
Iron	76 [a]	1	117 [b]	2	101 [b]	2
Zinc	75 [a]	1	112 [b]	1	148 [c]	2
Vitamin B1	71 [a]	1	114 [b]	1	141 [c]	2
Vitamin B2	69 [a]	1	147 [b]	2	184 [c]	2
Vitamin B3	63 [a]	1	92 [b]	1	103 [c]	1
Vitamin C	73 [a]	2	132 [b]	3	99 [c]	2
Vitamin A	63 [a]	1	96 [b]	1	88 [c]	2
Vitamin D	41 [a]	1	86 [b]	2	101 [c]	2

[a,b,c]: Different letters in superscripts indicate significant difference with other cells in the same row.

Table 4. Anthropometric variables in the different dairy consumption groups and prevalence of malnutrition after corrections for confounders †.

	<1 Dairy Consumption/Day		1 Dairy Consumption/Day		≥2 Dairy Consumptions/Day	
	Mean	SE	Mean	SE	Mean	SE
Age (years)	7.8 [a]	0.1	6.3 [b]	0.1	7.1 [c]	0.1
Height (cm)	114.6 [a]	0.1	115.9 [b]	0.1	117.1 [c]	0.1
Weight (kg)	22.2 [a]	0.2	22.8 [b]	0.1	23.2 [b]	0.2
BMI (kg/m²)	16.0 [a]	0.1	16.0 [a]	0.1	16.1 [a]	0.1
HAZ	−1.09 [a]	0.02	−0.84 [b]	0.02	−0.63 [c]	0.02
WAZ	−0.90 [a]	0.03	−0.73 [b]	0.03	−0.50 [c]	0.03
BAZ	−0.26 [a]	0.03	−0.25 [a]	0.03	−0.17 [a]	0.03
Stunted (%)	21.4 [a]		15.2 [b]		10.0 [c]	
Underweight (%)	18.0 [a]		15.0 [ab]		12.0 [b]	
Thinness (%)	6.9 [a]		8.3 [a]		7.9 [a]	
Overweight (%)	6.7 [a]		6.7 [a]		7.9 [a]	
Obese (%)	7.3 [a]		6.9 [a]		7.3 [a]	

† Except for age, all values are corrected for differences in age, sex, residence, education level of the mother, income quintile and country. Stunted is defined as HAZ <−2 SD; underweight as WAZ <−2 SD, and thinness as BAZ <−2 SD. Overweight and obesity are defined as BAZ > +2 SD and +3 SD, respectively, for children aged <5 years and >+1 SD and +2 SD, respectively, for children aged ≥5 years. [a,b,c]: Different letters in superscripts indicate significant difference with other cells in the same row.

One or ≥2 consumption of dairy per day was associated with a lower risk of being stunted and children who had ≥2 dairy consumptions per day were less likely to be underweight (Table 5). Dairy consumption was not significantly associated with the risk of being thin, overweight or obese (Table 5).

In Table 6, the sample sizes, mean blood values and prevalence are shown for anaemia, iron deficiency, vitamin A deficiency, and vitamin D insufficiency. One or ≥2 dairy consumptions per day were neither associated with the prevalence of anaemia which was around 11%–13% in the three groups nor with the prevalence of iron deficiency, with or without correction for inflammation even though there is a trend for a lower prevalence in the 1 and ≥2 dairy consumption groups. In contrast, the prevalence of vitamin A deficiency and vitamin D insufficiency were significant lower in children drinking 1 or ≥2 dairy consumptions per day. For vitamin A deficiency, the prevalence in the group of 1 dairy consumption per day was 3.9% while it was 7.5% in the group of <1 dairy consumption per day. For vitamin D insufficiency, the prevalence was 39.4% and 53.8%, respectively. Consequently, the odds of being vitamin A deficient or vitamin D insufficient were lower in the groups of 1 or ≥ 2 dairy consumptions per day.

Table 5. Odds ratio (OR) with 95% confidence interval (CI) for being stunted, underweight, thin, overweight or obese in relation to dairy consumption category.

	Stunted		Underweight		Thinness †		Overweight †		Obese †	
	OR	95% CI	OR	95% CI	OR	95% CI	OR	95% CI	OR	95% CI
<1 dairy consumption/day	1	-	1	-	1	-	1	-	1	-
1 dairy consumption/day	0.7 *	0.6, 0.9	0.9	0.7, 1.1	1.3	1.0, 1.6	1.0	0.8, 1.2	0.9	0.7, 1.2
≥ 2 dairy consumptions/day	0.5 *	0.4, 0.6	0.7 *	0.6, 0.9	1.2	0.9, 1.6	1.2	1.0, 1.6	1.1	0.8, 1.4

Data are corrected for confounding effect of age, sex, urban/rural, education of mother, income quintile, energy intake and country. Stunted is defined as HAZ < -2 SD; underweight as WAZ < -2 SD, and thinness as BAZ < -2 SD. Overweight and obesity are defined as BAZ $> +2$ SD and $+3$ SD, respectively, for children aged <5 years and $>+1$ SD and $+2$ SD, respectively, for children aged ≥ 5 years. † Reference category is 'normal weight'. * $p < 0.05$.

Table 6. Mean blood values and prevalence of anaemia, iron deficiency, vitamin A deficiency, and vitamin D insufficiency in the different dairy consumption groups and odds ratios for having a micronutrient deficiency.

	n	<1 Dairy Consumption/Day		1 Dairy Consumption/Day		≥ 2 Dairy Consumptions/Day	
		Mean	SE	Mean	SE	Mean	SE
Hb (g/L)	4149	126 [a]	0	126 [a]	0	127 [a]	0
Ferritin (µg/L)	3041	48.5 [a]	1.6	50.2 [ab]	1.5	55.1 [b]	1.4
Ferritin (µg/L) †	2861	45.7 [a]	1.4	46.4 [a]	1.4	49.6 [a]	1.5
Retinol (µmol/L)	3024	1.15 [a]	0.02	1.19 [a]	0.02	1.22 [a]	0.02
25 Hydroxyvitamin D (nmol/L)	1987	51.6 [a]	1.3	58.7 [b]	1.2	57.0 [b]	0.9
Anaemia		13.1 [a]		11.6 [a]		10.9 [a]	
Iron deficiency †		6.6 [a]		4.9 [a]		4.1 [a]	
Vitamin A deficiency		7.5 [a]		3.9 [b]		2.9 [b]	
Vitamin D insufficiency		53.8 [a]		39.4 [b]		40.6 [b]	
		ODDS	95% CI	ODDS	95% CI	ODDS	95% CI
Anaemia		1	-	0.8	0.6, 1.2	0.8	0.5, 1.1
Iron deficiency †		1	-	0.7	0.4, 1.3	0.6	0.3, 1.2
Vitamin A deficiency		1	-	0.5 *	0.3, 0.9	0.4 *	0.2, 0.7
Vitamin D deficiency		1	-	0.5 *	0.4, 0.7	0.6 *	0.4, 0.8

Hb: haemoglobin. Anaemia is defined as Hb concentrations <110 g/L for subjects <5 years, <115 g/L for subjects aged 5–11.9 years, and <120 g/L for subjects aged ≥ 12 years. Iron deficiency is defined as serum ferritin concentrations <12 µg/L for children <5 years and <15 µg/L for children ≥ 5 years. Serum retinol concentration <0.70 µmol/L is an indicator for vitamin A deficiency, whereas 25(OH)D concentration <50 nmol/L was used as an indicator for vitamin D insufficiency. † After correction for inflammation. [a,b] Different letters in superscript indicate significant difference with other cells in the same row. * $p < 0.05$. Data are corrected for the confounding effects of age, sex, and residence.

4. Discussion

The present study shows that incidence of dairy consumption was positively associated with the nutritional status of 1–12-year-old children in the SEANUTS population of Indonesia, Malaysia, Thailand, and Vietnam based on anthropometric indices. Children were less likely to be stunted or underweight when dairy was part of their daily diet. Stunting is associated with increased morbidity and impacts cognitive development [23,24]. It is also a risk factor for chronic diseases in adulthood [25].

Previous intervention and observational studies have shown a positive effect of milk and dairy products on the growth of preschool and school-aged children [26–29]. As early as 1928, it was reported that milk supplementation in 5–14-year-old Scottish children resulted in approximately 20% more height gain compared to children who received a biscuit as control [26]. Another study that followed the effect of a school milk programme in 6–9-year-old Malaysian primary school children showed that there was a reduction in underweight, stunting, and wasting after two years [27]. In Indonesia, it was shown that supplementation of fortified milk to 6–59 month old children was associated with a lower risk of stunting [29]. A meta-analysis of 12 trials examining the association between dairy consumption and height showed that supplementation of approximately 245 mL milk on a daily basis resulted in an additional 0.4 cm growth per year [28]. Our current results confirm the positive association between dairy consumption and growth.

Recently, it was hypothesized that insufficiency in essential amino acids may be an important limiting factor in linear growth [30]. When specific amino acids, especially the essential ones, are deficient in the children's diet, protein and lipid synthesis and cellular growth is negatively affected [31]. Dairy is known to provide all essential amino acids. Moreover, dairy protein has a high protein-digestibility-corrected amino acid score (PDCAAS) [12] indicating that the amino acids are easily bioavailable for digestion, absorption, and utilization by the body. This may be the mechanism behind the association between dairy consumption and lower prevalence and risk of stunting. Further analyses of the dietary intake data of SEANUTS showed that stunted children had a lower intake of total protein compared to normal height children (data not shown). Moreover, intake of animal protein was also lower (data not shown), which is also linked to stunting [32,33].

The association between dairy and overweight/obesity is more complicated than dairy and linear growth. A systematic review of 19 studies in both children and adults by Louie et al. [34] showed results ranging from dairy having a protective effect against weight gain (nine studies), to no impact (seven studies), or to even increasing the risk of weight gain (three studies) and the authors, therefore, stated that it is difficult making firm conclusions. Our data showed no difference in overweight/obesity prevalence between dairy consumers and non-dairy consumers and also the odds for being overweight or obese did not differ between the three groups.

The prevalence of vitamin A deficiency and vitamin D insufficiency in the group of 1 or ≥ 2 dairy consumptions per day was lower than in the group with <1 dairy consumption per day. Moreover, the former were also found to be less likely vitamin A or vitamin D deficient (Table 6). A possible explanation could be that dairy consumption is associated with healthier food choices and better total diet quality in general [35] resulting in better intakes of vitamin A and D. On the other hand, although cow's milk does not naturally contain high levels of these vitamins, today's trend is that many dairy products in Indonesia, Malaysia, Thailand, and Vietnam, especially those in powder formats and those targeted for children, are often fortified with micronutrients such as vitamin A, B2, and D. Vitamin D insufficiency is a major issue in many countries, also in the SEANUTS countries, despite the abundance of sun light available in the Southeast Asian region [7,36,37]. Therefore, dietary vitamin D intake, either via foods naturally rich in vitamin D such as oily fish and eggs, or via vitamin D fortified foods, might become more and more important. The relatively high percentages of vitamin D insufficiency in the groups of dairy consumers may warrant evaluation of fortification policies and practices by government and manufacturers [38].

No significant differences were found in anaemia and iron deficiency between the three groups, which is not surprising as dairy is not a good dietary source for iron. In contrast, a trial in Vietnam showed a decrease in anaemia prevalence from 46.7% to 9.3% and from 43.7% to 19.2% in the 7–8-year-old children after 6 months of consuming fortified milk and regular milk, respectively [39]. A reason for these different findings could be that the anaemia prevalence in the SEANUTS cohort was much lower than in the children studied by Lien et al. [39]. Another reason could be the type of milk consumed in the present study, whereby UHT milk was the format most commonly consumed, which is normally not iron-fortified while powder milk and especially growing up milk powder are fortified with iron.

Although the prevalence of lactose intolerance is higher in the Asian region compared to for example Western Europe, it is not a clinical issue in younger children. For adults and older children, most who have been diagnosed with lactase deficiency can often tolerate consuming some dairy products. Dairy formats such as yoghurt can be an alternative for normal milk products as fermented milk products are better tolerated by individuals who are lactose-intolerant [12,40]. For This reason, the possible higher risk of being lactose intolerant should not be a contra-indication for consuming dairy as prevention for stunting or micronutrient deficiencies.

The current study has its limitations as it was not designed to study the relationship between nutritional status and dairy consumption. Also, different methodologies were used to assess dairy consumption. Furthermore, local food composition databases might not be up to date in a fast changing market of dairy products and may differ between countries.

5. Conclusions

In conclusion, the results showed that children who consumed dairy were less likely to be stunted or underweight and less likely to be vitamin A deficient or vitamin D insufficient. Future studies should focus on the status of other micronutrients like B vitamins or zinc as more and more data are emerging that those deficiencies are prevalent in the Asian region [41,42]. On the other hand, more intervention studies should be conducted for a better understanding of the role of dairy and how to improve the nutritional status of children. Then, in relation to public health, national policies should consider the availability and accessibility of dairy to its population to support the healthy growth and development of children.

Author Contributions: Formal analysis, P.D.; Investigation, C.N.H., E.S., J.N.A. and S.S. (Sayamon Senaprom); Supervision, K.L.N.B., S.S. (Sandjaja Sandjaja), B.K.P. and N.R.; Writing—original draft, I.K.; Writing—review and editing, M.B.

Funding: This research was funded by FrieslandCampina.

Acknowledgments: The authors thank the research teams of each of the countries involved as well as the parents/carers, children involved in the study for their willingness to participate.

Conflicts of Interest: The results of the study will be used by FrieslandCampina but it had no influence on the outcome of the study. None of the other authors or the research institutes had any conflicts of interest.

References

1. United Nations. The Millennium Development Goals Report 2015. Available online: http://www.un.org/millenniumgoals/2015_MDG_Report/pdf/MDG%202015%20Summary%20web_english.pdf (accessed on 8 September 2015).

2. United Nations Children's Fund; World Health Organisation; The World Bank; UNICEF-WHO-World Bank. *Joint Child Malnutrition Estimates*; UNICEF: New York, NY, USA; WHO: Geneva, Switzerland; The World Bank: Washington, DC, USA, 2012.

3. Sandjaja, S.; Budiman, B.; Harahap, H.; Ernawati, F.; Soekatri, M.; Widodo, Y.; Sumedi, E.; Rustan, E.; Sofia, G.; Syarief, S.N.; et al. Food consumption and nutritional and biochemical status of 0.5–12-year-old Indonesian children: The SEANUTS study. *Br. J. Nutr.* **2013**, *110*, S11–S20. [CrossRef] [PubMed]

4. Poh, B.K.; Ng, B.K.; Siti Haslinda, M.D.; Nik Shanita, S.; Wong, J.E.; Budin, S.B.; Ruzita, A.T.; Ng, L.O.; Khouw, I.; Norimah, A.K. Nutritional status and dietary intakes of children aged 6 months to 12 years: Findings of the Nutrition Survey of Malaysian Children (SEANUTS Malaysia). *Br. J. Nutr.* **2013**, *110*, S21–S35. [CrossRef] [PubMed]

5. Rojroongwasinkul, N.; Kijboonchoo, K.; Wimonpeerapattana, W.; Purttiponthanee, S.; Yamborisut, U.; Boonpraderm, A.; Kunapan, P.; Thasanasuwan, W.; Khouw, I. SEANUTS: The nutritional status and dietary intakes of 0.5–12-year-old Thai children. *Br. J. Nutr.* **2013**, *110*, S36–S44. [CrossRef] [PubMed]

6. Le Nguyen, B.K.; Le Thi, H.; Nguyen Do, V.A.; Tran Thuy, N.; Nguyen Huu, C.; Thanh Do, T.; Deurenberg, P.; Khouw, I. Double burden of undernutrition and overnutrition in Vietnam in 2011: Results of the SEANUTS study in 0·5-11-year-old children. *Br. J. Nutr.* **2013**, *110*, S45–S56. [CrossRef] [PubMed]

7.	Poh, B.K.; Rojroongwasinkul, N.; Le Nguyen, B.K.; Sandjaja, A.T.R.; Yamborisut, U.; Hong, T.N.; Ernawati, F.; Deurenberg, P.; Parikh, P. 25-hydroxy-vitamin D demography and the risk of vitamin D insufficiency in the South East Asian Nutrition Surveys (SEANUTS). *Asia Pac. J. Clin. Nutr.* **2016**, *25*, 538–548. [CrossRef] [PubMed]

8.	Food and Agricultural Organization. Plates, Pyramids, Planet. Developments in National Healthy and Sustainable Dietary Guidelines: A State of Play Assessment. Available online: http://www.fao.org/3/a-i5640e.pdf (accessed on 19 May 2018).

9.	Koo, H.C.; Poh, B.K.; Lee, S.T.; Chong, K.H.; Bragt, M.C.E.; Abd Talib, R. Are Malaysian children achieving dietary guideline recommendations? *Asia Pac. J. Public Health* **2016**, *28*, 8S–20S. [CrossRef] [PubMed]

10.	Pereira, P.C. Milk nutritional composition and its role in human health. *Nutrition* **2014**, *30*, 619–627. [CrossRef] [PubMed]

11.	Michaelsen, K.F. Cow's milk in the prevention and treatment of stunting and wasting. *Food Nutr. Bull.* **2013**, *34*, 249–251. [CrossRef] [PubMed]

12.	Food and Agriculture Organization. Milk and Dairy Products in Human Nutrition. 2013. Available online: http://www.fao.org/docrep/018/i3396e/i3396e.pdf (accessed on 8 September 2015).

13.	Le Nguyen, B.K.; Burgers, M.R.; Nguyen Huu, C.; Bui Van, T.; Nguyen Dinh, D.; Deurenberg, P.; Schaafsma, A. Nutrient intake in Vietnamese preschool and school-aged children is not adequate: The role of dairy. *Food Nutr. Bull.* **2016**, *37*, 100–111. [CrossRef]

14.	Widodo, Y.; Sandjaja, S.; Sumedi, E.; Khouw, I.; Deurenberg, P. The effect of socio-demographic variables and dairy use on the intake of essential macro- and micronutrients in 0.5–12-year-old Indonesian children. *Asia Pac. J. Clin. Nutr.* **2016**, *25*, 356–367. [CrossRef] [PubMed]

15.	Hoppe, C.; Mølgaard, C.; Michaelsen, K.F. Cow's milk and linear growth in industrialized and developing countries. *Annu. Rev. Nutr.* **2006**, *26*, 131–173. [CrossRef] [PubMed]

16.	Schaafsma, A.; Deurenberg, P.; Calame, W.; van den Heuvel, E.G.H.M.; van Beusekom, C.; Hautvast, J.; Sandjaja; Poh, B.K.; Rojroongwasinkul, N.; Le Nguyen, B.K.; et al. Design of the South East Asian Nutrition Survey (SEANUTS): A four-country multistage cluster design study. *Br. J. Nutr.* **2013**, *110*, S2–S10. [CrossRef] [PubMed]

17.	World Health Organization. *WHO Child Growth Standards: Length/Height-for-Age, Weight-for-Age, Weight-for-Length, Weight-for Height and Body Mass Index-for-Age*; Methods and Development; World Health Organization: Geneva, Switzerland, 2006; Available online: http://www.who.int/childgrowth/publications/technical_report_pub/en/ (accessed on 28 December 2015).

18.	De Onis, M.; Onyango, A.W.; Borghi, E.; Siyam, A.; Nishida, C.; Siekmann, J. Development of a WHO growth reference for school-aged children and adolescents. *Bull. World Health Organ.* **2007**, *85*, 660–667. [CrossRef] [PubMed]

19.	World Health Organization. *Haemoglobin Concentrations for the Diagnosis of Anaemia and Assessment of Severity*; Vitamin and Mineral Nutrition Information System; World Health Organization: Geneva, Switzerland, 2011; Available online: http://www.who.int/vmnis/indicators/haemoglobin (accessed on 7 September 2015).

20.	World Health Organization. *Serum Ferritin Concentrations for the Assessment of Iron Status and Iron Deficiency in Populations*; Vitamin and Mineral Nutrition Information System; World Health Organization: Geneva, Switzerland, 2011; Available online: http://www.who.int/vmnis/indicators/serum_ferritin.pdf (accessed on 9 September 2015).

21.	World Health Organization. *Global Prevalence of Vitamin A Deficiency in Populations at Risk 1995–2005*; WHO Global Database on Vitamin A Deficiency; World Health Organization: Geneva, Switzerland, 2009; Available online: http://www.who.int/vmnis/vitamina/prevalence/en/ (accessed on 7 September 2015).

22.	Misra, M.; Pacaud, D.; Petryk, A.; Collett-Solberg, P.F.; Kappy, M. Vitamin D deficiency in children and its management: Review of current knowledge and recommendations. *Pediatrics* **2008**, *122*, 398–417. [CrossRef] [PubMed]

23.	Black, R.E.; Allen, L.H.; Bhutta, Z.A.; Caulfield, L.E.; de Onis, M.; Ezzati, M.; Mathers, C.; Rivera, J. Maternal and child undernutrition: Global and regional exposures and health consequences. *Lancet* **2008**, *371*, 243–260. [CrossRef]

24.	Grantham-McGregor, S.; Cheung, Y.B.; Cueto, S.; Glewwe, P.; Richter, L.; Strupp, B. Developmental potential in the first 5 years for children in developing countries. *Lancet* **2007**, *369*, 60–70. [CrossRef]

25. DeBoer, M.D.; Lima, A.A.M.; Oria, R.B.; Scharf, R.J.; Moore, S.R.; Luna, M.A.; Guerrant, R.L. Early childhood growth failure and the developmental origins of adult disease: Do enteric infections and malnutrition increase risk for the metabolic syndrome? *Nutr. Rev.* **2012**, *70*, 642–653. [CrossRef] [PubMed]

26. Orr, J.B. Influence of amount of milk consumption on the rate of growth of school children. *Br. Med. J.* **1928**, *1*, 140–141. [CrossRef] [PubMed]

27. Chen, S.T. Impact of a school milk programme on the nutritional status of school children. *Asia Pac. J. Public Health* **1989**, *3*, 19–25. [CrossRef] [PubMed]

28. De Beer, H. Dairy products and physical stature: A systematic review and meta-analysis of controlled trials. *Econ. Hum. Biol.* **2012**, *10*, 299–309. [CrossRef] [PubMed]

29. Semba, R.D.; Moench-Pfanner, R.; Sun, K.; de Pee, S.; Akhter, N.; Rah, J.H.; Campbell, A.A.; Badham, J.; Bloem, M.W.; Kraemer, K. Consumption of micronutrient-fortified milk and noodles is associated with lower risk of stunting in preschool-aged children in Indonesia. *Food Nutr. Bull.* **2011**, *32*, 347–353. [CrossRef] [PubMed]

30. Semba, R.D.; Shardell, M.; Sakr Ashour, F.A.; Moaddel, R.; Trehan, I.; Maleta, K.M.; Ordiz, M.I.; Kraemer, K.; Khadeer, M.A.; Ferrucci, L.; et al. Child stunting is associated with low circulating essential amino acids. *EBioMedicine* **2016**, *6*, 246–252. [CrossRef] [PubMed]

31. Laplante, M.; Sabatini, D.M. mTOR signalling in growth control and disease. *Cell* **2012**, *149*, 274–293. [CrossRef] [PubMed]

32. Darapheak, C.; Takano, T.; Kizuki, M.; Nakamura, K.; Seino, K. Consumption of animal source foods and dietary diversity reduce stunting in children in Cambodia. *Int. Arch. Med.* **2013**, *6*, 29. [CrossRef] [PubMed]

33. Muslimatun, S.; Wiradnyani, L.A.A. Dietary diversity, animal source food consumption and linear growth among children aged 1–5 years in Bandung, Indonesia: A longitudinal observational study. *Br. J. Nutr.* **2016**, *116*, S27–S35. [CrossRef] [PubMed]

34. Louie, J.C.Y.; Flood, V.M.; Hector, D.J.; Rangan, A.M.; Gill, T.P. Dairy consumption and overweight and obesity: A systematic review of prospective cohort studies. *Obes. Rev.* **2011**, *12*, e582–e592. [CrossRef] [PubMed]

35. Maillot, M.; Rehm, C.D.; Vieux, F.; Rose, C.M.; Drewnowski, A. Beverage consumption patterns among 4–19 y old children in 2009-14 NHANES show that the milk and 100% juice pattern is associated with better diets. *Nutr. J.* **2018**, *17*, 54. [CrossRef] [PubMed]

36. Khor, G.L.; Chee, W.S.S.; Shariff, Z.M.; Poh, B.K.; Arumugam, M.; Rahman, J.A.; Theobald, H.E. High prevalence of vitamin D insufficiency and its association with BMI-for-age among primary school children in Kuala Lumpur, Malaysia. *BMC Public Health* **2011**, *11*, 95. [CrossRef] [PubMed]

37. Palacios, C.; Gonzalez, L. Is vitamin D deficiency a major global public health problem? *J. Steroid Biochem. Mol. Biol.* **2014**, *144*, 138–145. [CrossRef] [PubMed]

38. Al-Daghri, N.M.; Aljohani, N.; Al-Attas, O.S.; Krishnaswamy, S.; Alfawaz, H.; Al-Ajlan, A.; Alokail, M.S. Dairy products consumption and serum 25-hydroxyvitamin D level in Saudi children and adults. *Int. J. Clin. Exp. Pathol.* **2015**, *8*, 8480–8486. [PubMed]

39. Lien, D.T.K.; Nhung, B.T.; Khan, N.C.; Hop, L.T.; Nga, N.T.Q.; Hung, N.T.; Kiers, J.; Shigeru, Y.; te Biesebeke, R. Impact of milk consumption on performance and health of primary school children in rural Vietnam. *Asia Pac. J. Clin. Nutr.* **2009**, *18*, 326–334.

40. Lomer, M.C.E.; Parkes, G.C.; Sanderson, J.D. Review article: Lactose intolerance in clinical practice—Myths and realities. *Aliment. Pharm. Therap.* **2008**, *27*, 93–103. [CrossRef] [PubMed]

41. Allen, L.H. How common is vitamin B-12 deficiency. *Am. J. Clin. Nutr.* **2009**, *89*, 693S–696S. [CrossRef] [PubMed]

42. Akhtar, S. Zinc status in South Asian population—An update. *J. Health Popul. Nutr.* **2013**, *31*, 139–149. [CrossRef] [PubMed]

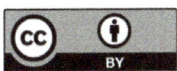

MDPI

Article

Bovine Lactoferrin Modulates Dendritic Cell Differentiation and Function

Olaf Perdijk [1], R. J. Joost van Neerven [1,2], Erik van den Brink [1], Huub F. J. Savelkoul [1] and Sylvia Brugman [1,*]

[1] Cell Biology and Immunology Group, Wageningen University, P.O. Box 338, 6708 WD Wageningen, The Netherlands; olaf.perdijk@wur.nl (O.P.); joost.vanneerven@wur.nl (R.J.v.N.); erik.vandenbrink@wur.nl (E.v.d.B.); huub.savelkoul@wur.nl (H.F.J.S.)

[2] FrieslandCampina, P.O. Box 1551, 3800 BN Amersfoort, The Netherlands

* Correspondence: sylvia.brugman@wur.nl; Tel.: +31-3178-2729

Received: 16 May 2018; Accepted: 26 June 2018; Published: 29 June 2018

Abstract: Lactoferrin is an abundant glycoprotein in bovine milk that has immunomodulatory effects on human cells. Bovine lactoferrin (LF) binds lipopolysaccharides (LPS) with high affinity and is postulated to act via TLR4-dependent and -independent mechanisms. It has been shown that LF modulates differentiation of human monocytes into tolerogenic dendritic cells. However, in a previous study, we showed that LPS also mediates differentiation into tolerogenic dendritic cells (DC). Since LF binds LPS with high affinity, it remains to be investigated whether LF or LPS is mediating these effects. We, therefore, further investigated the LPS-independent effect of LF on differentiation of human monocytes into dendritic cells (DC). Human monocytes were isolated by magnetic cell sorting from freshly isolated PBMCs and cultured for six days in the presence of IL-4 and GM-CSF with or without LF or proteinase K treated LF to generate DC. These immature DC were stimulated for 48 h with LPS or Poly I:C + R848. Cell surface marker expression and cytokine production were measured by flow cytometry. DC differentiated in the presence of LF produced higher IL-6 and IL-8 levels during differentiation and showed a lower expression of CD1a and HLA-DR. These LFDCs showed to be hyporesponsive towards TLR ligands as shown by their semi-mature phenotype and reduced cytokine production. The effect of LF was abrogated by proteinase K treatment, showing that the functional effects of LF were not mediated by LPS contamination. Thus, LF alters DC differentiation and dampens responsiveness towards TLR ligands. This study indicates that LF can play a role in immune homeostasis in the human GI tract.

Keywords: bovine lactoferrin; moDC; DC differentiation; semi-mature phenotype; hyporesponsive; LPS

1. Introduction

Bovine lactoferrin (LF) is an abundant glycoprotein in cow's milk that is 69% identical to human lactoferrin at the protein level [1]. LF is an extensively researched protein that has been shown to exert antimicrobial and antiviral activity [2]. The involved anti-pathogenic mechanisms, which are mostly investigated in vitro, range from depriving iron, antimicrobial activity by bioactive peptides and decoy receptor activity. These mechanisms may underlie the protective effect against sepsis by LF supplementation in very low birth weight (VLBW) infants [3–7]. LF was shown to protect against sepsis in VLBW infants in either breast fed or formula fed, showing the need for additional supplementation [3]. Subsequent analysis of this study showed that LF inhibits the progression of invasive fungal infections [4], indicating immunomodulatory effects of LF. In line with these findings, LF was shown to induce the prevalence of regulatory T cells in VLBW infants [6]. Although these studies indicate an immunoregulatory role of LF in humans, little mechanistic evidence is available to date.

In infants, LF ends up in the intestine intact and is only partly hydrolysed into bioactive peptides with antibacterial activity [8]. Moreover, intact human lactoferrin was found in stool and urine of VLBW infants and resisted trypsin and chemotrypsin treatment in vitro [9]. LF was shown to largely resists gastric hydrolysis in vivo in adults [10]. However, LF is completely degraded in the small intestine of adults [11]. Thus LF may, in contrast to adults, retain its bioactivity throughout the gastro-intestinal tract and may even become systemically available in infants [9,12,13]. This could be explained by lower concentrations of proteases in the small intestine in infants compared to adults [14]. Additionally, breast milk contains protease inhibitors, which may limit degradation of milk proteins in the GI tract of infants [15].

LF has specific domains that bind iron with high affinity, a high isoelectric point (pI around 9) and an overall nett positive charge with high cationic peptide regions, which is crucial for its bactericidal activity [16]. Due to these biochemical properties, LF may bind multiple receptors (e.g., intelectin-1 and DC-SIGN) with low affinity [1,17,18]. LF was shown to bind the human lactoferrin receptor (i.e., intelectin-1) on Caco-2 cells and, dependent on the concentration, induce proliferation or differentiation of these epithelial cells [19].

Additionally, LF is known for its binding activity to lipopolysaccharides (LPS). Binding of LF to LPS may result in neutralisation of LPS, which is hypothesized to play an important role in the immune regulatory role of LF [20]. In contrast, LF was shown to activate monocytes during DC differentiation, which resulted in diminished TLR activation [21]. Similarly, human LF was shown to induce the differentiation into anergic macrophages that were hyporesponsive towards TLR ligands [22]. However, LF binds LPS with a high binding affinity [23]. Since LPS induces differentiation of monocytes into tolerogenic DC as well [24], it is of interest to investigate the true immunomodulatory potential of LPS-free LF. A previous study showed that LPS-free LF induces the expression of pro-inflammatory cytokines on porcine derived macrophages in a TLR4-independent manner [25]. It is however unknown whether this TLR4-independent signaling of LF affects the functionality of human monocytes and dendritic cells. We therefore investigated whether LF, independently of bound LPS, is capable of inducing differentiation of human monocytes into tolerogenic dendritic cells.

2. Materials and Methods

2.1. Isolation of Bovine Lactoferrin

The whey fraction from bovine colostrum was collected after spinning the milk at 100,000 g for 45 min (Ultracentrifuge Avanti J301, Beckman Coulter, Brea, CA, USA). This casein and fat-free fraction was stored at $-20\,^{\circ}$C until further use. These whey proteins were thawed and diluted with washing buffer containing 0.01 M KH_2PO_4 and 0.1 M NaCl, pH 6.5. Samples were centrifuged at 23,500 g for 20 min and the supernatant was carefully collected through a filter paper to remove casein traces. Ion exchange chromatography (Akta Purifier, Pharmacia, Stockholm, Sweden) was used to isolate LF from the whey proteins. The Hiprep SP FF 16/10 column was preconditioned by rinsing the column with 100 mL washing buffer (3 mL/min; 12 mS/cm) and elution buffer (3 mL/min; 85 mS/cm). Whey proteins were loaded on the preconditioned column with a flow rate of 3 mL/min (HiLoad P50 pump, Pharmacia). After the complete volume of whey protein has run over the column, it was connected to the AKTA. Unbound matrix proteins were washed from the column with washing buffer (3 mL/min). Bovine lactoferrin was eluted from the column using an increasing gradient of 0.1–1 M NaCl. The preparation was desalted and concentrated on a 10 kDa Ultracel PLGC membrane using an Ultrafiltration Cell model 8200 (Amicon/Millipore).

2.2. Isolation and Culturing of Monocyte-Derived DC

Peripheral blood mononuclear cells (PBMCs) were isolated by density centrifugation from buffy coats obtained from healthy anonymous donors (Sanquin blood bank, Nijmegen, The Netherlands) as described previously [24]. A written informed consent was provided before blood collection. In short,

1:1 diluted blood in phosphate buffered saline (PBS) (Mg^{2+} and Ca^{2+} free, Lonza, BE17-516F, Basel, Switzerland) was loaded on Ficoll-Paque (Amersham Bioscience, Uppsala, Sweden) and centrifuged for 20 min at 500 g without brake. The PBMC layer was collected and washed three times with PBS. Cells were spun down and the pellet was resuspended with anti-human CD14 magnetic beads (BD Biosciences, 557769, Franklin Lakes, NJ, USA). CD14+ cells were isolated on a separation magnet (BD IMagnet, BD Biosciences) according to the manufacturer's instructions. 100,000 monocytes per well were cultured in 96 cells wells flat bottom plates in RPMI 1640 (Gibco, Carlsbad, CA, USA, 22409-015) and 10% FCS (Gibco, 10270-106), normocin (100 µg/mL, Invivogen, anti-nr-1, San Diego, CA, USA), penicillin and streptomycin (100 U/mL, Gibco, 14150-122). Monocytes were differentiated into dendritic cells by culturing them for six days in the presence of 20 ng/mL IL-4 (Peptrotech; 200-04, Rocky Hill, CT, USA) and GM-CSF (Peprotech; 300-03, Rocky Hill, CT, USA) with or without 10 µg/mL, 250 µg/mL bovine lactoferrin (FC) or 10 nM VitD3 (Sigma-Aldrich, D1530, St. Louis, MO, USA). After six days, immature DC were matured with 1 µg/mL LPS (*Escherichia coli*, Sigma, L2880, St. Louis, MO, USA) or 3 µg/mL R848 (Invivogen: tlrl-r848-5) and 20 µg/mL Poly I:C (Sigma, P1530) for 48 h.

2.3. Isolation and Staining of moDC

After 6 days (immature-) or 8 days (mature-) moDC were incubated on ice (while shaking) for 30 min in ice cold FACS buffer (PBS (Lonza, BE17,516F) containing 0.5% BSA fraction V (Roche, 10735086002, Basel, Switzerland), 2.0 mM EDTA (Merck, 108418, Kenalworth, NJ, USA) and 0.05 NaN_3) to facilitate the detachment of DC from the surface. Surface marker expression was analysed by using fluorochrome-conjugated antibodies directed against CD14 (FITC; BD Biosciences, 555397), CD86 (V450; BD Biosciences, 560357), CD83 (FITC; BD Biosciences, 556910), HLA-DR (APCef780; eBiosciences, 47-9956-42, San Diego, CA, USA), CD80 (PE-Cy5; BD Biosciences, 559370), PD-L1 (PE-Cy7; BD Biosciences, 558017), CD1a (PerCP/Cy5-5; Biolegend, 300130, San Diego, CA, USA). 10 µg/mL of human Fc Block (BD Bioscience, 554220) was added to the antibody mixture to block non-specific binding. Compensation beads (eBiosciences, 01-2222-41) stained with single antibodies were run for every experiment. Cells were washed with 200 µL FACS buffer and stained by incubating the antibody mixture for 30 min in the dark at 4 °C. Before measuring DRAQ7 (Abcam; ab109202, Cambridge, UK) was added and incubated for 10 min in the dark to stain nonviable cells. Cells were resuspended in 100 µL FACS buffer and acquired on a BD FACS Canto II (BD Biosciences) and analysed using the FlowJo software V10.

2.4. Quantification of Cytokine Levels in Supernatants

Levels of IL-8, IL-6, IL-10, TNF-α and IL-12p70 were measured in the supernatants of moDC cultures using cytometric bead array technique (BD Biosciences). Individual flex-sets for IL-8 (558277), IL-6 (558276), TNF-α (560112), IL-10 (558274) or IL-12p70 (558283) were run according to the manufacturer's instructions.

2.5. Proteinase K Treatment and SDS-Page

LF was treated with 100 µg/mL proteinase K for 1 h at 46 °C followed by 10 min on 95 °C to inactivate the enzyme activity. 1 µg of LF and proteinase K treated LF were loaded on a SDS-page gel (Mini-PROTEAN TGX Precast SDS-page gel, Biorad, Berkeley, CA, USA) and run on 120 V for 1 h. The gel was stained with GelCode (Thermo Scientific, 24590, Waltham, MA, USA) according to the manufacturer's instructions.

2.6. LPS Detection

LF and Triton X-114 treated LF was tested for LPS contamination by a recombinant factor C LAL assay that was performed according to the manufacturers recommendations (EndoZyme recombinant factor C assay, Hyglos; 609050, Bernried am Starnberger See, Germany).

2.7. Triton X-114 Treatment

LPS was removed from LF by an optimized Triton X-114 method (Amresco, cat. # M114, Solon, OH, USA) [26]. In short, 2% v/v Triton X-114 was added to the sample and the mixture was stirred for 30 min at 4 °C and thereafter transferred to a 41 °C water bath for 10 min. The micelles were spun down by centrifugation for 10 min at 20,000 g at 25 °C. The upper layer was collected and treated with 10 mg/mL Bio-beads SM-2 (cat. # 152-8920) under constant stirring at 4 °C to remove Triton X-114 traces.

2.8. TLR4 Reporter Assay

HEK-293 cells expressing human TLR4, CD14 and MD-2 and harbouring a pNIFTY construct (Invivogen, Toulouse, France) were grown on selective medium containing DMEM and Glutamax (Fisher Emergo, Landsmeer, The Netherlands) supplemented with 10% FCS, 100 µg/mL penicillin/streptomycin (Sigma, St. Louis, MO, USA), Zeozin (50 µg/mL), Normocin (100 µg/mL) and HygroGold (45 µg/mL) (Invitrogen, Carlsbad, CA, USA) in an atmosphere of 5% CO_2 at 37 °C. HEK-293 cells were seeded at 3×10^5 cells/mL and cultured overnight before stimulation the next day. NF-κB activation was measured after 24 h stimulation by adding Bright-Glo™ (Promega, Fitchburg, MA, USA) substrate to cells. The plate was shaken and luminescence was measured using a spectramax M5 (Molecular Devices, Sunnyvale, CA, USA).

2.9. Statistics

Data was assessed for normality using a D'Agistino and Pearson omnibus test. A repeated measures ANOVA with Tukey's multiple comparison test or Friedman test with Dunn's multiple comparison post-hoc test was performed for normal and non-normal distributed data, respectively. Data is represented as mean ± standard error of the mean (SEM). Graphpad Prism V. 5.0 was used for all statistical analyses.

3. Results

Monocytes were differentiated into monocyte-derived DC (moDC) in the presence or absence of LF. Upon differentiation into moDC, monocytes lost CD14 expression and gained CD1a expression. Although LFDC were negative for CD14, a lower percentage of cells gained CD1a expression (Figure 1A). LFDC showed a higher expression of CD86 and PD-L1 (Figure 1B,C) and a significantly lower expression of HLA-DR when differentiated in the presence of 250 µg/mL LF (Figure 1D). These phenotypical changes induced by LF during differentiation were accompanied by a dose-dependent increase in IL-8 production (Figure 1E) and increase in IL-6 production when cultured in the presence of 250 µg/mL LF (Figure 1F). Interestingly, in contrast to the profound effects of LF during the differentiation of monocytes into moDC, LF did not induce phenotypic changes on moDC that were already differentiated (Figure S1). Moreover, moDC stimulated with LF or LF + Poly I:C and R848 for two days did not show phenotypic changes compared to moDC or moDC + Poly I:C and R848, respectively.

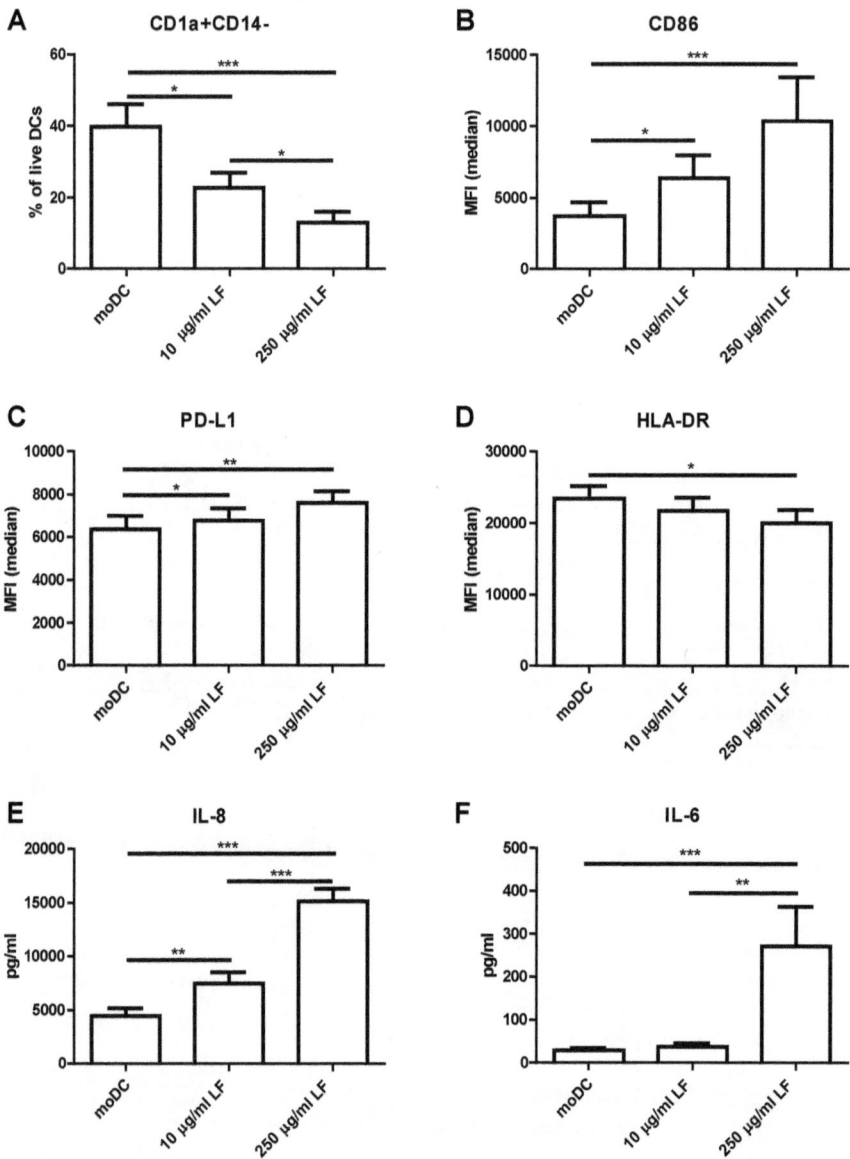

Figure 1. LF modulates DC differentiation. Monocytes were differentiated into moDC by culturing them for six days in the presence of IL-4 and GM-CSF with or without LF (10 or 250 μg/mL LF). (**A**) The percentage CD1a+CD14− DC and the median fluorescent intensity (MFI) of (**B**) CD86, (**C**) PD-L1 and (**D**) HLA-DR was shown. The production of (**E**) IL-8 and (**F**) IL-6 was measured in the supernatant by CBA. The mean ± SEM of four independent experiments with 12 different donors was shown. Significance is indicated by *** = $p < 0.001$, ** = $p < 0.01$ and * = $p < 0.05$.

Next, we investigated the responsiveness of LFDC by stimulating the cells with LPS. LFDC showed to be hyporesponsive towards LPS as observed by the reduced induction of the maturation marker CD83 (Figure 2A) and costimulatory molecules CD86 (Figure 2B), PD-L1 (Figure 2C) and

CD80 (Figure S2A) upon LPS stimulation. HLA-DR expression was lower on mature LFDC compared to mature moDC (Figure 2D). In line with their phenotype, LFDC also produced lower cytokine levels, showing a lower production of IL-10 (Figure 2E), IL-6 (Figure S2B), TNF (Figure S2C) and abrogated levels of IL-12p70 (Figure 2F). Since DC were differentiated and subsequently stimulated in the presence of LF, we wanted to exclude the possibly that the hyporesponsiveness towards LPS was caused by neutralisation of LPS by LF. We showed that the surface marker expression was unaffected by replacing $\frac{3}{4}$ of the medium and that the cells were also hyporesponsive towards R848 and Poly:IC stimulation, indicating that the effect was not mediated by LPS neutralisation (Figure S3).

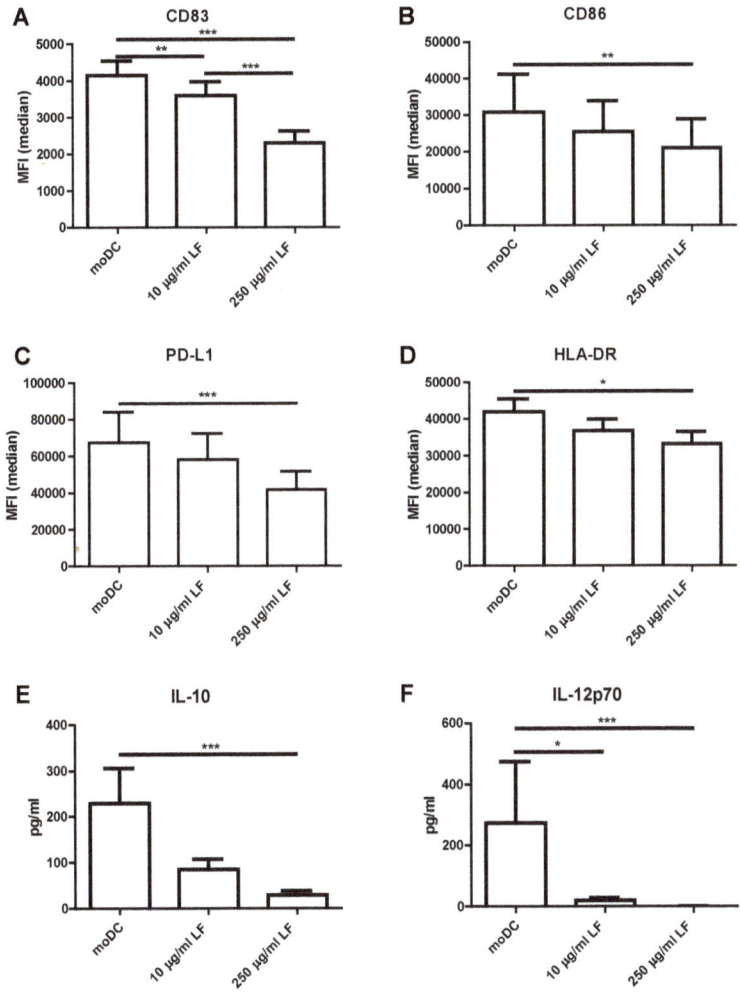

Figure 2. LFDC are hyporesponsive for LPS stimulation. Immature DC that were cultured in the presence or absence of LF were stimulated with 1 µg/mL LPS for 48 h. (**A**) The median fluorescent intensity (MFI) of (**A**) CD83, (**B**) CD86, (**C**) PD-L1 and (**D**) HLA-DR was shown. The production of (**E**) IL-10 and (**F**) IL-12p70 was measured in the supernatant by CBA. The mean ± SEM of four independent experiments with 12 different donors was shown. Significance is indicated by *** = $p < 0.001$, ** = $p < 0.01$ and * = $p < 0.05$.

LF is reported to bind LPS and has been postulated to induce immunomodulation via TLR4-dependent mechanisms. However, previously we showed that low concentrations of LPS can also LPS induce these phenotypic changes. We therefore measured the concentration of LPS in LF by an endozyme LAL assay. LF used in this study showed concentrations of 2.6 EU LPS/mg LF (Figure S4A). We therefore applied an optimized Triton X-114 method [26] to reduce LPS levels. This method reduced the endotoxin levels to 0.58 EU LPS/mg LF (Figure S4A). Despite this five-fold decrease in LPS levels, the immunomodulatory activity of LF remained the same (Figure S4). Nevertheless, we have previously shown that low concentrations of LPS induce endotoxin tolerance [24]. We therefore wanted to be absolutely certain that the functional effects of LF were not mediated by LPS. Therefore, we treated LF with proteinase K to degrade the protein and release any potentially bound endotoxins. We confirmed that LF was completely degraded after proteinase K treatment as observed on SDS-page gel (Figure S5A), Additionally, we showed by using a TLR4 reporter assay that the NF-κB inducing capacity of LPS was unaltered by proteinase K treatment (Figure S5B), indicating that the LPS released from bound to LF remains functional. Interestingly, the dose-dependent increase of CD86 (Figure 3A) and PD-L1 (Figure S6B) and decreased CD1a (Figure 3B) expression induced by LF was reduced to moDC levels after proteinase K treatment. Similarly, the LF induced production of IL-6 (Figure 3C) and IL-8 (Figure S6A) during DC differentiation was abrogated after degradation of the protein. Thus, the LF-induced phenotype on immature DC was completely abolished by proteinase K treatment of the protein, showing that the effect is mediated by LF and not by LPS. In line with these findings, the responsiveness towards LPS of LFDC was completely restored to that of moDC upon proteinase K treatment as shown by the expression of CD86 (Figure 3D), CD83 (Figure 3E), CD80 and PD-L1 (Figure S7A,B) and the production of cytokines such as IL-6 (Figure 3F), IL-12p70, TNF and IL-10 (Figure S7D–F).

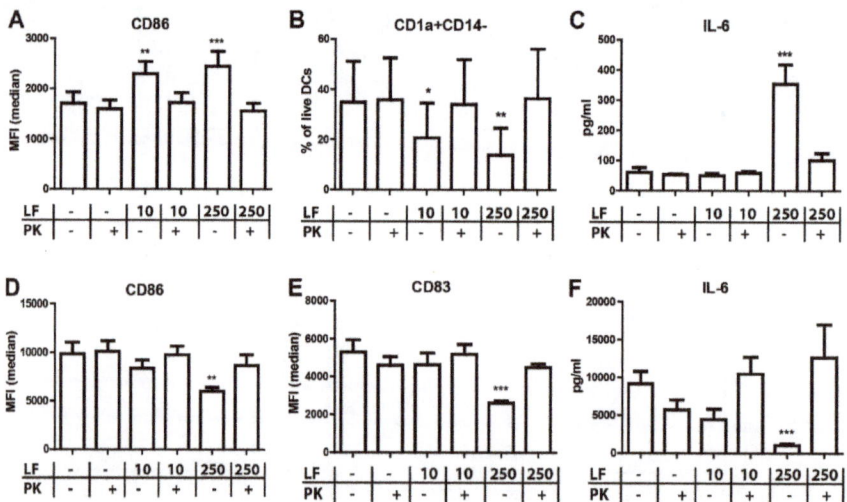

Figure 3. Proteinase K treatment of LF restores responsiveness towards LPS. (**A–C**) monocytes were cultured in the presence of IL-4 and GM-CSF with or without LF or proteinase K treated LF. (**D,E**) These immature DC were subsequently stimulated with 1 µg/mL LPS for 48 h. The median fluorescent intensity (MFI) of (**A,D**) CD86 and (**E**) CD83 and (**B**) the percentage CD1a+CD14− DC was shown. (**C,F**) The production IL-6 was measured in the supernatant by CBA. The mean ± SEM of 3 different donors was shown. Significance is indicated by *** = $p < 0.001$, ** = $p < 0.01$ and * = $p < 0.05$.

4. Discussion

In this paper, we show that LF modulates human DC differentiation and function. Additionally, we show that its immunomodulatory capacity is not mediated by LPS. With this study, we confirm and expand on the study of Puddu et al. (2011), that showed that LF is capable of inducing differentiation into tolerogenic DC [21]. Since trace amounts of LPS can already induce a tolerogenic phenotype [24], it is necessary to assess that LF and not LPS is responsible for the effect. Here, we show that LF alters the differentiation of monocytes into DC, resulting in a phenotypical distinct DC type which is hyporesponsive towards several TLR ligands.

It has been proposed that the GI tract is in a constant state of low-grade inflammation or "primed homeostasis" due to the constant exposure to commensal bacteria and microbial products in which monocytes are recruited toward the GI tract [27,28]. In line with this thought, a local micro-environment comprised of dietary and microbial factors may steer monocyte differentiation. We therefore investigated the effect of LF on monocyte differentiation into DC. It is well established that monocytes lose CD14 expression and gain CD1a expression during differentiation into moDC. In the presence of LF, DC lose CD14 expression and gain less CD1a expression compared to conventional differentiated moDC. CD1a is an important functional marker for immature DC. Moreover, CD1a+ DC produce higher IL-12p70 levels and lower IL-10 levels upon stimulation and show a lower internalisation capacity compared to CD1a-DC [29,30]. Potential explanations for the reduced CD1a expression on LFDC can be induction of PPARγ activity [30], differentiation into more macrophage-like cells due to IL-6-mediated autocrine M-CSF production [31], or inhibition of GM-CSF signalling [32]. Interestingly, an embryonic fibroblast cell line transfected with the human lactoferrin gene showed inhibited GM-CSF levels upon stimulation [33]. LF is, in contrast to moDC, internalised into the nucleus of human monocytes [21]. This finding makes it appealing to speculate about direct effect of internalised LF on the GM-CSF promotor in monocytes. Additionally, LF induces the production of IL-6 and IL-8 within 24 h of differentiation (data not shown). Although IL-6 has been shown to be an important cytokine capable of modulating DC differentiation [18] and boosting autocrine G-CSF production [31], Puddu et al. (2011) showed that the effects of LF are not mediated by IL-6. In line with these findings we show that IL-6 production was not elevated if monocytes are differentiated in the presence of 10 μg/mL LF and yet this concentration is sufficient to induce DC that are hyporesponsive towards TLR ligands.

LFDC produced much lower cytokine levels and upregulated costimulatory molecules markers to a lesser extent compared to moDC upon contact with TLR ligands. Moreover, they showed a semi-mature (CD83int CD86int) phenotype, which is postulated to induce polarisation of naive T cells in regulatory T cells [34]. Thus, LF induces the differentiation of monocytes into more tolerogenic DC. In contrast to the effect of LF on monocytes, we show that LF does not induce phenotypical changes on human moDC nor modulate Poly I:C and R848-induced inflammation. These findings are in line with previous research, showing internalisation of LF into the nucleus of human monocytes and not in moDC [21]. Their findings propose that the uptake of LF is mediated by a receptor expressed on human monocytes that is not expressed on moDC, which could explain the distinct effect of LF on both cell types. LF binds to intelectin-1 (i.e., intestinal lactoferrin receptor), which is expressed on epithelial cells [19]. To date, no evidence suggests expression of intelectin-1 on myeloid cells. LF also binds DC-SIGN which is expressed on monocytes and moDC [18]. However, the observed effects are also not likely mediated via DC-SIGN since its expression increases upon differentiation into DC [35]. Additionally, it has been suggested that LF binds with low affinity to several other receptors (e.g., RAGE and MNR). Interestingly, human LF was also shown to bind to soluble CD14 [36]. Since CD14 expression is lost upon differentiation of monocyte into moDC, it is tempting to speculate that our phenotypic changes are induced via CD14. However, LF in concentration used in this study did not activate NF-κB on CD14-MD-2:TLR4 expressing HEK cells (data not shown). Recently, CD14 was shown to be essential for endocytosis of the TLR4 complex [37], showing that its function is more than just facilitating LPS to bind TLR4. We therefore hypothesize that LF:LPS complexes can be internalized on monocytes in a unknown CD14-mediated manner.

This study shows, in line with the literature, that bovine LF, as well as human LF, induces differentiation of monocytes into hyporesponsive DC [21] and macrophages [22], respectively. However, due to the high binding affinity of LF to LPS, it is essential to investigate whether LPS or LF is responsible for this tolerogenic phenotype. Importantly, we showed that our sample did contain traces of LPS as measured by a LAL assay. In this assay, a recombinant factor C protein is used to detect LPS, which binds the lipid A part of the molecule [38]. LF was also shown to bind the lipid A part of the molecule [23], which could shield LPS from binding TLR4 and apparently not factor C. According to the LPS contamination measured in our sample (i.e., 2.6 EU/mg), the concentrations of LF used in our study of 0.25 mg/mL and 0.01 mg/mL, thus, contain 0.65 EU and 0.026 EU, respectively. We have shown that LPS contamination of >0.5 EU induces the differentiation into tolerogenic DC [24]. The concentrations of LPS measured in LF in this study could, thus, theoretically explain the tolerogenic DC phenotype. Nevertheless, we demonstrated that the effects of LF are lost upon proteinase K treatment and that Triton X-114-treated LF shows the same immunomodulatory capacity compared to non-treated LF. We thereby exclude the possibility that effects of LF are mediated by endotoxin tolerance. This finding is in line with earlier research showing that the induced expression of pro-inflammatory genes in porcine macrophages is mediated in a TLR4-independent manner [25].

This study adds on to the current understanding of the role of LF in immune regulation. Additionally, LF is well-known for its anti-pathogenic activity. Hence, LF supplementation to infants and immunocompromised individuals has been studied to investigate its efficacy against inflammatory conditions. Moreover, several clinical studies in children have been conducted with LF, all showing no adverse effects of LF supplementation [39]. LF supplementation to breast milk or infant formulas has been shown to reduce the incidence of sepsis VLWB infants [3–7]. These VLWB infants often suffer from excessive gut inflammation and have an impaired epithelial barrier functioning, which may result in necrotizing enterocolitis [40]. Additionally, several studies show that LF fortification to early life nutrition may alleviate symptoms of viral infections [41–44]. Moreover, LF supplementation to children <5 years of age and to infants in the first year of life showed a reduction of the incidence of rotaviral gastroenteritis [41] and lower respiratory tract infections [42]. Similarly, LF supplementation to infant nutrition resulted in a lower incidence of symptoms of respiratory illness (e.g., running nose, coughing, wheezing) compared to infants receiving non-fortified formula [43]. LF supplementation has also been investigated for its additive effect in HIV therapy in children by measuring several immune parameters and viral titers. Interestingly, phagocytic activity, CD14/TLR2 expression and IL-12p70/IL-10 ratio in CD14+ was increased in children receiving LF supplementation [44]. Thus, apart from functioning as a direct anti-pathogenic protein, LF may inhibit infections by its immunomodulatory capacity. Since, LF is poorly digested in the GI tract of infants and a fraction of the protein is taken up intact and reaches the circulation [9,12,13], it may impact the functionality of monocytes and DC in vivo. Larger cohorts should validate the protective effect of LF supplementation against viral infections and sepsis and investigate its immunomodulatory potential in vivo.

5. Conclusions

Taken together, our results show that LF inhibits DC differentiation which hampers their responsiveness towards TLR ligands. Additionally, we showed that these effects are diminished after degrading the protein, formally showing that the LF-induced differentiation of monocytes into hyporesponsive DC is not mediated by endotoxin tolerance. This study indicates that LF may promote immune homeostasis in the gastrointestinal tract.

Supplementary Materials: The following are available online at http://www.mdpi.com/2072-6643/10/7/848/s1. Figure S1: LF does not modulate immature DC activation. Monocytes were differentiated into moDC by culturing them for six days in the presence of IL-4 and GM-CSF. These immature DC were stimulated with 20 µg/mL Poly I:C and 3 µg/mL R848 in the presence or absence of LF. The median fluorescent intensity (MFI) of (A)

Nutrients **2018**, *10*, 848

CD8, (B) CD86, (D) HLA-DR, (E) PD-L1, (F) CD80 and the percentage of CD83 + CD86 + DC was shown. The expression of three individual donors with mean and standard deviation was shown in a scatter plot. Figure S2: LFDC are hyporesponsive for LPS stimulation. Immature DC that were cultured in the presence or absence of LF were stimulated with 1 μg/mL LPS for 48 h. (A) The median fluorescent intensity (MFI) of (A) CD80 was shown. The production of (B) IL-6 and (C) TNF was measured in the supernatant by CBA. The mean ± SEM of four independent experiments with 12 different donors was shown. Significance is indicated by *** = $p < 0.001$, ** = $p < 0.01$ and * = $p < 0.05$. Figure S3: hyporesponsiveness of LFDC is not mediated by decoy activity. Immature DC that were cultured in the presence or absence of LF were stimulated with 1 μg/mL LPS (A)without or (B) with replacing $\frac{3}{4}$ of the medium or (C) 20 μg/mL Poly I:C and 3 μg/mL R848 for 48 h. (A) The median fluorescent intensity (MFI) of (A) CD80 was shown. The mean ± SEM 3 different donors was shown. Figure S4: DC modulatory activity of LF is not reduced by Triton X-114 treatment. (A) an Endozyme LAL assay was used to detect LPS in LF before or after applying an optimised Triton X-114 method. Immature DC were cultured in the presence or absence of Triton X-114 treated or non-treated LF. (A) The percentage CD1a+ CD14− DC was shown on immature DC. These immature DC were stimulated with 1 μg/mL LPS for 48 h. Median fluorescent intensity (MFI) of (C) CD83 and (D) CD86 was shown. The production of (E) IL-10 and (F) IL-12p70 was measured in the supernatant by CBA. The mean ± SEM of 3 different donors was shown. Significance is indicated by *** = $p < 0.001$, ** = $p < 0.01$ and * = $p < 0.05$. Figure S5: Proteinase K treatment does not affect NF-κB activation via TLR4 by LPS. (A) 1 μg/mL LF was loaded before and after proteinase K treatment on SDS-PAGE gel. (B) LPS, proteinase K treated LPS and heated LPS was tested for its NF-κB activation in a TLR4 reporter assay. Figure S6: proteinase K treatment of LF abrogates its effect on DC differentiation. Monocytes were cultured in the presence of IL-4 and GM-CSF with or without LF or proteinase K treated LF. (A) The production of IL-8 was measured in the supernatant by CBA. The median fluorescent intensity (MFI) of (B) PD-L1 and (C) HLA-DR was shown. The mean ± SEM of 3 different donors was shown. Figure S7: proteinase K treatment of LF restores responsiveness towards LPS. Monocytes were cultured in the presence of IL-4 and GM-CSF with or without LF or proteinase K treated LF for six days and subsequently stimulated with 1 μg/mL LPS for 48 h. The median fluorescent intensity (MFI) of (A) CD80, (B) PD-L1 and (C) HLA-DR was shown. The production of (D) TNF, (E) IL-10 and (F) IL-12p70 was measured in the supernatant by CBA. The mean ± SEM of 3 different donors was shown. Significance is indicated by *** = $p < 0.001$, ** = $p < 0.01$ and * = $p < 0.05$.

Author Contributions: O.P. and E.v.d.B. conducted and designed the experiments; O.P. analyzed the data; O.P., R.J.J.v.N., S.B. and H.F.J.S. contributed to interpretation of the results and writing process of the paper. All authors approve the final version of the paper.

Funding: This work was supported by the Netherlands Organization of Scientific Research (NWO) as part of the technology foundation STW (project number 13017).

Acknowledgments: The authors would like to thank Wim Mengerink and Evelien Kramer for isolation of bovine lactoferrin.

Conflicts of Interest: R.J.J.v.N. is an employee of FrieslandCampina.

References

1. Liao, Y.; Jiang, R.; Lonnerdal, B. Biochemical and molecular impacts of lactoferrin on small intestinal growth and development during early life. *Biochem. Cell Biol.* **2012**, *90*, 476–484. [CrossRef] [PubMed]
2. Brock, J.H. Lactoferrin—50 years on. *Biochem. Cell Biol.* **2012**, *90*, 245–251. [CrossRef] [PubMed]
3. Manzoni, P.; Rinaldi, M.; Cattani, S.; Pugni, L.; Romeo, M.G.; Messner, H. Bovine lacoferrin supplementation for prevention of late-onset sepsis in very low-birth-weight neonates. *J. Am. Med. Assoc.* **2009**, *302*, 1421–1428. [CrossRef] [PubMed]
4. Manzoni, P.; Stolfi, I.; Messner, H.; Cattani, S.; Laforgia, N.; Romeo, M.G.; Bollani, L.; Rinaldi, M.; Gallo, E.; Quercia, M.; et al. Bovine lactoferrin prevents invasive fungal infections in very low birth weight infants: A randomized controlled trial. *Pediatrics* **2011**. [CrossRef] [PubMed]
5. Ochoa, T.J.; Zegarra, J.; Cam, L.; Llanos, R.; Pezo, A.; Cruz, K.; Zea-Vera, A.; Cárcamo, C.; Campos, M.; Bellomo, S. Randomized Controlled Trial of Lactoferrin for Prevention of Sepsis in Peruvian Neonates Less than 2500 g. *Pediatr. Infect. Dis. J.* **2015**, *34*, 571–576. [CrossRef] [PubMed]
6. Akin, I.M.; Atasay, B.; Dogu, F.; Okulu, E.; Arsan, S.; Karatas, H.D.; Ikinciogullari, A.; Turmen, T. Oral lactoferrin to prevent nosocomial sepsis and necrotizing enterocolitis of premature neonates and effect on T-regulatory cells. *Am. J. Perinatol.* **2014**, *31*, 1111–1120. [CrossRef] [PubMed]
7. Manzoni, P.; Meyer, M.; Stolfi, I.; Rinaldi, M.; Cattani, S.; Pugni, L.; Romeo, M.G.; Messner, H.; Decembrino, L.; Laforgia, N.; et al. Bovine lactoferrin supplementation for prevention of necrotizing enterocolitis in very-low-birth-weight neonates: A randomized clinical trial. *Early Hum. Dev.* **2014**, *90*, S60–S65. [CrossRef]

8. Bellamy, W.; Takase, M.; Wakabayashi, H.; Kawase, K.; Tomita, M. Antibacterial spectrum of lactoferricin B, a potent bactericidal peptide derived from the *N*-terminal region of bovine lactoferrin. *J. Appl. Bacteriol.* **1992**, *73*, 472–479. [CrossRef] [PubMed]

9. Goldman, A.S.; Garza, C.; Schanler, R.J.; Goldblum, R.M. Molecular forms of lactoferrin in stool and urine from infants fed human milk. *Pediatr. Res.* **1990**, *27*, 252–255. [CrossRef] [PubMed]

10. Troost, F.J.; Steins, J.; Saris, W.H.M.; Brummer, R.-J.M. Gastric Digestion of Bovine Lactoferrin In Vivo in Adults. *J. Nutr.* **2001**, *131*, 2101–2104. [CrossRef] [PubMed]

11. Troost, F.J.; Saris, W.H.M.; Brummer, R.-J.M. Orally ingested human lactoferrin is digested and secreted in the upper gastrointestinal tract in vivo in women with ileostomies. *J. Nutr.* **2002**, *132*, 2597–2600. [CrossRef] [PubMed]

12. Kitagawa, H.; Yoshizawa, Y.; Yokoyama, T.; Takeuchi, T.; Talukder, M.J.R.; Shimizu, H.; Ando, K.; Harada, E. Persorption of bovine lactoferrin from the intestinal lumen into the systemic circulation via the portal vein and the mesenteric lymphatics in growing pigs. *J. Vet. Med. Sci.* **2003**, *65*, 567–572. [CrossRef] [PubMed]

13. Fischer, R.; Debbabi, H.; Blais, A.; Dubarry, M.; Rautureau, M.; Boyaka, P.N.; Tome, D. Uptake of ingested bovine lactoferrin and its accumulation in adult mouse tissues. *Int. Immunopharmacol.* **2007**, *7*, 1387–1393. [CrossRef] [PubMed]

14. Dallas, D.C.; Underwood, M.A.; Zivkovic, A.M.; German, J.B. Digestion of Protein in Premature and Term Infants. *J. Nutr. Disord. Ther.* **2012**, *2*, 112. [CrossRef] [PubMed]

15. Lindberg, T.; Ohlsson, K.; Weström, B. Protease inhibitors and their relation to protease activity in human-milk. *Pediatr. Res.* **1982**, *16*, 479–483. [CrossRef] [PubMed]

16. Steijns, J.M.; van Hooijdonk, A.C.M. Occurrence, structure, biochemical properties and technological characteristics of lactoferrin. *Br. J. Nutr.* **2000**, *84*, 11–17. [CrossRef]

17. Suzuki, Y.A.; Lopez, V.; Lönnerdal, B. Mammalian lactoferrin receptors: Structure and function. *Cell. Mol. Life Sci.* **2005**, *62*, 2560–2575. [CrossRef] [PubMed]

18. Groot, F.; Geijtenbeek, T. Lactoferrin prevents dendritic cell-mediated human immunodeficiency virus type 1 transmission by blocking the DC-SIGN-gp120 interaction. *J. Virol.* **2005**, *79*, 3009–3015. [CrossRef] [PubMed]

19. Lönnerdal, B.; Jiang, R.; Du, X. Bovine lactoferrin can be taken up by the human intestinal lactoferrin receptor and exert bioactivities. *J. Pediatr. Gastroenterol. Nutr.* **2011**, *53*, 606–614. [CrossRef] [PubMed]

20. Puddu, P.; Latorre, D.; Valenti, P.; Gessani, S. Immunoregulatory role of lactoferrin-lipopolysaccharide interactions. *BioMetals* **2010**, *23*, 387–397. [CrossRef] [PubMed]

21. Puddu, P.; Latorre, D.; Carollo, M.; Catizone, A.; Ricci, G.; Valenti, P.; Gessani, S. Bovine lactoferrin counteracts Toll-Like receptor mediated activation signals in antigen presenting cells. *PLoS ONE* **2011**, *6*, e22504. [CrossRef] [PubMed]

22. Wisgrill, L.; Wessely, I.; Spittler, A.; Förster-Waldl, E.; Berger, A.; Sadeghi, K. Human lactoferrin attenuates the proinflammatory response of neonatal monocyte-derived macrophages. *Clin. Exp. Immunol.* **2018**, 315–324. [CrossRef] [PubMed]

23. Elass-Rochard, E.; Roseanu, A.; Legrand, D.; Trif, M.; Salmon, V.; Motas, C.; Montreuil, J.; Spik, G. Lactoferrin-lipopolysaccharide interaction: Involvement of the 28–34 loop region of human lactoferrin in the high-affinity binding to Escherichia coli 055B5 lipopolysaccharide. *Biochem. J.* **1995**, *312*, 839–845. [CrossRef] [PubMed]

24. Perdijk, O.; van Neerven, R.J.J.; Meijer, B.; Savelkoul, H.F.J.; Brugman, S. Induction of human tolerogenic dendritic cells by 3'-sialyllactose via TLR4 is explained by LPS contamination. *Glycobiology* **2018**, *28*, 126–130. [CrossRef] [PubMed]

25. Zemankova, N.; Chlebova, K.; Matiasovic, J.; Prodelalova, J.; Gebauer, J.; Faldyna, M. Bovine lactoferrin free of lipopolysaccharide can induce a proinflammatory response of macrophages. *BMC Vet. Res.* **2016**, *12*, 251. [CrossRef] [PubMed]

26. Teodorowicz, M.; Perdijk, O.; Verhoek, I.; Govers, C.; Savelkoul, H.F.J.; Tang, Y.; Wichers, H.; Broersen, K. Optimized Triton X-114 assisted lipopolysaccharide (LPS) removal method reveals the immunomodulatory effect of food proteins. *PLoS ONE* **2017**, *12*, e0173778. [CrossRef] [PubMed]

27. Ginhoux, F.; Jung, S. Monocytes and macrophages: Developmental pathways and tissue homeostasis. *Nat. Rev. Immunol.* **2014**, *14*, 392–404. [CrossRef] [PubMed]

28. Bain, C.C.; Mowat, A.M.I. The monocyte-macrophage axis in the intestine. *Cell. Immunol.* **2014**, *291*, 41–48. [CrossRef] [PubMed]

29. Cernadas, M.; Lu, J.; Watts, G.; Brenner, M.B. CD1a expression defines an interleukin-12 producing population of human dendritic cells. *Clin. Exp. Immunol.* **2009**, *155*, 523–533. [CrossRef] [PubMed]

30. Gogolak, P.; Rethi, B.; Szatmari, I.; Lanyi, A.; Dezso, B.; Nagy, L.; Rajnavolgyi, E. Differentiation of CD1a⁻ and CD1a⁺ monocyte-derived dendritic cells is biased by lipid environment and PPARγ. *Blood* **2007**, *109*, 643–652. [CrossRef] [PubMed]

31. Chomarat, P.; Banchereau, J.; Davoust, J.; Karolina Palucka, A. IL-6 switches the differentiation of monocytes from dendritic cells to macrophages. *Nat. Immunol.* **2000**, *1*, 510–514. [CrossRef] [PubMed]

32. Roy, K.C.; Bandyopadhyay, G.; Rakshit, S.; Ray, M.; Bandyopadhyay, S. IL-4 alone without the involvement of GM-CSF transforms human peripheral blood monocytes to a CD1a^{dim}, CD83⁺ myeloid dendritic cell subset. *J. Cell Sci.* **2004**, *117*, 3435–3445. [CrossRef] [PubMed]

33. Penco, S.; Pastorino, S.; Bianchi-Scarrà, G.; Garrè, C. Lactoferrin down-modulates the activity of the granulocyte macrophage colony-stimulating factor promoter in interleukin-1 beta-stimulated cells. *J. Biol. Chem.* **1995**, *270*, 12263–12268. [CrossRef] [PubMed]

34. Nikolic, T.; Roep, B.O. Regulatory multitasking of tolerogenic dendritic cells—Lessons taken from vitamin D3-treated tolerogenic dendritic cells. *Front. Immunol.* **2013**, *4*. [CrossRef] [PubMed]

35. Relloso, M.; Puig-Kroger, A.; Pello, O.M.; Rodriguez-Fernandez, J.L.; de la Rosa, G.; Longo, N.; Navarro, J.; Munoz-Fernandez, M.A.; Sanchez-Mateos, P.; Corbi, A.L. DC-SIGN (CD209) expression is IL-4 dependent and is negatively regulated by IFN, TGF-β, and anti-inflammatory agents. *J. Immunol.* **2002**, *168*, 2634–2643. [CrossRef] [PubMed]

36. Baveye, S.; Elass, E.; Fernig, D.G.; Blanquart, C.; Mazurier, J.; Legrand, D. Human lactoferrin interacts with soluble CD14 and inhibits expression of endothelial adhesion molecules, E-selectin and ICAM-1, induced by the CD14-lipopolysaccharide complex. *Infect. Immun.* **2000**, *68*, 6519–6525. [CrossRef] [PubMed]

37. Zanoni, I.; Ostuni, R.; Marek, L.R.; Barresi, S.; Barbalat, R.; Barton, G.M.; Granucci, F.; Kagan, J.C. CD14 Controls the LPS-Induced Endocytosis of Toll-like Receptor 4. *Cell* **2011**, *147*, 868–880. [CrossRef] [PubMed]

38. Koshiba, T.; Hashii, T.; Kawabata, S.I. A structural perspective on the interaction between lipopolysaccharide and factor C, a receptor involved in recognition of gram-negative bacteria. *J. Biol. Chem.* **2007**, *282*, 3962–3967. [CrossRef] [PubMed]

39. Ochoa, T.J.; Pezo, A.; Cruz, K.; Chea-Woo, E.; Cleary, T.G. Clinical studies of lactoferrin in children. *Biochem. Cell Biol.* **2012**, *90*, 457–467. [CrossRef] [PubMed]

40. Neu, J.; Walker, A.W. Necrotizing enterocolitis. *N. Engl. J. Med.* **2011**, *110*, 255–264. [CrossRef] [PubMed]

41. Egashira, M.; Takayanagi, T.; Moriuchi, M.; Moriuchi, H. Does daily intake of bovine lactoferrin-containing products ameliorate rotaviral gastroenteritis? *Acta Paediatr. Int. J. Paediatr.* **2007**, *96*, 1242–1244. [CrossRef] [PubMed]

42. King, J.C., Jr.; Cummings, G.E.; Guo, N.; Trivedi, L.; Readmond, B.X.; Keane, V.; Feigelman, S.; De, W.R. A double-blind, placebo-controlled, pilot study of bovine lactoferrin supplementation in bottle-fed infants. *J. Pediatr. Gastroenterol. Nutr.* **2007**, *44*, 245–251. [CrossRef] [PubMed]

43. Chen, K.; Chai, L.; Li, H.; Zhang, Y.; Xie, H.M.; Shang, J.; Tian, W.; Yang, P.; Jiang, A.C. Effect of bovine lactoferrin from iron-fortified formulas on diarrhea and respiratory tract infections of weaned infants in a randomized controlled trial. *Nutrition* **2016**, *32*, 222–227. [CrossRef] [PubMed]

44. Zuccotti, G.V.; Vigano, A.; Borelli, M.; Saresella, M.; Giacomet, V.; Clerici, M. Modulation of innate and adaptive immunity by lactoferrin in human immunodeficiency virus (HIV)-infected, antiretroviral therapy-naïve children. *Int. J. Antimicrob. Agents* **2007**, *29*, 353–355. [CrossRef] [PubMed]

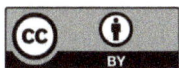

nutrients

MDPI

Article

Effect of Supplementation of a Whey Peptide Rich in Tryptophan-Tyrosine-Related Peptides on Cognitive Performance in Healthy Adults: A Randomized, Double-Blind, Placebo-Controlled Study

Masahiro Kita [1],*, Kuniaki Obara [1], Sumio Kondo [2], Satoshi Umeda [3] and Yasuhisa Ano [1]

[1]   Research Laboratories for Health Science & Food Technologies, Kirin Company, Ltd., Yokohama 1-13-5, Japan; k-obara@kirin.co.jp (K.O.); Yasuhisa_Ano@kirin.co.jp (Y.A.)
[2]   Kensyokai Medical Corporation, Osaka 2-12-16, Japan; s.kondo@drc-web.co.jp
[3]   Department of Psychology, Keio University, Tokyo 2-15-45, Japan; umeda@flet.keio.ac.jp
*   Correspondence: Masahiro_Kita@kirin.co.jp; Tel.: +81-45-330-9007

Received: 6 June 2018; Accepted: 11 July 2018; Published: 13 July 2018

Abstract: Background: Previous epidemiological and clinical studies have shown that dairy products have beneficial effects on cognitive decline and dementia. Enzymatic digestion of whey protein produces a whey peptide rich in tryptophan-tyrosine-related peptides which improve cognitive performance in mice. We evaluated the effects of whey peptides on cognitive functions in healthy adults in a randomized, double-blind, placebo-controlled design. **Methods:** 101 healthy adults (45 to 64 years), with a self-awareness of cognitive decline received either whey peptide or placebo supplements for 12 weeks. Changes in cognitive function were assessed using neuropsychological tests at 6 and 12 weeks after the start of supplementation. **Results:** Verbal fluency test (VFT) score changes tended to be higher in the whey peptide group compared with the placebo at 12 weeks. Subgroup analysis classified by the degree of subjective fatigue showed that changes in the VFT as well as the Stroop and subjective memory function tests between baseline and 6 weeks of intervention were significantly better in subjects with high-level fatigue from the whey peptide group as compared to the placebo group. Conclusions: Intake of whey peptide might improve cognitive function in healthy middle- and older-aged adults with high subjective fatigue levels. Further studies will elucidate the relationship among cognitive improvement, whey peptides, and psychological fatigue.

Keywords: dairy food; whey peptide; cognitive function

1. Introduction

With the rapid increase in the world's aging population, the number of people suffering with dementia and cognitive decline is rapidly increasing. The United Nations estimates that the number of people aged over 60 years will reach 1.4 billion by 2030, and 2.1 billion by 2050 [1]. The number of patients with dementia is estimated to reach 130 million by 2050 [2]. At present, there is no effective therapy for dementia, and thus preventive approaches are receiving increasing attention.

Recent epidemiological and clinical studies have suggested that consumption of dairy products, including yogurt and cheese, may reduce the risk of cognitive decline in later life [3]. A prospective cohort study surveyed more than 1000 Japanese subjects in a local community and showed that frequent intake of milk and dairy products is associated with a lower risk of cognitive decline and dementia [4]. In addition, a retrospective cross-sectional study in Australia revealed that intake of low-fat dairy products is beneficial for social functioning and memory function [5]. A clinical trial using a sample of twin pairs showed that high intake of dairy products was associated with better short-term memory scores, using the Wechsler memory scale, in men [6]. We previously demonstrated that intake of a dairy product fermented with *Penicillium candidum*, i.e., Camembert cheese, had preventive effects against Alzheimer's disease pathology in a mouse model [7]. It is concluded that the consumption of dairy products is associated with the prevention of cognitive decline and that some of the ingredients in the dairy products are beneficial to cognitive function [8]; however, the underlying mechanism and responsible agents have not yet been elucidated.

Whey, the supernatant of yogurt and a byproduct of cheese, is rich in protein and consists of β-lactalbumin, α-lactoglobulin, immunogloblin, bovine serum albumin, and other minor proteins. Whey protein is a globally consumed food material and is well known for its health benefits, such as its reducing effects on body weight, blood glucose, and blood pressure [9]. In addition, recent clinical trials revealed that whey protein improves cognitive functions and mood status: an intake of 20 g whey protein improved memory performance in stress-vulnerable subjects aged from 18 to 35 years old [10]. Whey protein also reduced depressive symptoms in stress-vulnerable subjects under conditions of stress [11]. In healthy elderly subjects, the intake of 50.5 g whey protein improved delayed paragraph recall [12], but this quantity is not easily consumed in everyday life. We previously demonstrated that some whey peptides, produced through specific enzymatic digestion, improved spatial working memory, episodic memory, and attention in an experiment using scopolamine-induced amnesia model mice and aged mice [13]. The memory improvements were more pronounced in mice which received whey peptide compared with mice which received whey protein: tryptophan-tyrosine (WY)-related peptides, especially the glycine–threonine–tryptophan–tyrosine (GTWY) peptide, were identified for their involvement in the improved cognitive performance. Whey protein did not show any memory improvement effects when used at the same dose as the whey peptide rich in WY-related peptides, suggesting that the whey peptide has greater memory improvement effects than whey protein These studies suggest that intake of whey peptides rich in WY-related peptides could improve cognitive performance in middle aged and older people; however, the effect of whey peptides has not been elucidated. The present study is the first clinical demonstration to evaluate the effects of whey peptides rich in WY-related peptides, which are not whey protein itself but are in fact the result of enzymatic digestion of whey protein, on cognitive function in middle aged and older people in a randomized, placebo-controlled, double-blind, parallel-group comparative study.

2. Materials and Methods

2.1. Subjects

We recruited 101 healthy Japanese-speaking adults, aged from 45 to 65 years, with a self-awareness of carelessness and forgetfulness; in particular adults that tended to forget the names of people and objects. Subjects with relatively low neuropsychological test scores were preferentially included. Exclusion criteria included: (1) visual or hearing impediments; (2) suspected dementia (Hasegawa Dementia Rating Scale-Revised; HDS-R $\leq$ 20); (3) anamnesis of cranial nerve disease; (4) current treatment for cognitive function; (5) diagnosis of depressive disorder or depressive symptoms; (6) diagnosed menopausal symptoms or hormone treatment; (7) frequent irregular lifestyle, such as shift work; (8) high habitual consumption of alcohol (>20 g/day); (9) use of cigarettes; (10) experience of the same neuropsychological tests within the prior year; (11) regular consumption of drugs or health foods affecting cognitive functions (>once a week); (12) regular consumption of protein supplements (>once a week); (13) anamnesis of severe disease requiring regular treatment; (14) allergy or sensitivity to milk; (15) pregnancy or breastfeeding; (16) participation in other clinical trials; (17) blood donation within 3 months; (18) unhealthy status as determined during clinical examination; (19) classification of unsuitability by the principal investigator for other reasons. Inclusion and exclusion criteria were checked during the screening session by the questionnaire and clinical examination.

Based on the pilot study, we calculated a sample size of 44 to detect differences of 0.86 in the word recall test with a power of 0.80 and a significance level of 0.05 (two-sided α level). An assumption of a 10% withdrawal rate required at least 50 subjects in each group.

2.2. Experimental Supplements

The test formula consisted of 6 tablets containing a total of 1 g of whey peptide, which included 1.6 mg of GTWY peptide; the tablets were ingested by the test group every day for 12 weeks. Whey peptide was purchased from Megmilk Snow Brand Co., Ltd. (Tokyo, Japan). The placebo group ingested tablets substituted with an equivalent amount of maltodextrin every day for 12 weeks. The test and placebo tablets were the same size and shape and were indistinguishable by taste. Using amnesia model mice, we previously evaluated that 1 g of whey peptide, which is much lower than the amount of whey protein in the previous clinical studies (>20 g) [10,11], displayed an equivalent memory improvement to 1.6 mg of GTWY peptide.

2.3. Procedures

This study was performed using a randomized, placebo-controlled, double-blind, parallel group comparative design. Figure 1 shows the screening procedure for the 101 subjects. Questionnaires for the inclusion/exclusion criteria, the HDS-R, and clinical examinations for safety assessments were performed as part of the first screening step and neuropsychological tests and subjective psychological assessments were performed in the second screening step. Selected subjects were then randomly allocated using the table of random numbers in a 1:1 ratio to the whey peptides group or placebo group under the stratification of the median of the score of the 5 min-delayed word recall and delayed story recall. The person generating the table of random numbers was not involved in determining subject eligibility, data collection, or analysis. Both research staff and subjects were blinded to the group allocation until the completion of data analysis. Neuropsychological tests and subjective psychological assessments were repeated at 6 and 12 weeks of tablet ingestion. Clinical examinations for safety assessment were also performed at 12 weeks. Subjects were instructed to maintain their regular lifestyles and avoid taking any drugs, health functional foods, and protein supplements which could affect the neuropsychological tests during the study. Compliance was monitored by interview, subject diary, and number of ingested tablets. On the day of the neuropsychological tests, subjects were instructed to completely avoid food and beverages containing caffeine and to avoid ingesting other food and beverages, except water, for 4 hours prior to the tests. Subjects were instructed to ingest the study tablets 30 minutes before the start of the neuropsychological tests. The data were collected at Kensyokai Medical Corporation (Osaka, Japan) between June 2017 and December 2017, and the study was conducted by the contract research organization, TTC Co., Ltd. (Tokyo, Japan).

2.4. Neuropsychological Tests

Memory function was evaluated using word and story recall tests, and a verbal fluency test (VFT). The word recall test was conducted according to the Hamamatsu Higher Brain Function Scale which assesses short-term memory [14]. Subjects were given seven words and asked to verbally recall them immediately and then 5 and 20 min after they were given. The story recall test was conducted according to the Japanese version of the Rivermead Behavioural Memory Test (RBMT) which also assesses short-term memory [15]. Subjects were given a short story and asked to verbally recall it immediately and 20 min later. The VFT was used to assess long-term memory; subjects were asked to verbally name as many items as they could beginning with "a" (phonemic fluency task) and as many animals as possible (semantic fluency task) in one minute [16]. The Stroop test, digit span, and paced auditory serial addition test (PASAT) were used to evaluate attention and executive functions. For the Stroop test, subjects named words and colors (step 1, read the words printed in black; step 2, read the color of the printed circle; step 3, read words when it has been printed in a different-colored font, e.g., subjects should say red when it has been printed in blue font; step 4, read the print color of words that can be seen in step 3, e.g., subjects should say blue where the word "red" has been printed in blue font). Error numbers and reading time were measured [17]. Digit span (forward) test and PASAT were conducted according to the clinical assessment for attention (CAT) [18]. In the digit span test, which assessed working memory, subjects repeated numbers in increasing spans in forward sequences. The PASAT assessed updating and shifting attention: single digits were introduced every 2 s, and subjects added the new digit to the one immediately prior to it.

2.5. Subjective Psychological Assessment

Subjective mental fatigue from the neuropsychological test was assessed using a 100-mm visual analog scale (VAS) before and after the neuropsychological tests. The VAS consisted of a 100-mm line drawn from "not at all" to "most", and subjects indicated the degree of fatigue at that moment on the line [19]. Previous reports defined high-level fatigue as a greater than 20-mm VAS score [20,21]. The subjective mood status during one week was assessed using the Profile of Mood States (second edition short version; POMS2), which consists of subscales of anger–hostility (AH), confusion–bewilderment (CB), depression–dejection (DD), fatigue–inertia (FI), tension–anxiety (TA), vigor–activity (VA), friendliness (F), and total mood disturbance (TMD). Every POMS2 score was normalized to the T-score which is the score adjusted to the normal distribution (generation average: 50, and standard deviation: 10) and shows the degree of difference from the generation average [22]. To evaluate subjective memory performance, the Japanese version of the everyday memory checklist (EMC), composed of 13 four-point scaled items, was used to assesses memory impairments in an individual's daily life [23].

2.6. Safety Assessment

Safety assessments were performed by clinical examinations and included blood collection (white blood cell (WBC), red blood cell (RBC), hemoglobin (Hb), hematocrit (Ht), platelet (PLT), total protein (TP), albumin (Alb), total bilirubin (TB), direct bilirubin (D-B), indirect bilirubin (I-B), alkaline phosphatase (ALP), aspartate aminotransferase (AST), alanine aminotransferase (ALT), lactate dehydrogenase (LD), γ-glutamyl transpeptidase (γ-GT), total cholesterol (TC), triglyceride (TG), HDL-cholesterol (HDL-C), LDL-cholesterol (LDL-C), urea nitrogen (UN), creatinine (Cr), uric acid (UA), Na, K, CL, glucose (GLU)), urine collection (protein, glucose, uric occult blood), body weight, blood pressure, and pulse measurements. Adverse events were reported in the subject's diary and supervised by the principal investigator.

2.7. Statistical Analysis

The results were expressed as means ± standard deviation (SD). Statistical comparisons were performed using IBM SPSS Statistics 23 (IBM, New York, NY, USA) and Microsoft Excel 2010 (Microsoft, Redmond, WA, USA). Comparisons of all results, except for EMC, were examined with paired *t*-tests (between baseline and after intervention), and unpaired *t*-tests (between groups). EMC results were analyzed using the Wilcoxon signed-rank test (between baseline and after intervention), and Mann–Whitney *u*-tests (between groups). Multiple comparisons were not employed because this study was exploratory.

2.8. Ethics and Registration

The study was conducted in accordance with the Declaration of Helsinki, and approved by the ethics committee of Kensyokai Medical Corporation (Osaka, Japan). Written informed consent was obtained from all participants. The study was registered on 5 June 2017 in the database of the University Hospital Medical Information Network (UMIN) prior to enrollment (Registration No. UMIN000027644; Registration title. A study for the effect of intake of ingredients derived from animal on cognitive functions).

3. Results

3.1. Baseline Characteristics of the Study Groups

The flow of subjects through the experimental procedure is described in Figure 1. Following the first screening step, 242 subjects were included, and 64 subjects were excluded due to withdrawal of participation ($n = 8$), not meeting inclusion criteria ($n = 1$), suspected dementia ($n = 3$), anamnesis of cranial nerve disease ($n = 1$), high habitual alcohol consumption ($n = 5$), regular consumption of supplements affecting cognitive functions ($n = 6$), anamnesis of severe disease ($n = 4$), classification as unhealthy on clinical examination ($n = 31$), and unsuitability as per the principal investigator ($n = 5$). At the second screening step, 141 subjects were excluded due to withdrawal of participation ($n = 5$), not meeting inclusion criteria (relatively low neuropsychological test score) ($n = 59$), participation in other clinical trials ($n = 1$), anamnesis of severe disease ($n = 1$), and unsuitability as per the principal investigator ($n = 75$). The remaining 101 subjects were randomly allocated into either the whey peptides group or the placebo group for 12 weeks. Two subjects in the whey peptides group withdrew from the study due to whey peptides-unrelated health reasons, and one subject in the placebo group withdrew due to participation in another clinical trial, disclosed after allocation. Finally, 98 subjects completed all tests and were analyzed; their characteristics are shown in Table 1.

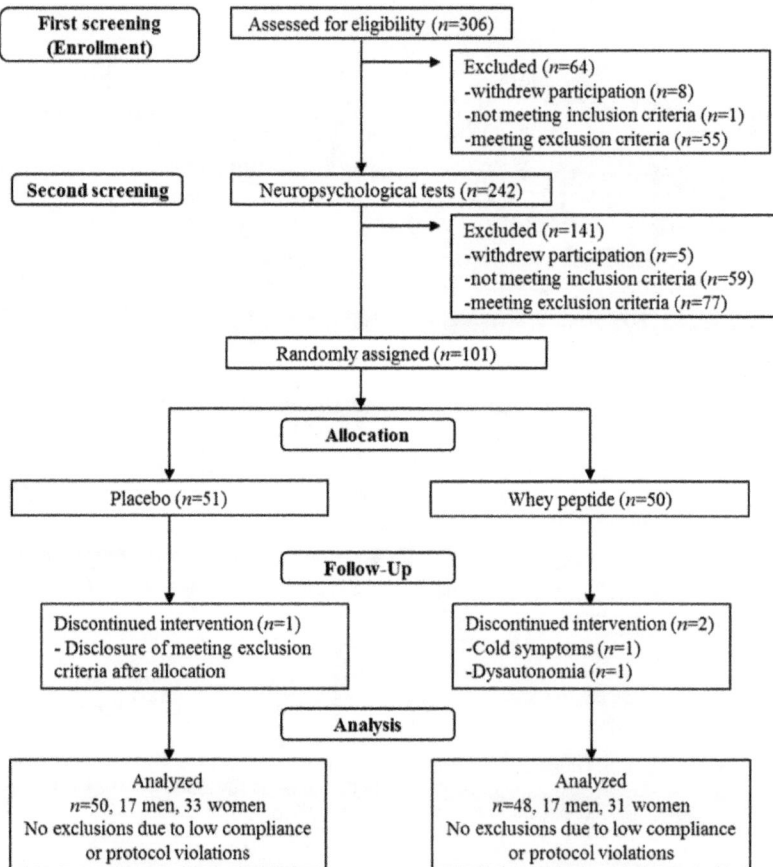

Figure 1. The flow of subjects.

Out of 306 subjects who were screened for the inclusion and exclusion criteria, 101 subjects were included in the study. The subjects were randomly allocated into the whey peptide (n = 50) or placebo (n = 51) group. Two subjects in the whey peptide and one subject in the placebo group dropped out of the study during intervention, and thus finally 48 subjects in the whey peptide and 50 subjects in the placebo group were analyzed.

Table 1. Characteristics of the analyzed subjects at baseline (week 0).

Characteristics	Placebo (n = 50)	Whey Peptide (n = 48)	p-Value
Age	51.8 ± 5.2	52.3 ± 4.3	0.568
Male/female	17/33	17/31	1.000
Body mass index (kg/m^2)	21.35 ± 2.04	21.11 ± 2.10	0.564
Education years	14.1 ± 1.8	14.5 ± 2.0	0.406
HDS-R score	28.4 ± 1.5	28.5 ± 1.8	0.678

Data are the mean $\pm$ SD. The p-values were calculated using unpaired t-tests, except for the male/female p-value which was calculated using the χ^2 test. HDS-R: Hasegawa Dementia Rating Scale-Revised.

3.2. Subjective Psychological Assessment

The baseline scores of the POMS2, VAS, and EMC before intervention are shown in Table 2. There were no significant differences in the POMS2, VAS, and EMC scores between groups before and after intervention, except V-A and F scores. These results suggest that psychological and cognitive fatigue, evaluated by VAS, were induced by the series of neuropsychological tests; however, no psychological improvement between the groups was measured after whey peptide intake.

Table 2. Subjective psychological assessments at baseline (week 0).

Psychological Status	Placebo (n = 50)	Whey Peptide (n = 48)	p-Value
POMS2			
AH	45.9 ± 9.1	45.5 ± 8.7	0.842
CB	48.8 ± 7.6	48.2 ± 8.4	0.707
DD	46.9 ± 6.0	46.3 ± 7.3	0.663
FI	45.2 ± 7.9	44.2 ± 8.9	0.547
TA	47.8 ± 7.4	46.4 ± 7.9	0.360
VA	47.2 ± 8.3	53.0 ± 10.2	0.002
F	48.8 ± 8.9	53.3 ± 9.5	0.019
TMD	47.2 ± 6.9	45.0 ± 8.6	0.159
VAS (after-before)	19.1 ± 16.1	20.6 ± 18.1	0.661
EMC	13.0 ± 4.8	12.8 ± 4.6	0.826

Data are presented as the mean $\pm$ SD. Unpaired t-tests were performed for the POMS2 and VAS. The Mann–Whitney u-test was performed for EMC. POMS2: Profile of Mood States (second edition short version); VAS: visual analog scale; EMC: everyday memory checklist; AH: anger–hostility; CB: confusion–bewilderment; DD: depression–dejection; FI: fatigue–inertia; TA: tension–anxiety; VA: vigor–activity; F: friendliness; TMD: total mood disturbance.

3.3. Neuropsychological Tests (Full Analysis Set (FAS))

The neuropsychological test measurements at weeks 0 (baseline), 6, and 12, in addition to the changes from baseline are shown in Table 3 (memory) and Table 4 (attention and executive functions). The changes in VFT (words beginning with "a") at 12 weeks of intervention from baseline tended to be higher in the whey peptide group compared with the placebo group (p = 0.094). In the VFT (animal), the scores were significantly increased at 6 weeks of intervention compared to baseline in the whey peptide group (p = 0.012) but there were no significant changes in the placebo group. These results suggest that whey peptide intake may affect long term memory retrieval rather than short term memory, however, there were no significant differences between the groups in the neuropsychological tests.

Table 3. Changes in neuropsychological tests assessing memory function.

Test		Group	Week 0 (Baseline)	Week 6	Week 12
Word recall					
Immediate recall	Score	P	4.2 ± 0.9	4.8 ± 0.9 **	5.1 ± 1.1 **
		W	4.4 ± 1.0	5.1 ± 0.9 **	5.2 ± 1.0 **
	Changes from baseline	P		0.7 ± 1.3	0.9 ± 1.1
		W		0.8 ± 1.2	0.8 ± 1.3
5-min delayed recall	Score	P	3.6 ± 1.1	4.9 ± 1.3 **	5.3 ± 1.2 **
		W	3.7 ± 1.1	4.7 ± 1.5 **	5.1 ± 1.4 **
	Changes from baseline	P		1.3 ± 1.4	1.7 ± 1.3
		W		1.0 ± 1.9	1.4 ± 1.7
20-min delayed recall	Score	P	4.3 ± 1.2	5.3 ± 1.3 **	5.6 ± 1.4 **
		W	4.2 ± 1.2	5.1 ± 1.6 **	5.4 ± 1.4 **
	Changes from baseline	P		1.0 ± 1.8	1.3 ± 1.6
		W		0.9 ± 1.8	1.2 ± 1.7
Story recall					
Immediate recall	Score	P	15.93 ± 2.53	17.65 ± 3.03 **	17.56 ± 2.77 **
		W	15.51 ± 2.55	16.58 ± 2.64 *	16.92 ± 2.52 **
	Changes from baseline	P		1.72 ± 3.71	1.63 ± 3.63
		W		1.07 ± 3.08	1.41 ± 3.38
20-min delayed recall	Score	P	14.39 ± 3.05	16.59 ± 3.45 **	16.63 ± 2.81 **
		W	14.44 ± 2.50	15.88 ± 3.00 **	16.83 ± 2.53 **
	Changes from baseline	P		2.20 ± 3.83	2.24 ± 3.65
		W		1.44 ± 3.51	2.40 ± 3.66
VFT (verbal fluency test)					
Beginning with "a"	Score	P	12.1 ± 3.3	13.1 ± 3.6 *	13.7 ± 3.8 **
		W	11.4 ± 4.1	13.2 ± 3.9 **	14.1 ± 4.1 **
	Changes from baseline	P		1.0 ± 2.8	1.7 ± 3.1
		W		1.9 ± 3.3	2.8 ± 3.1
Animal	Score	P	19.5 ± 4.4	19.6 ± 4.7	20.9 ± 3.9 *
		W	18.3 ± 4.1	19.4 ± 4.0 *	20.1 ± 4.6 **
	Changes from baseline	P		0.2 ± 3.7	1.4 ± 3.9
		W		1.2 ± 3.2	1.9 ± 3.9

Data are presented as the mean ± SD for the placebo (P) (n = 50) and whey peptide (W) groups (n = 48). * $p < 0.05$, ** $p < 0.01$, performed by paired *t*-tests (vs. baseline).

Table 4. Changes in neuropsychological tests assessing attention and executive functions.

Test		Group	Week 0 (Baseline)	Week 6	Week 12
Stroop test					
Step 3 error numbers	Score	P	0.0 ± 0.1	0.2 ± 0.9	0.1 ± 0.3
		W	0.1 ± 0.3	0.0 ± 0.2	0.1 ± 0.3
	Changes from baseline	P		0.1 ± 0.9	0.1 ± 0.3
		W		0.0 ± 0.4	0.0 ± 0.5
Step 3 reading time (second)	Score	P	45.6 ± 7.1	42.9 ± 8.1 **	41.0 ± 7.5 **
		W	44.8 ± 10.7	42.4 ± 9.6 **	40.9 ± 7.8 **
	Changes from baseline	P		−2.7 ± 6.0	−4.6 ± 6.9
		W		−2.4 ± 5.8	−3.9 ± 8.2
Step 4 error numbers	Score	P	0.1 ± 0.3	0.1 ± 0.4	0.2 ± 0.7
		W	0.2 ± 0.5	0.2 ± 0.4	0.2 ± 0.6
	Changes from baseline	P		0.0 ± 0.4	0.1 ± 0.7
		W		0.0 ± 0.6	0.0 ± 0.6
Step 4 reading time (second)	Score	P	59.5 ± 15.4	53.5 ± 9.9 **	50.8 ± 12.0 **
		W	57.2 ± 11.4	52.0 ± 10.1 **	49.7 ± 8.5 **
	Changes from baseline	P		−6.1 ± 10.8	−8.7 ± 12.4
		W		−5.2 ± 6.8	−7.5 ± 7.1

Table 4. *Cont.*

Test		Group	Week 0 (Baseline)	Week 6	Week 12
Digit Span					
Spans	Score	P	6.1 ± 1.1	6.4 ± 1.2 *	6.6 ± 1.4 **
		W	6.2 ± 1.2	6.3 ± 1.1	6.6 ± 1.1*
	Changes from baseline	P		0.3 ± 1.0	0.5 ± 1.1
		W		0.1 ± 1.1	0.4 ± 1.1
PASAT (paced auditory serial addition test)					
Accuracy (%)	Score	P	68.8 ± 16.0	77.4 ± 16.6 **	83.1 ± 11.7 **
		W	70.0 ± 16.0	76.4 ± 14.8 **	78.4 ± 19.6 **
	Changes from baseline	P		8.6 ± 12.3	14.2 ± 11.8
		W		6.4 ± 12.7	8.4 ± 18.1

Data are presented as the mean $\pm$ SD for the placebo (P) ($n = 50$) and whey peptide (W) ($n = 48$) groups. * $p < 0.05$, ** $p < 0.01$, performed by paired t-tests (vs. baseline).

3.4. Subgroup Analysis by the Degree of Fatigue

The change in VAS scores between before and after the neuropsychological tests indicated that the series of cognitive tasks induced psychological fatigue in subjects. The VAS score levels differed among the subjects, and therefore subjects were classified into two subgroups of high-level and low-level fatigue, similar to previous reports [20,21]. Previous reports defined high-level fatigue as a VAS greater than 20 mm.

In the high-level fatigue subgroup, the increase in the number of recalled words beginning with "a" in the VFT at 6 weeks from baseline was significantly higher in the whey peptide group compared with the placebo group ($p = 0.023$). In addition, the number of recalled words beginning with "a" at 6 and 12 weeks and the number of animal words recalled at 6 weeks were significantly increased from baseline in the whey peptide group, whereas the scores did not change in the placebo group (Table 5 and Figure 2A).

The reduction in error numbers in the Stroop test (step 3), was significantly lower at 6 weeks in the high fatigue whey peptide group compared with the high fatigue placebo group ($p = 0.047$); at 12 weeks the reduction in error numbers tended to be lower in the whey peptide group compared with the placebo group ($p = 0.080$, Table 5 and Figure 2B). These results suggest that whey peptide intake for 6 weeks improves long-term memory retrieval, attention, and executive functions in subjects vulnerable to psychological fatigue.

Table 5. Changes of word numbers in VFT and error numbers in the Stroop test from baseline (week 0) in the high and low fatigue subgroups, classified using the VAS.

Test		Group	Week 6	Week 12	Week 6	Week 12
VFT			**High fatigue**		**Low fatigue**	
Beginning with "a"	Changes from baseline	P	1.0 ± 3.7	1.3 ± 3.6	1.1 ± 2.2 *	2.0 ± 2.8 **
		W	3.3 ± 2.5 **,#	2.6 ± 3.0 **	0.9 ± 3.5	2.8 ± 3.2 **
Animal	Changes from baseline	P	-0.6 ± 4.2	0.5 ± 3.7	0.7 ± 3.3	2.0 ± 3.9 **
		W	1.3 ± 2.6 *	0.8 ± 4.5	1.1 ± 3.6	2.5 ± 3.4 **
Stroop test			**High fatigue**		**Low fatigue**	
Step 3 error numbers	Changes from baseline	P	0.1 ± 0.3	0.0 ± 0.2	0.2 ± 1.1	0.1 ± 0.4
		W	-0.1 ± 0.3 #	-0.1 ± 0.3	0.0 ± 0.4	0.1 ± 0.5
Step 4 error numbers	Changes from baseline	P	0.1 ± 0.4	0.3 ± 1.0	0.0 ± 0.4	0.0 ± 0.4
		W	-0.1 ± 0.2	0.0 ± 0.5	0.0 ± 0.7	0.0 ± 0.7

Data are presented as the mean $\pm$ SD for the placebo (P) ($n = 21$) and whey peptide (W) ($n = 19$) groups classified into the high fatigue subgroup, and placebo ($n = 29$) and whey peptide ($n = 29$) groups in the low fatigue subgroup. # $p < 0.05$ performed using unpaired t-tests. * $p < 0.05$, ** $p < 0.01$, performed using paired t-tests (vs. baseline).

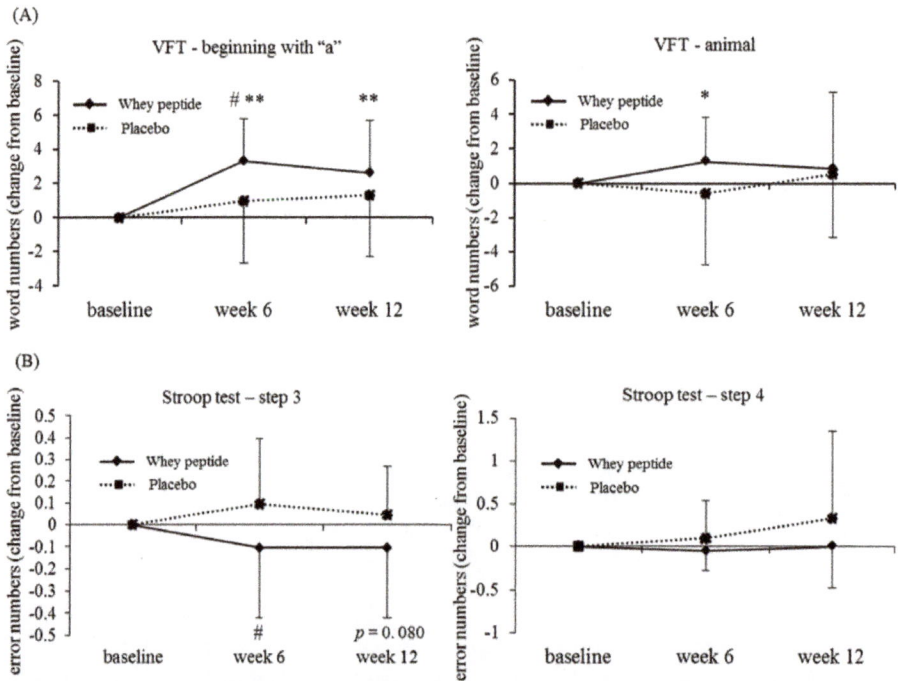

Figure 2. Changes of word numbers in the VFT (**A**) and error numbers in the Stroop test—step 3 (**B**) from baseline in the high fatigue subgroup, classified by the VAS. The solid line shows the whey peptide group (*n* = 19) and the dotted line shows the placebo group (*n* = 21). The data represent mean, and error bars indicate SD. The *p*-values and # show between group differences, performed using unpaired *t*-tests, # *p* < 0.05. * *p* < 0.05; ** *p* < 0.01 performed using paired *t*-tests (vs. baseline).

In addition to the neuropsychological tests, the EMC scores, which give a subjective measure of memory failure in everyday life, were significantly lower in the high fatigue whey peptide group compared with the high fatigue placebo group at 12 weeks. In addition, the EMC score was significantly decreased compared to baseline in the whey peptide group at 12 weeks, but not in the placebo group (Figure 3).

In the low-level fatigue subgroup, there were no significant differences between the whey peptide and placebo groups in the neuropsychological test results, except the word recall test: immediate recall was significantly higher in the whey peptide group compared with the placebo group at 6 weeks (5.2 (whey peptide group), 4.8 (placebo), *p* = 0.040, data not shown).

Subjects were also classified into fatigue-level subgroups using the FI scores from the POMS2 test, which indicates fatigue level in subjects in the week that tests are performed. The average test score is set as 50, therefore subjects with an FI score more than or equal to 50 at baseline were defined as the high fatigue subgroup. The changes in number of recalled words beginning with "a" and animal names were significantly higher or tended to be higher in the high fatigue whey peptide group compared with the high fatigue placebo group at 6 weeks (*p* = 0.047 and *p* = 0.072, respectively) (Table 6 and Figure 4).

EMC

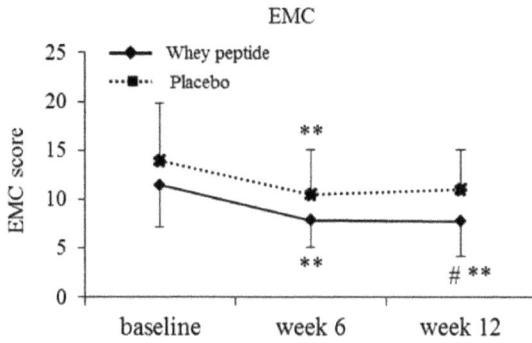

Figure 3. Changes in the EMC scores in the high fatigue subgroup, classified using the VAS. The solid line shows the whey peptide group (n = 19) and the dotted line shows the placebo group (n = 21). The data represent mean, and error bars indicate SD. # $p < 0.05$ between groups performed using the Mann–Whitney u-test. ** $p < 0.01$ performed using the Wilcoxon signed-rank test (vs. baseline).

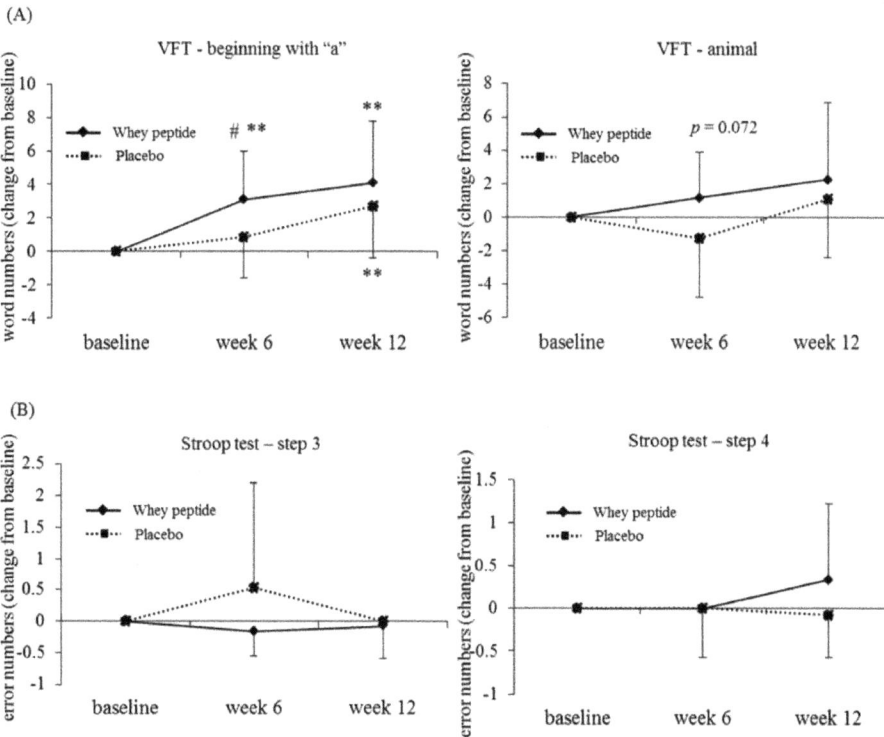

(A)

(B)

Figure 4. Changes of word numbers in the VFT and error numbers in the Stroop test from baseline in the high-fatigue subgroup, classified using POMS2. The solid line shows the whey peptide group (n = 12) and the dotted line shows the placebo group (n = 13). The data represent mean, and error bars indicate SD. The p-values and # show between group differences, performed using unpaired t-tests, # $p < 0.05$. ** $p < 0.01$ performed using paired t-tests (vs. baseline).

Table 6. Changes of word numbers in the VFT and error numbers in the Stroop test from baseline (week 0) in the high and low fatigue subgroups, classified using the POMS2 FI score.

Test		Group	Week 6	Week 12	Week 6	Week 12
VFT			High fatigue		Low fatigue	
Beginning with "a"	Changes from baseline	P	0.8 ± 2.4	2.7 ± 3.1 **	1.1 ± 3.0 *	1.3 ± 3.1 *
		W	3.1 ± 2.9 **,#	4.1 ± 3.7 **	1.4 ± 3.4 *	2.3 ± 2.8 **
Animal	Changes from baseline	P	-1.2 ± 3.5	1.1 ± 3.5	0.7 ± 3.7	1.5 ± 4.0 *
		W	1.2 ± 2.7	2.3 ± 4.6	1.2 ± 3.3 *	1.7 ± 3.7 **
Stroop test			High fatigue		Low fatigue	
Step 3 error numbers	Changes from baseline	P	0.5 ± 1.7	0.0 ± 0.0	0.0 ± 0.2	0.1 ± 0.4
		W	-0.2 ± 0.4	-0.1 ± 0.5	0.0 ± 0.3	0.0 ± 0.4
Step 4 error numbers	Changes from baseline	P	0.0 ± 0.6	-0.1 ± 0.5	0.0 ± 0.4	0.2 ± 0.8
		W	0.0 ± 0.0	0.3 ± 0.9	-0.1 ± 0.7	-0.1 ± 0.5 #

Data are presented as the mean $\pm$ SD for the placebo (P) ($n = 13$) and the whey peptide (W) ($n = 12$) groups classified into the high fatigue subgroup, and placebo ($n = 37$) and the whey peptide (W) ($n = 36$) groups in the low fatigue subgroup. # $p < 0.05$ performed using the unpaired t-test. * $p < 0.05$, ** $p < 0.01$ performed using the paired t-test (vs. baseline).

3.5. Safety Assessment and Compliance

In order to evaluate the safety of whey peptide used in this study, we conducted safety assessments using subject diaries in 101 subjects (whole subjects after allocation) and clinical assessments in 98 subjects (final number of subjects completing the analysis): 74 adverse events occurred in the placebo group (30 subjects/51 subjects), and 63 adverse events occurred in the whey peptide group (25 subjects/50 subjects). None of the adverse events were severe and were judged to have no association with whey peptide by the principal investigator. Slight changes to some of the clinical assessment values from baseline were detected but these were judged to have no clinical significance by the principal investigator. Compliance with this trial was high, with a tablet consumption rate of 91.7–102.4%. The changes in clinical assessments are shown in supplementary Tables S1–S3.

4. Discussion

This is the first reported evaluation of the effects of whey peptide on cognitive performance in middle- and older-aged volunteers in a randomized, double-blind, placebo-controlled trial. The low dropout rate (3%) during the interventions and no exclusions during the analysis increases the reliability of this study. Whey peptide intake tended to improve the VFT score, reflecting fluent semantic memory retrieval in middle- and older-aged healthy subjects with self-awareness of cognitive decline. In the full analysis set, there was no significant improvement in neuropsychological tests between the groups.

Subgroup analysis, stratified for subjective fatigue, revealed that the intakes of whey peptides for 6 weeks improved the fluent semantic memory retrieval (VFT), and attention and executive function (Stroop test) in the subjects with high fatigue. In these tests, the improvements were significant after 6 weeks of whey peptide intake but not significant after 12 weeks. It is suggested that repeated memory and attention assessments might increase the learning effects at week 12, resulting in a reduction in the difference between placebo and whey peptide group at week 12 compared with week 6. According to previous reports [20,21], subjects with high fatigue levels were classified as those with over 20-mm changes in their VAS before and after neuropsychological testing at week 0 of the intervention. Since subjects are required to concentrate for about one hour during the neuropsychological tests, those experiencing fatigue are considered to be vulnerable to psychological or cognitive fatigues. In addition to the neuropsychological test results, subjective memory conditions in daily life, measured by EMC, were also improved in the high fatigue subgroup. The fatigue levels indicated by the VAS score in the present study reflect the fatigue induced by the neuropsychological test, which indicates a short-term acute condition; the fatigue levels indicated by POMS2 reflect the fatigue in the subject's daily life for as recently as one week, which indicates a long-term condition. Whey peptide intake could improve fluent semantic memory retrieval, attention and executive function in subjects with both acute and chronic psychological fatigue. However, it should be noted that VAS and POMS2 are subjective scales. Subjective fatigue is affected by multiple physical and psychological conditions, so, we could not clearly assert "fatigue", and further study will elucidate this issue.

In the present study, whey peptide intake improved the phonemic verbal fluency of the VFT and error numbers in the Stroop test. VFT is often included in clinical practice to diagnose the cognitive impairment of neurodegenerative disorders, such as Alzheimer's disease, and in research to measure verbal ability and lexical retrieval ability [24]. Phonemic verbal fluency, including words beginning with a specific letter, is closely associated with the frontal cortex, especially the dorsolateral prefrontal cortex (dlPFC); sematic words, including objects such as animals, are associated with the temporal cortex [25,26]. Neuroimaging studies revealed that phonemic fluency tests activate the neurons in the dlPFC [25]. The Stroop test is used to evaluate inhibition of executive function, which is composed of inhibition, updating/shifting and working memory [27]. In the present study, the functions of inhibition, updating/shifting, and working memory were measured using the Stroop test, PASAT, and digit span, respectively. Inhibition of executive function is closely associated with conditions of the prefrontal cortex, especially the dlPFC, and anterior cingulate cortex (ACC). Functional magnetic resonance imaging revealed that dlPFC and ACC play important roles in the implementation of control and performance monitoring in incongruent stimuli, respectively [28]. The evidence suggests that whey peptide intake may improve the function of the frontal cortex, especially the dlPFC, and ACC. Psychological and cognitive fatigue induced by cognitive tasks in the present study are common symptoms in neurological disorders (e.g., dementia, mild traumatic brain injury) and aging, which are associated with executive functions and conditions of the PFC and ACC [29–31]. Subjects with high fatigue levels might be sensitive to the effects of whey peptides in certain neuropsychological tests, e.g., the VFT and Stroop test which are related to PFC and ACC performance.

We previously demonstrated that the whey peptide used in the present study improves long-term episodic memory and spatial working memory in amnesia model mice and aged mice and identified GTWY peptides as an ingredient to improve cognitive function [13]. Short-term oral administration of GTWY peptides increased dopamine levels in the brains of mice. The dopaminergic system in the PFC is crucial for cognitive function, including attention, executive function, learning, and memory function [32,33]; intake of whey peptide rich in GTWY peptides might improve the fluency and executive functions via dopaminergic activation in the PFC. In addition to dopaminergic activation, some whey peptides have anti-oxidant and anti-inflammatory activity [34,35]. Thus, reduction of oxidative stress and inflammation might contribute to the beneficial effects of whey peptide in this study. Further clinical studies to evaluate the effects of whey peptides on cerebral activity, oxidative stress, or inflammatory markers will be conducted to elucidate the underlying mechanisms.

There are some limitations in this study: firstly, the fatigue scales evaluated in the present study are subjective methods, which might be affected by other psychological conditions other than fatigue; further studies measuring biochemical fatigue markers (e.g., salivary amylase) should be conducted in order to distinguish fatigue from other psychological conditions. Secondly, multiple comparisons were not employed, so there is a risk of α-errors. Further studies should confirm the results obtained in this study. Thirdly, we could not dissociate the chronic effects of whey peptide from the acute effects: further studies are required to dissociate these effects.

5. Conclusions

In the present study, the effects of daily whey peptide intake on cognitive functions in healthy middle- and older-aged people were evaluated. It is suggested that whey peptide improves some cognitive functions in people with a high level of subjective fatigue. Our results support previous epidemiological and preclinical findings which suggested that intake of whey peptide in daily life might be beneficial to cognitive function.

Supplementary Materials: The following are available online at http://www.mdpi.com/2072-6643/10/7/899/s1, Table S1: Clinical assessment of the changes in blood parameters, Table S2: Clinical assessment of the changes in urine parameters, Table S3: Changes in weight, blood pressure, and pulse.

Author Contributions: M.K., K.O., S.U. and Y.A. designed this study; S.K. conducted this study as principal investigator; M.K. and Y.A. wrote the manuscript; and M.K. assumed primary responsibility for the final content. All authors read and approved the final manuscript.

Funding: This study was funded by the Kirin Company, Limited.

Acknowledgments: We thank Yutaka Miura for valuable discussions about the present experimental design. We also thank Yuichiro Nakano, Junji Watanabe, and Keiko Kobayashi for the preparation of the test tablets used in this experiment.

Conflicts of Interest: The funder designed this study and supplied the test tablets and placebo. The funder had no role in data collection nor data analysis. This manuscript was prepared by the members of the funder. The funder decided to publish the results.

References

1. Department of Economic and Social Affairs United Nations. *World Population Prospects: Key Findings and Advance Tables—The 2015 Revision*; United Nations Publications: New York, NY, USA, 2015.
2. Prince, M.; Wimo, A.; Guerchet, M.; Ali, G.C.; Wu, Y.T.; Prina, M. World Alzheimer Report 2015 The Global Impact of Dementia. An Analysis of Prevalence, Incidence, Cost and Trends. Alzheimer's Disease International publications. Available online: https://www.alz.co.uk/research/WorldAlzheimerReport2015.pdf. (accessed on 25 January 2018).
3. Ano, Y.; Nakayama, H. Preventive effects of dairy products on dementia and the underlying mechanisms. *Int. J. Mol. Sci.* **2018**, *19*, 1927. [CrossRef] [PubMed]
4. Ozawa, M.; Ninomiya, T.; Ohara, T.; Doi, Y.; Uchida, K.; Shirota, T.; Yonemoto, K.; Kitazono, T.; Kiyohara, Y. Dietary patterns and risk of dementia in an elderly Japanese population: The Hisayama Study. *AJCN* **2013**, *97*, 1076–1082. [CrossRef] [PubMed]
5. Crichton, G.E.; Murphy, K.J.; Bryan, J. Dairy intake and cognitive health in middle-aged South Australians. *Asia Pac. J. Clin. Nutr.* **2010**, *19*, 161–171. [PubMed]
6. Ogata, S.; Tanaka, H.; Omura, K.; Honda, C.; Hayakawa, K. Association between intake of dairy products and short-term memory with and without adjustment for genetic and family environmental factors: A twin study. *Clin. Nutr.* **2016**, *35*, 507–513. [CrossRef] [PubMed]
7. Ano, Y.; Ozawa, M.; Kutsukake, T.; Sugiyama, S.; Uchida, K.; Yoshida, A.; Nakayama, H. Preventive effects of a fermented dairy product against Alzheimer's disease and identification of a novel oleamide with enhanced microglial phagocytosis and anti-inflammatory activity. *PLoS ONE* **2015**, *10*, e0118512. [CrossRef] [PubMed]
8. Camfield, D.A.; Owen, L.; Scholey, A.B.; Pipingas, A.; Stough, C. Dairy constituents and neurocognitive health in ageing. *Br. J. Nutr.* **2011**, *106*, 159–174. [CrossRef] [PubMed]
9. Kiyosawa, I. Progress in Recent Reesearches on the Whey Protein Concentrates and their Functional Properties (Japanese). *Milk Sci.* **2002**, *51*, 13–26.
10. Markus, C.R.; Olivier, B.; de Haan, E.H. Whey protein rich in alpha-lactalbumin increases the ratio of plasma tryptophan to the sum of the other large neutral amino acids and improves cognitive performance in stress-vulnerable subjects. *AJCN* **2002**, *75*, 1051–1056. [CrossRef] [PubMed]
11. Markus, C.R.; Olivier, B.; Panhuysen, G.E.; Van Der Gugten, J.; Alles, M.S.; Tuiten, A.; Westenberg, H.G.; Fekkes, D.; Koppeschaar, H.F.; de Haan, E.E. The bovine protein alpha-lactalbumin increases the plasma ratio of tryptophan to the other large neutral amino acids, and in vulnerable subjects raises brain serotonin activity, reduces cortisol concentration, and improves mood under stress. *AJCN* **2000**, *71*, 1536–1544. [CrossRef] [PubMed]
12. Kaplan, R.J.; Greenwood, C.E.; Winocur, G.; Wolever, T.M. Dietary protein, carbohydrate, and fat enhance memory performance in the healthy elderly. *AJCN* **2001**, *74*, 687–693. [CrossRef] [PubMed]
13. Ano, Y.; Ayabe, T.; Kutsukake, T.; Ohya, R.; Uchida, S.; Yamada, K.; Takashima, A.; Nakayama, H. Novel lacto-peptides in fermented dairy products improve memory function and cognitive decline. *Neurobiol. Aging* **2018**, under review.

14. Imamura, Y.; Uemura, K. Functional localization in prefrontal area by hamamatsu higher brain function scale (Japanese). *Japan. J. Neuropsychol.* **1996**, *12*, 99–105.

15. Kazui, H.; Watamori, T.; Honda, R.; Tokimasa, A.; Hirono, N.; Mori, E. Nihonban Rivermead Behavioural Memory Test (RBMT) no yuuyousei no kentou (Japanese). *Adv. Neurol. Sci.* **2002**, *46*, 307–318.

16. Borkowski, J.G.; Benton, A.L.; Spreen, O. Word fluency and brain damage. *Neuropsychologia* **1967**, *5*, 135–140. [CrossRef]

17. Stroop, J.R. Studies of interference in serial verbal reactions. *J. Exp. Psychol.* **1935**, *18*, 643–662. [CrossRef]

18. Kato, M. The development and standardization of Clinical Assessment for Attention (CAT) and Clinical Assessment for Spontaneity (CAS) (Japanese). *Higher Brain Function Res.* **2006**, *26*, 310–319. [CrossRef]

19. Japanese Society of Fatigue Science. Available online: http://www.hirougakkai.com (accessed on 27 February 2017).

20. Verhoeven, E.W.; Kraaimaat, F.W.; van de Kerkhof, P.C.; van Weel, C.; Duller, P.; van der Valk, P.G.; van den Hoogen, H.J.; Bor, J.H.; Schers, H.J.; Evers, A.W. Prevalence of physical symptoms of itch, pain and fatigue in patients with skin diseases in general practice. *Br. J. Dermatol.* **2007**, *156*, 1346–1349. [CrossRef] [PubMed]

21. Rat, A.C.; Pouchot, J.; Fautrel, B.; Boumier, P.; Goupille, P.; Guillemin, F. Factors associated with fatigue in early arthritis: Results from a multicenter national French cohort study. *Arthrit. Care Res.* **2012**, *64*, 1061–1069.

22. Heuchert, J.P.; McNair, D.M. *Profiles of Mood States*, 2nd ed.; Kaneko syobo: Tokyo, Japan, 2015.

23. Kazui, H.; Watamori, T.S.; Honda, R.; Mori, E. The validation of a Japanese version of the Everyday Memory Checklist (Japanese). *Brain Nerve* **2003**, *55*, 317–325. [PubMed]

24. Cottingham, M.E.; Hawkins, K.A. Verbal fluency deficits co-occur with memory deficits in geriatric patients at risk for dementia: Implications for the concept of mild cognitive impairment. *Behav. Neurol.* **2010**, *22*, 73–79. [CrossRef] [PubMed]

25. Alvarez, J.A.; Emory, E. Executive function and the frontal lobes: A meta-analytic review. *Neuropsychol. Rev.* **2006**, *16*, 17–42. [CrossRef] [PubMed]

26. Troyer, A.K.; Moscovitch, M.; Winocur, G.; Alexander, M.P.; Stuss, D. Clustering and switching on verbal fluency: The effects of focal frontal- and temporal-lobe lesions. *Neuropsychologia* **1998**, *36*, 499–504. [CrossRef]

27. Miyake, A.; Friedman, N.P.; Emerson, M.J.; Witzki, A.H.; Howerter, A.; Wager, T.D. The unity and diversity of executive functions and their contributions to complex "frontal lobe" tasks: A latent variable analysis. *Cogn. Psychol.* **2000**, *41*, 49–100. [CrossRef] [PubMed]

28. MacDonald, A.W.; Cohen, J.D.; Stenger, V.A.; Carter, C.S. Dissociating the role of the dorsolateral prefrontal and anterior cingulate cortex in cognitive control. *Science* **2000**, *288*, 1835–1838. [CrossRef] [PubMed]

29. Lin, F.; Roiland, R.; Heffner, K.; Johnson, M.; Chen, D.G.; Mapstone, M. Evaluation of objective and perceived mental fatigability in older adults with vascular risk. *J. Psychosom. Res.* **2014**, *76*, 458–464. [CrossRef] [PubMed]

30. DeLuca, J.; Genova, H.M.; Capili, E.J.; Wylie, G.R. Functional neuroimaging of fatigue. *Phys. Med. Rehabil. Clin. N. Am.* **2009**, *20*, 325–337. [CrossRef] [PubMed]

31. Wylie, G.R.; Genova, H.M.; DeLuca, J.; Dobryakova, E. The relationship between outcome prediction and cognitive fatigue: A convergence of paradigms. *Cogn. Affect. Behav. Neurosci.* **2017**, *17*, 838–849. [CrossRef] [PubMed]

32. Arnsten, A.F.; Li, B.M. Neurobiology of executive functions: Catecholamine influences on prefrontal cortical functions. *Biol. Psychiatry* **2005**, *57*, 1377–1384. [CrossRef] [PubMed]

33. Puig, M.V.; Rose, J.; Schmidt, R.; Freund, N. Dopamine modulation of learning and memory in the prefrontal cortex: Insights from studies in primates, rodents, and birds. *Front. Neural Circ.* **2014**, *8*, 93. [CrossRef] [PubMed]

34. Sugawara, K.; Takahashi, H.; Kashiwagura, T.; Yamada, K.; Yanagida, S.; Homma, M.; Dairiki, K.; Sasaki, H.; Kawagoshi, A.; Satake, M.; et al. Effect of anti-inflammatory supplementation with whey peptide and exercise therapy in patients with COPD. *Respir. Med.* **2012**, *106*, 1526–1534. [CrossRef] [PubMed]

35. Madadlou, A.; Abbaspourrad, A. Bioactive whey peptide particles: An emerging class of nutraceutical carriers. *Clin. Rev. Food Sci. Nutr.* **2018**, *58*, 1468–1477. [CrossRef] [PubMed]

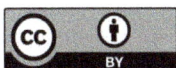

nutrients

MDPI

Article

Metabolism of Caprine Milk Carbohydrates by Probiotic Bacteria and Caco-2:HT29–MTX Epithelial Co-Cultures and Their Impact on Intestinal Barrier Integrity

Alicia M. Barnett [1,2,*], Nicole C. Roy [1,2,3], Adrian L. Cookson [2,4] and Warren C. McNabb [2]

[1]   Food Nutrition & Health Team, AgResearch Ltd., Palmerston North 4442, New Zealand; nicole.roy@agresearch.co.nz
[2]   Riddet Institute, Massey University, Palmerston North 4442, New Zealand; adrian.cookson@agresearch.co.nz (A.L.C.); W.Mcnabb@massey.ac.nz (W.C.M.)
[3]   High-Value Nutrition National Science Challenge, Auckland 1142, New Zealand
[4]   Food Assurance Team, AgResearch Ltd., Hopkirk Institute, Palmerston North 4474, New Zealand
*   Correspondence: alicia.barnett@agresearch.co.nz; Tel.: +64-6-351-8174

Received: 19 June 2018; Accepted: 20 July 2018; Published: 23 July 2018

Abstract: The development and maturation of the neonatal intestine is generally influenced by diet and commensal bacteria, the composition of which, in turn, can be influenced by the diet. Colonisation of the neonatal intestine by probiotic *Lactobacillus* strains can strengthen, preserve, and improve barrier integrity, and adherence of probiotics to the intestinal epithelium can be influenced by the available carbon sources. The goal of the present study was to examine the role of probiotic lactobacilli strains alone or together with a carbohydrate fraction (CF) from caprine milk on barrier integrity of a co-culture model of the small intestinal epithelium. Barrier integrity (as measured by trans epithelial electrical resistance (TEER)), was enhanced by three bacteria/CF combinations (*Lactobacillus rhamnosus* HN001, *L. plantarum* 299v, and *L. casei* Shirota) to a greater extent than CF or bacteria alone. Levels of occludin mRNA were increased for all treatments compared to untreated co-cultures, and *L. plantarum* 299v in combination with CF had increased mRNA levels of *MUC4*, *MUC2* and *MUC5AC* mucins and MUC4 protein abundance. These results indicate that three out of the four probiotic bacteria tested, in combination with CF, were able to elicit a greater increase in barrier integrity of a co-culture model of the small intestinal epithelium compared to that for either component alone. This study provides additional insight into the individual or combined roles of microbe–diet interactions in the small intestine and their beneficial contribution to the intestinal barrier.

Keywords: caprine milk carbohydrates; in vitro studies; small intestinal epithelium; barrier integrity; probiotic lactobacilli bacteria

1. Introduction

Milk is the first food for all mammals [1] and provides the nutritional needs for normal growth and development of the rapidly growing offspring [2]. Milk has a complex chemical composition which can be influenced by the diet, environmental conditions and the stage of lactation, and can also vary between animal species [1]. For example, the average protein, lipid and lactose profile of human milk is 1.2%, 4.4% and 6.8%, respectively, whilst that of caprine milk is 3.4%, 3.9% and 4.4%, respectively [2]. Together with lactose, oligosaccharides are the main contributor to the carbohydrate profile of milk, and in human milk there are 5–8 g/L of oligosaccharides [3]. In comparison caprine milk has 0.25–0.3 g/L of oligosaccharides, which although less than human milk, has an overall profile of neutral and acidic oligosaccharide structures which is more similar to human milk than either bovine or ovine milk [3].

Milk in early age has multifunctional roles beyond simply nutrition within the gastrointestinal tract by assisting in the establishment of a symbiotic microbiota [1], aiding in the development of the immune system, stimulating cellular growth and inducing epithelial barrier maturation [4]. At birth, although the gastrointestinal tract has all the cellular and structural features of the adult intestine [5], the epithelial barrier is functionally immature, and as such, there is increased risk of injury and inflammation caused by the movement of toxins and bacteria from the lumen [6]. The intestinal barrier is comprised of a single layer of epithelial cells known as the intrinsic barrier and the extrinsic mucus barrier [7–9]. Important components of the intrinsic barrier are the intercellular junctional complexes [10]. Occludin is an integral membrane protein that contributes to the tight junction (TJ) complex and interacts with tight junction protein (TJP)-1 and TJP2, which in turn interacts with the cytoskeleton [11]. The TJ structure can be altered in response to stimuli, such as growth factors, pathogenic/commensal bacteria, and dietary components leading to an increase or decrease in permeability [12]. Dietary components, such as fructo-oligosaccharides, can directly promote barrier protective effects by activating host cell signalling and the induction of select TJs in the intestine [13].

Intestinal development and barrier maturation after birth is not only influenced by dietary intake, but also by the colonisation by mutualistic microorganisms [14]. Bacterial colonisation is initiated in utero [15], but establishment of the intestinal microbiota after birth is influenced by the mode of delivery and the environment [16]. The establishment of a microbiota that is protective to the infant [17] may aid in barrier integrity via modulation of host gene expression and mucin secretion [18–20], whereas abnormal bacterial colonisation may disrupt this process and contribute to the development of host diseases [21]. Diet plays a major role in selecting for initial colonisers of the intestine [17], for example; milk oligosaccharides which are composed of 3–10 monosaccharide residues [22] are not-digested by infants, but instead pass unabsorbed into the large intestine where they selectively stimulate the growth and/or activity of specific bacterial genera such as bifidobacteria and lactobacilli [23,24]. In addition to the beneficial effects exerted by such oligosaccharides on the commensal microbiota, they are generally considered to improve the survival, adherence, transient colonisation and subsequent proliferation of probiotic micro-organisms [25,26]. However, few reports have focused on the influence of such substrates on the adherence of probiotic bacteria in the small intestine.

Determining the adherence or persistence of dietary probiotics in the intestine is largely dependent on measurements of the microbial composition in faecal samples, mainly because obtaining samples directly from the small intestine is difficult due to the highly invasive intubation methods used. At best the measurement in faecal samples reflects the microbial composition of the large intestine, which differs substantially from that of the small intestine. For example, anaerobic bacteria from the families Bacteriodaceae and Clostridiaceae are found in high abundance in the large intestine [27], whilst in the small intestine, fast-growing facultative anaerobes such as Lactobacillaceae and Enterobacteriaceae are dominant families of the microbial community, which "tolerate the combined effects of bile acids and antimicrobials while still effectively competing with both the host and other bacteria for the simple carbohydrates that are available in this region of the gastrointestinal tract" [27]. Studies of orally administered lactic acid bacteria have demonstrated that the lactic acid bacterial counts in the small intestine increase after ingestion [28–31]. Evidence indicates that particular *Lactobacillus* probiotic strains can strengthen and preserve the intestinal barrier in an in vitro model of necrotising enterocolitis [32], increase the expression of genes involved in TJ formation [33], and increase barrier integrity of intestinal epithelial cell (IEC) monolayers as measured by trans epithelial electrical resistance (TEER) [34–36]. In addition, probiotics may provide protective effects for the intestinal barrier by actively secreting soluble mediators [37], facilitating TJ formation [38], and inducing mucin gene expression with a resultant change in the mucus layer composition which may occur as a direct response to bacterial adhesion to the epithelium [39]. From in vitro investigations using IECs such as mono-cultures of Caco-2 cells [34], mono-cultures of HT29 (and various sub-clones) [40], and co-cultures of Caco-2:HT29–MTX cells [41] it has been determined that adherence of probiotics can be both species and strain specific [42] and dependent on the carbon source present in their growth medium [43]. For example, a study undertaken by Wickramasinghe et al. [44] determined that there was a higher rate of adhesion of *Bifidobacterium infantis* ATCC 15697 to Caco-2 cells when grown with human milk oligosaccharides than when cultured in lactose [44]. These studies provided the evidence of the protective effects of some probiotics on epithelial barrier maturation and the ability of prebiotic substrates to enhance the survival and transient colonisation of probiotic bacteria in the intestinal tract.

In this study, we hypothesised that a carbohydrate fraction (CF) from caprine milk in combination with known probiotic bacterial strains would increase the barrier integrity of a co-culture model of the small intestinal epithelium when compared to either the CF or bacteria alone. A representative co-culture model of the small intestine which incorporated both absorptive enterocytes (Caco-2) and mucin secreting goblet cells (HT29–MTX), in a ratio similar to that of the small intestine (90:10 Caco-2:HT29–MTX) [45] was used because this would typically be the first site of probiotic interaction with the host's intestinal cells and the site at which the host and the microbiota (probiotics) compete for the simple carbohydrates found in milk such as lactose, glucose and galactose. Additionally, because milk oligosaccharides are not absorbed or directly utilised by cells of the small intestine, these components of milk have the potential to influence the adherence and therefore the overall persistence of probiotic bacterial strains in the small intestine. The epithelial barrier integrity (as measured by TEER), the expression levels of genes that encode for TJs and mucins, and the abundance of mucin proteins were measured after 3 h, to determine if selected probiotic bacterial strains in combination with CF had a greater enhancing effect on barrier integrity, when compared to either component alone. A 3 h time point was used in this study as this reflects the transit time of digesta through the small intestine (15 min to 5 h) and as such is biologically relevant. A comparison of the effects on the barrier integrity of the co-culture model could help elucidate the distinct responses of intestinal cells to the combined or specific effects of probiotics or the CF.

2. Materials and Methods

2.1. Composition of Carbohydrate Fraction (CF) and Stock Solutions

The CF used in this study was kindly provided by Caroline Thum (AgResearch, Grasslands, Palmerston North, NZ) [46]. The carbohydrate composition of the CF (as a percentage of total carbohydrates) used in this study was: 25.6% oligosaccharides, 0.4% galacto-oligosaccharides, 46.1% lactose, 12% glucose and 15.9% galactose [47].

In addition to CF, a sugar combination (galactose, glucose and lactose (all from BDH, Global Science, Auckland, NZ)) as well as the monosaccharide galactose and the disaccharide lactose were used at comparable concentrations to that found in the CF. Also two acidic oligosaccharides, 3' and 6' sialyl lactose (both from Carbosynth, Berkshire, UK) were used.

The CF and selected carbohydrates for all experiments were suspended in phosphate buffered saline (PBS, pH 7.2), and filter sterilised (0.22 μm filters; Millipore Australia Pty Ltd., Sydney, Australia). For use in IEC assays, stock carbohydrate solutions were diluted with Dulbecco's Modified Eagles Medium (DMEM; Life Technologies, Penrose, Auckland, NZ). CF was used at a final concentration of 4 mg/mL because this concentration of CF has previously been shown to increase TEER, and *MUC2* and *MUC5AC* mucin gene and protein abundance of 90:10 Caco-2:HT29–MTX co-cultures [47]. The sugar combination, galactose and lactose were used at final concentrations (comparable to those found in the CF) of 3 mg/mL, 0.6 mg/mL and 1.8 mg/mL respectively, whilst 3' and 6' sialyl lactose were both used at 1 mg/mL.

2.2. IEC Co-Culture Conditions

The human colon adenocarcinoma cell line HT29 (HTB-38; ATCC, Manassas, VA, USA) previously adapted with 10^{-7} M methotrexate (MTX) was kindly provided by Rachel Anderson

(AgResearch, Grasslands, Palmerston North, NZ) and further adapted with 10^{-6} M MTX as described previously [48,49]. The human colorectal adenocarcinoma cell line Caco-2 (HTB-37) was obtained from the ATCC at passage 18. The HT29–MTX and Caco-2 cells were used in experiments from passage 18–25 and 28–33 respectively.

Caco-2 and HT29–MTX cells were cultured separately in tissue culture flasks (Corning, Lindfield, Sydney, Australia) in DMEM supplemented with 10% (*v/v*) foetal bovine serum (FBS; Life Technologies, Auckland, NZ) and 1% (*v/v*) Penicillin-Streptomycin (Pen-Strep; 10,000 units/mL Penicillin and 10 mg/mL Streptomycin; Sigma-Aldrich, Auckland, NZ) as described previously [47].

Both Caco-2 and HT29–MTX cells were subcultured when they reached 80% confluence, and re-seeded at a 1:5 dilution into new 75 cm^2 flasks (Corning). The cultures were maintained at 37 °C in a 5% CO_2, 95% air/water saturated atmosphere, with the medium being replaced every 48 h.

For experimental studies, Caco-2 and HT29–MTX cells were stained with trypan blue, counted using the Countess automated cell counter (Life Technologies), suspended at a ratio of 90:10 (Caco-2:HT29–MTX) to simulate the cellular configuration of the small intestine [45] and seeded at a density of 6.3×10^4 cells per cm^2. Co-cultures of IECs were cultured for 21 days. Twenty four hours prior to their use in experiments (day 20 post-seeding) the co-cultures were washed as described previously [47], replenished with serum- and antibiotic-free medium (DMEM) to eliminate any interference from extraneous proteins or hormones [50] and incubated for 24 h.

2.3. Bacterial Strains and Culture Conditions

Four probiotic lactobacilli strains used in this study were originally isolated from human, dairy or food origins; *L. rhamnosus* Goldin and Garbach (LGG; American Type Culture Collection (ATCC) 53103—healthy human faecal sample), *L. plantarum* 299v (Lp299v; Deutsche Sammlung von Mikroorganismen (DSM) 9843—healthy human intestinal mucosa), *L. rhamnosus* HN001 (HN001; Danisco New Zealand Ltd, Auckland, NZ—dairy—cheddar cheese), and *L. casei* Shirota (LcS; Yakult New Zealand, Auckland, NZ—food). These strains were chosen as they are all Generally Recognised As Safe (GRAS) by the United States Food and Drug Administration (FDA) and as such have published data showing their efficacy in in vitro models, animal models, and controlled human trials. For more information refer to the FDA website using the GRAS notice numbers: 231 (LGG), 685 (Lp299v), 288 (HN001), and 429 (LcS). Strains were stored in deMan, Rogosa and Sharpe (MRS) broth (Acumedia, MI, USA) containing 35% glycerol at −80 °C and propagated twice in MRS broth prior to use. All strains were grown overnight at 37 °C in anaerobic broth (MRS flushed with oxygen-free CO_2) using Hungate culture tubes (16 mm diameter, 125 mm long; BellCo glass, Vineland, NJ, USA) sealed with butyl rubber stoppers. For all studies, the bacterial strains were used at stationary growth phase. The time taken for bacteria to enter stationary phase was determined by constructing growth curves by measuring optical density at 600 nm (OD600) using an Ultrspec 1100 pro photometer (Amersham Biosciences, Auckland, NZ) at intervals during growth.

2.4. Bacterial Growth with CF and Selected Carbohydrates

The growth characteristics of each probiotic were assessed in triplicate using Hungate tubes containing DMEM-supplemented with the selected carbohydrate substrate. DMEM was used as the basal media because it is the same media that the Caco-2:HT29–MTX (90:10) co-cultures are typically cultured with. Briefly, 30 µL of stationary phase bacteria from MRS broth cultures was inoculated into the test media. All cultures were incubated in a 5% CO_2, 95% air/water saturated atmosphere at 37 °C. The growth of the bacteria was monitored by measuring optical density at 600 nm at hourly intervals post inoculation, and assessed after 3 h. Prior to absorbance measurements the incubated tubes were inverted three times to suspend any sedimented bacterial cells. The arithmetical median was calculated from all single OD readings and absorbance values at time zero were subtracted from each time point for respective Hungate tubes.

2.5. IEC and Bacterial Cell Co-Cultures

Bacteria from stationary phase cultures were washed by diluting 1:5 in PBS, following centrifugation at 2492× *g* for 5 min (11180/13190 rotor, Sigma 3-18K centrifuge) and re-suspension in DMEM or DMEM supplemented with CF. Approximately 10^7 colony forming units (CFU) were added to each well as ascertained by plate counts.

Caco-2:HT29–MTX (90:10) co-cultures in 24-well tissue-culture plates (Corning), were prepared 24 h prior (day 20 post-seeding) to the adhesion assay as described in Section 2.2. On the day of the assay the co-cultures were gently washed four times with PBS, and to appropriate wells, bacteria-supplemented medium was added and plates incubated at 37 °C in a 5% CO_2 atmosphere for 3 h.

2.6. Adhesion Assays to IEC Co-Cultures

Following incubation, the growth medium was removed, and the co-cultures were gently washed 4 times with PBS to remove any non-adherent bacteria, and lysed with 1 mL of PBS containing 1% (*v*/*v*) Triton X-100 (Sigma-Aldrich) to release adherent bacteria. The lysates were serially diluted with PBS and bacteria enumerated on MRS agar plates as described previously [34]. To determine original CFU/mL aliquots of the experimental inocula were retained, diluted, and plated on MRS agar. To account for variaions in the orginal inocula between strains the results were expressed as adherent bacteria as a percentage of the original inoculum, (CFU/mL of recovered adherent bacteria ÷ CFU/mL of inoculum) × 100. Each adhesion assay was conducted independently in triplicate over two successive passages of IECs.

2.7. Measurement of Metablic Activity of IEC Co-Cultures

The metabolic activity of Caco-2:HT29–MTX (90:10) co-cultures was quantified by absorbance at 450 nm with a reference wavelength of 650 nm (FlexStation 3 Benchtop Multi-Mode Microplate Reader; Molecular Devices, Sunnyvale, CA, USA) using the 4–[3–(4–Iodophenyl)–2–(4–nitrophenyl)–2H–5–tetrazolio]–1,3 benzene disulfonate (Wst-1) colourimetric assay (Roche, Auckland, NZ). In 96-well tissue-culture plates (Corning), post-confluent (21 days post-seeding) Caco-2:HT29–MTX (90:10) co-cultures were incubated for 3 h in carbohydrate-supplemented DMEM media. Additional wells in each plate containing medium and Wst-1 reagent only (without cells) were processed in parallel and used as reference blanks [51,52]. Each substrate was tested in 10 replicates, over three successive passages of IECs. The metabolic activity of the Caco-2:HT29–MTX (90:10) co-cultures was expressed as absorbance (A450 nm–A650 nm).

2.8. TEER Assay

The TEER assays were undertaken as described in [47]. Briefly, Caco-2 and HT29–MTX cells (90:10) were seeded onto 12 mm diameter, 0.4 μm^2 pore size, polyester (PET) Transwell inserts (Corning) and cultured as described in Section 2.2.

Post-confluent, differentiated co-cultures were prepared 24 h prior (day 20 post-seeding) to the TEER assay as described in Section 2.2. After 24 h incubation, initial resistance readings were obtained (EndOhm Culture cup connected to an EVOM voltohmmeter (World Precision Instruments, Sarasota, FL, USA)) for all co-cultures. The medium in the well was replaced with DMEM, and the medium in the Transwell insert was replaced with either DMEM (untreated) or DMEM supplemented with CF (4.0 mg/mL) with or without bacteria. The resistance across each cell monolayer was measured after 3 h, and the percentage change in TEER calculated as described previously [34]. Experiments were undertaken in triplicate (three successive passages of cells), each with three replicates per treatment.

2.9. Mucin Protein Quantification

The abundance of mucin proteins in cell lysate (CL) and spent media (SM) was determined by indirect enzyme linked immunosorbent assay (indirect ELISA) using MUC2 mouse mono-clonal antibody (clone 4A4, 1:250; Creative Biomart, New York, NY, USA), MUC4 mouse mono-clonal antibody (clone 5B12, 1:500; Abnova, Taipei, Taiwan) or MUC5AC mouse mono-clonal antibody (clone 2H7, 1:250; Abnova) and horseradish peroxidase-rabbit anti-mouse immunoglobulin G conjugate (Abcam, Cambridge, UK; 1:5000 dilution for MUC2 and MUC5AC and 1:10,000 dilution for MUC4) as described previously [47]. 3,31,5,51-tetramethylbenzidine (TMB) peroxidase solution (Invitrogen) was added for 0.5 h and stopped with 2N H_2SO_4 (Reagent grade sulphuric acid; Sigma-Aldrich). Using the well scan option on a FlexStation 3 Benchtop Multi-Mode Microplate Reader (Molecular Devices, Sunnyvale, CA, USA) the absorbance was read at 450 nm and the abundance of mucin proteins was calculated from standard curves using MUC2 (Creative Biomart, New York, NY, USA), MUC4 (Abnova) and MUC5AC (Abnova) recombinant proteins as standards. Experiments were undertaken in triplicate (three successive passages of cells), each with three replicates per treatment. Each sample was analysed in duplicate by indirect ELISA.

2.10. Quantification of mRNA of IEC Co-Cultures

The expression of mucin and TJ related genes in Caco-2:HT29–MTX (90:10) co-cultures was quantified using TaqMan quantitative real-time PCR (qPCR). All reagents were obtained from Applied Biosystems (Foster City, CA, USA) unless otherwise stated. The expression of these genes in reference samples (untreated controls) was also quantified. The genes quantified were; *MUC2, MUC4, MUC5AC, TJP1, TJP2,* and *OCLN.* (TaqMan assay IDs Hs.PT.56a.26485553, Hs.PT.56a.5039491, Hs.PT.56a.25473826, Hs.PT.58.39733148, Hs.PT.58.25666947 and Hs.PT.58.24465876 respectively).

Caco-2:HT29–MTX cells (90:10) were seeded into 12-well cell culture plates (Corning). Twenty days post-seeding monolayers were prepared as described in Section 2.2 After 24 h the SM was removed and monolayers washed gently four times with PBS. Pre-warmed, DMEM (untreated) or DMEM supplemented with 4.0 mg/mL CF was gently added to the monolayers either with or without the bacterial strains of interest and cultures incubated for 3 h.

After 3 h the SM was removed and monolayers lysed with 1 mL of Tri-reagent (Invitrogen). The total RNA from each well was isolated as described previously [47] using the RiboPure RNA isolation kit. The total RNA was stored at −80 °C overnight and quantified using a Nanodrop 1000 spectrophotometer (Thermo Fisher Scientific, Auckland, NZ). The integrity of the RNA was measured using an Agilent 2100 Bioanalyser (Agilent Technologies, Santa Clara, CA, USA) to ensure samples had an RNA integrity number (RIN) above 8.0 prior to downstream analysis.

For real-time PCR analysis, 1.5 µg of total RNA was reverse transcribed into cDNA using a high-capacity RNA-to-cDNA Kit (Applied Biosystems) according to the manufacturer's instructions. The cDNA was stored at −20 °C prior to the determination of the expression levels of the six genes, relative to the reference genes hypoxanthine phosphoribosyltransferase [53,54] (*HPRT1*; Hs.PT.39a.22214821), glyceraldehyde 3-phosphate dehydrogenase (*GAPDH*; Hs.PT.39a 22214836) and βeta-2-microglobulin (*B2M*; Hs.PT.58v.18759587) determined using TaqMan probes on the Rotor-Gene 6000 real-time thermal cycler (Corbett Life Science, Concord, Australia). The *ACTB* (Hs.PT.39a.22214847) reference gene was also evaluated but excluded from the final analysis as it did not meet the requirements of a reference gene in all the samples tested [55]. All PCRs (no template controls, untreated, and treated samples) were prepared as triplicate 10 µL reactions as described previously [55]. The thermal profile used was 95 °C for 180 s followed by 40 cycles 95 °C for 3 s and 60 °C for 30 s. The data were normalised to the reference genes and analysed for expression level changes using Relative Expression Software Tool (REST) 2009 software (version 2.0.13; Qiagen, Valencia, CA, USA). Experiments in triplicate were completed (three successive passages of cells), each with three replicates per treatment. Each sample was analysed in triplicate by qPCR.

2.11. Statistical Analysis

Data were first evaluated for normality with the Shapiro-Wilk test, and for equal variance with the Brown-Forsythe test using SigmaPlot 13.0b software. Data that were normally distributed but had heterogeneous variances, such as the bacterial growth and adherence data, were assessed by non-parametric tests, namely the Kruskall–Wallis test, followed by the Mann–Whitney U test. All TEER assay data were analysed for statistical significance, using a repeated measure ANOVA with SigmaPlot 13.0b software. The real-time PCR data was analysed using REST with efficiency correction [45]. For the Wst-1 metabolic activity bioassay and the ELISA protein abundance assay, treatments were compared using an analysis of variance (ANOVA), followed by the Holm–Sidak post-hoc method. Differences were considered statistically different at probability values less than 0.05.

3. Results and Discussion

The aim of this study was to determine the influence of specific combinations of probiotic bacteria and a CF from caprine milk on the barrier integrity of IEC co-cultures. The CF used in this study was a mixture of carbohydrates therefore we first sought to determine whether CF or individual CF components had contrasting impacts on the growth of four probiotic bacteria or the metabolic activity of the IECs. A pure preparation of oligosaccharides could not be obtained using our standard CF purification methods, therefore we used the acidic milk oligosaccharides 3′ and 6′ sialyl lactose as they represent 22% of the oligosaccharides found in the CF [47].

3.1. Selective Carbohydrate Fermentation by Probiotic Lactobacilli

The effect of carbohydrate substrate on the growth of all four probiotic *Lactobacillus* strains when cultured in DMEM (5% CO_2) was examined (Figure 1A–D). Only *L. rhamnosus* GG appeared able to utilise the acidic milk oligosaccharide 6′ sialyl lactose for growth compared to both the media control (DMEM) and CF (Figure 1A). The growth of the remaining three lactobacilli strains during culture in 3′ and 6′ sialyl lactose supplemented media was significantly lower than CF (Figure 1B–D).There was increased growth of *L. rhamnosus* HN001 during incubation with CF, sugar combination and galactose compared to the DMEM control (Figure 1B). Similarly, growth of *L. plantarum* 299v in CF was increased when compared to all other carbohydrate substrates investigated (Figure 1C) suggesting that *L. plantarum* 299v could utilise additional components such as the neutral oligosaccharide N-Acetyl-glucosaminyl-lactose or other acidic oligosaccharides that are present in the CF but not in the sugar combination. *L. plantarum* strain FUA3112 has previously been reported to metabolise neutral oligosaccharides [56].

3.2. Carbohydrates Do not Influence Metabolic Activity of IEC Co-Cultures

Incubation of monolayers with CF or selected carbohydrates for 3 h had no significant effect on the metabolic activity and thus proliferation rates, of post-confluent Caco-2:HT29–MTX (90:10) co-cultures when compared to the media control (DMEM) (Figure 2). A previous study by Kuntz et al. [57] reported that proliferation rates of HT29 and Caco-2 cells was inhibited by neutral oligosaccharides (2.3 and 0.2 mg/mL respectively) and acidic oligosaccharide (0.3 and 0.7 mg/mL respectively) isolated from human milk [57]. In contrast, 1 mg/mL lactose had no effect on the proliferation of primary human foetal intestinal cells [58], but proliferation of the same cell line was increased after exposure to whey produced from bovine colostrum [59] and complete human milk [60]. Thus, it could be suggested that treatment of IECs with purified preparations of neutral or acidic oligosaccharides inhibits cellular proliferation to a greater extent than IECs exposed to treatments comprised of a combination of carbohydrates such as the CF. How this relates to the mechanism of action was not determined in this study, but it is known that neutral and acidic oligosaccharides inhibit proliferation rates of IECs through alterations in epidermal growth factor receptor (EGFR) signalling and cell cycle regulators [58,61], and human milk increases proliferation through a unique tyrosine kinase pathway [60].

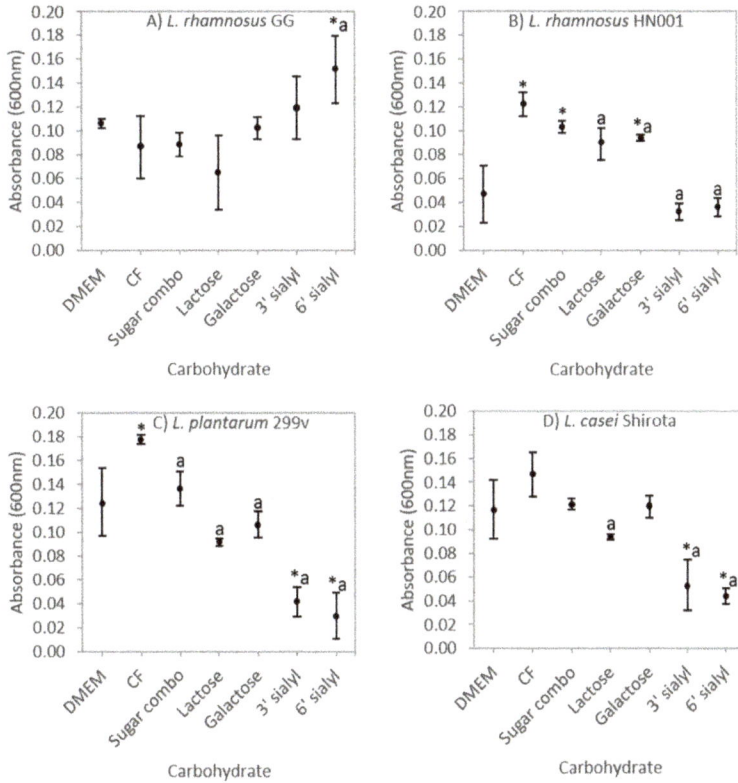

Figure 1. Ability of (**A**) *Lactobacillus rhamnosus* GG, (**B**) *L. rhamnosus* HN001, (**C**) *L. Plantarum* 299v, and (**D**) *L. casei* Shirota to ferment carbohydrates. Bacterial growth (absorbance 600 nm) in Dulbecco's Modified Eagles Medium (DMEM) or DMEM supplemented with a carbohydrate fraction from caprine milk (CF; 4 mg/mL) or selected carbohydrates (at comparable concentrations to those found in the CF—refer to text) as fermentable carbohydrate source as indicated and cultured for 3 h under 5% CO_2 atmospheric conditions. Values represent the mean absorbance (±S.D.); $n = 3$. * = significantly different ($P < 0.05$) to DMEM media control; a = significantly different ($P < 0.05$) to CF.

3.3. CF Modulates Bacterial Adherence to Caco-2:HT29–MTX (90:10) Co-Cultures

There was a marked species-specific difference in adherence of the four probiotic bacterial strains to Caco-2:HT29–MTX (90:10) co-cultures (Figure 3). This result is similar to that observed previously [62]. Although levels of adherence were modulated by the inclusion of CF in the media, only the adherence of *L. rhamnosus* HN001 was significantly reduced (Figure 3). Decreased adherence to the epithelial monolayers in CF-supplemented assay media, such as occurred for *L. rhamnosus* HN001, may have been related to the oligosaccharides in the CF being structurally similar to receptor sites of the IECs or mucus layer to which specific bacteria recognise and adhere. For some bacterial strains, oligosaccharides may act as a molecular receptor decoy inhibiting bacterial adherence [63]. Unfortunately the binding of oligosaccharides to the surface of probiotic bacteria or commensal bacteria is not well investigated, although there is a larger body of work studying glycan binding with pathogenic bacteria [64].

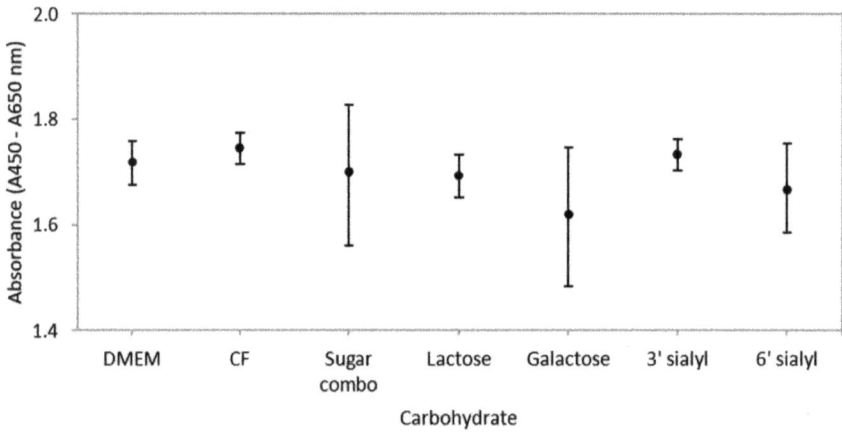

Figure 2. The metabolic activity of post-confluent (21 days post seeding) 90:10 Caco-2:HT29–MTX co-cultures after 3 h incubation with a carbohydrate fraction (CF) from caprine milk (CF; 4 mg/mL) and selected carbohydrates (at comparable concentrations to those found in the CF—refer to text) as determined from the Wst-1 assay. Values are means (±SEM) for three experiments (10 samples per treatment per experiment); $n = 3$. DMEM is the media control.

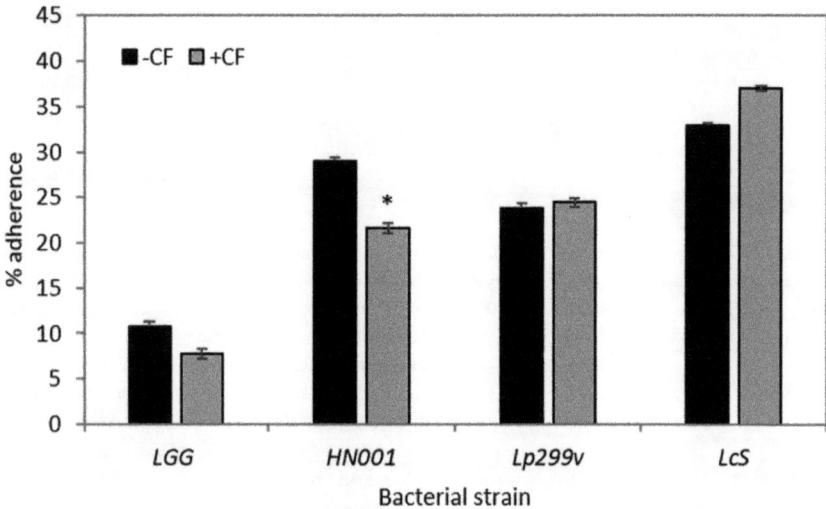

Figure 3. Influence of a carbohydrate fraction (CF) from caprine milk (CF; 4 mg/mL) on the adherence of bacteria (as percentage of inoculum) to 90:10 Caco-2:HT29–MTX co-cultures. Data are expressed as the means (±SEM) for three experiments (three samples per treatment per experiment); $n = 3$. * = Significantly different ($P < 0.05$) to respective bacteria only treated monolayers. LGG = *L. rhamnosus* GG; HN001 = *L. rhamnosus* HN001; Lp299v = *L. plantarum* 299v and LcS = *L. casei* Shirota.

Other strain specific observations have been reported previously for *Lactobacillus* strains; Kadlec et al. [25] reported that the prebiotic substance Orafti P95 increased the adherence of *L. rhamnosus* strain CCDM150 to Caco-2:HT29–MTX (90:10) co-cultures, but decreased the adherence of both *L. rhamnosus* strain CCDM289 and strain CCDM598 to the same co-cultures [25].

Adherence to intestinal surfaces, whether directly to IECs or the mucus layer, and temporary colonisation within the intestine, are considered to be defining activities of a probiotic [62]. For *Lactobacillus* species, both protein and non-protein mediated adherence mechanisms have been reported [65]. For example, *L. rhamnosus* GG possesses mucin binding proteins [66] which are known as one of the effector molecules involved in its adherence to the host [67]. Conversely, the cell surface of *L. rhamnosus* GG contains high molecular weight, galactose rich heteropolymeric exopolysaccharide molecules, which may negatively impact its adherence, possibly by shielding adhesion molecules [68,69]. The binding affinity of bacteria can be modulated by the presence of different sugars on the epithelial surface. For example *L. plantarum* 299v adheres to mannose residues on IECs [70,71]. Adherence of bacteria to biotic or abiotic surfaces can also be influenced by growth temperature, pH of the cultures and the specific growth phase of the bacteria themselves [72,73].

3.4. The Combination of CF and Probiotic Bacteria Increases TEER

After 3 h incubation the TEER of Caco-2:HT29–MTX (90:10) co-cultures was increased for all individual bacteria/CF combinations compared to untreated, CF and also to the respective bacteria only control, except for the *L. rhamnosus* GG/CF combination (Figure 4). Only co-cultures treated with *L. casei* Shirota had similar TEER compared to untreated (Figure 4).

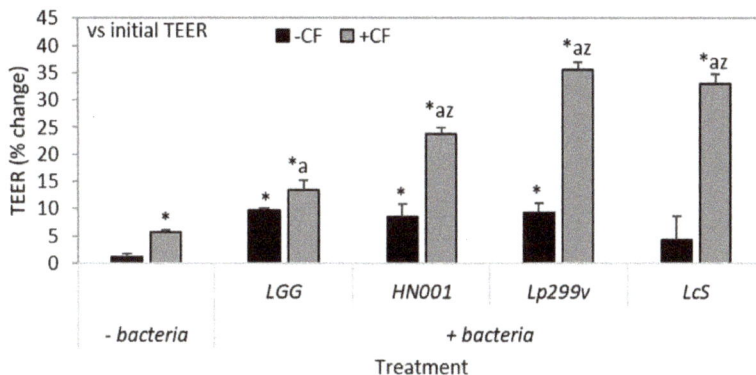

Figure 4. Influence of a carbohydrate fraction (CF) from caprine milk (CF; 4 mg/mL) and probiotic bacteria either alone or in combination on trans-epithelial electrical resistance (TEER) of 90:10 Caco-2:HT29–MTX co-cultures. The change in TEER as the percentage change after 3 h compared with initial TEER. Values are means (±SEM) for three experiments (three samples per treatment per experiment); $n = 3$. * = Significantly different ($P < 0.05$) to untreated monolayers; a = significantly different ($P < 0.05$) to CF treated monolayers; and z = significantly different ($P < 0.05$) to respective bacteria only treated monolayers. UNT = untreated; LGG = *L. rhamnosus* GG; HN001 = *L. rhamnosus* HN001; Lp299v = *L. plantarum* 299v and LcS = *L. casei* Shirota.

Similar to that of bacterial adherence, the effect of bacteria/CF combinations on TEER was strain-dependent (Figure 4). This observation is concordant with other studies where *L. plantarum* strain 299 had a greater effect on enhancing the TEER of Caco-2 cells compared to *L. plantarum* strain 299v [34]. In addition, a previous study using Caco-2 mono-cultures, determined that there were definite species- and sugar-dependent effects with fermentation of inulin based oligofructose [74,75] where the probiotic *B. lactis* Bb-12 exerted the most beneficial effects [75]. In another study, the synbiotic combination of resistant starch and *B. lactis* (strain unknown), protected against the development of colorectal cancer in rats, and was greater than the benefit of either component alone [76].

3.5. CF and Bacteria When Cultured Alone or in Combination Impacts on TJ Related Gene Expression

The ability of CF and probiotic lactobacilli either alone or in combination to alter the expression level of three TJ related genes of Caco-2:HT29MTX (90:10) co-cultures was quantified using qPCR. The mRNA expression of *OCLN*, but not *TJP1* or *TJP2*, was increased (fold change >1.5) by all bacterial strains, both alone and when in combination with CF, compared to untreated monolayers (Figure 5A,B), but not when compared to CF (Figure 5C) or their respective bacteria controls (Figure 5D). This result is in accordance with Orlando et al. [77] where incubation of Caco-2 cells with *L. rhamnosus* GG over a 6 h period increased *OCLN* expression levels. Increased expression or abundance of occludin is associated with protection of the epithelial barrier, whilst decreased occludin levels are associated with epithelial barrier dysfunction and increased epithelial permeability [11]. Additionally a study by Yan et al. [78] determined that the colonisation of neonatal mice with *L. rhamnosus* GG resulted in increased claudin 3 mRNA expression and TJP1 membrane localisation in the ileum, in addition to increased proliferation and differentiation of epithelial cells indicating that *L. rhamnosus* GG colonisation is beneficial for intestinal growth and development during early life and promotes intestinal functional maturation and tight junction formation [78].

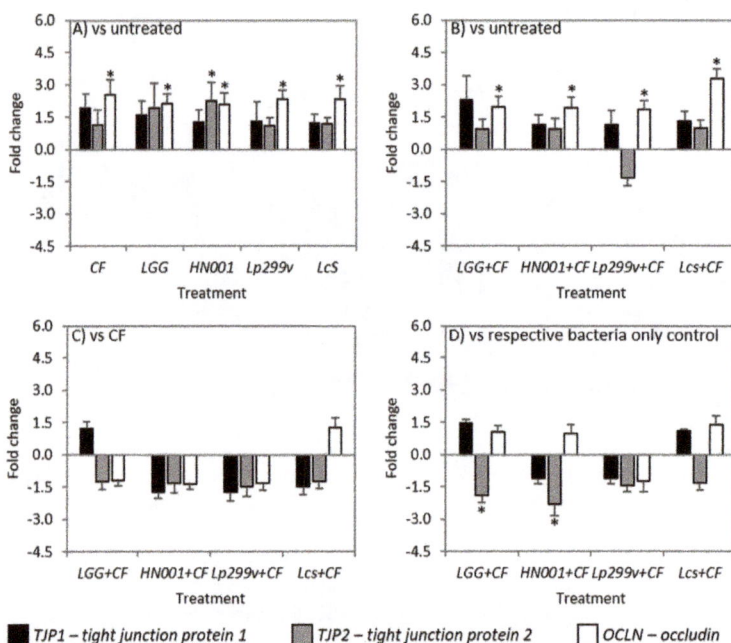

Figure 5. Fold change of *TJP1*, *TJP2*, and *OCLN* mRNA from Caco-2:HT29–MTX (90:10) co-cultures after 3 h incubation with (**A**) probiotic bacteria or a carbohydrate fraction (CF) relative to untreated co-cultures; (**B**) bacteria/CF combinations compared to untreated monolayers; (**C**) bacteria/CF combinations compared to monolayers incubated with CF; and (**D**) bacteria/CF combinations relative to bacteria only controls. Data are expressed as the mean fold change (±SEM) of three replicates across three independent experiments; $n = 3$ A statistically significant difference in fold change at ±1.5 is indicated by * ($P < 0.05$). LGG = *L. rhamnosus* GG; HN001 = *L. rhamnosus* HN001; Lp299v = *L. plantarum* 299v and LcS = *L. casei* Shirota.

In this study, levels of *TJP1* mRNA did not change as a result of any treatment (Figure 5A–D). This result is similar to those findings of Yang et al. [74] where the expression and abundance of *TJP1* were unchanged in IPEC-J2 cells after incubation with *L. reuteri* I5007. Caco-2:HT29–MTX (90:10) co-cultures incubated with *L. rhamnosus* HN001 had increased levels of *TJP2* mRNA compared to untreated (Figure 5A). Treatment of co-cultures with *L. rhamnosus* GG and *L. rhamnosus* HN001 in combination with CF resulted in decreased ($P < 0.05$) levels of *TJP2* mRNA compared to treatment of co-cultures with bacteria alone (Figure 5D).

Changes to other TJ components not measured in this study may also account for the observed increases in TEER. For example, the intracellular plaque protein cingulin, which binds directly to TJP1 as well as to actin filaments of the cytoskeleton [79], contributed to an increase in TEER of Caco-2 monolayers after treatment with *L. plantarum* MB452 [33]. Other important transmembrane TJ proteins such as claudin 1, also interact directly with TJP1, the upregulation of which was observed in jejunal epithelium of young piglets after treatment with *L. reuteri* I5007 [74]. Similarly, treatment of mice with *L. rhamnosus* GG increased the abundance levels of both claudin-1 and claudin-3 protein [80].

There are different mechanisms through which probiotic bacteria can enhance the intestinal barrier and include:

1. The secretion of bacterial proteins such as the p40 and p75 proteins secreted by *L. rhamnosus* GG [81], leading to the activation of protein kinase C (PKC) and the mitogen activated protein (MAP) kinases, extracellular signal-regulated kinases (ERK) 1/2 [36] and enhanced TJ expression;
2. Increased phosphorylation levels and activation of p38, MAPK, and ERK signalling pathways [82,83] resulting in a reorganisation of the TJ complex and an increase in the expression levels of TJ proteins, following treatment with the probiotic mix *VSL#3* [82];
3. Directly modulating the function of epithelial cells by increasing TEER with a corresponding increase in the expression of *TJP1* and *OCLN* after administration of live probiotic strains such as *L. rhamnosus* GG or *L. plantarum* [77,84]; and
4. An increase in occludin and TJP1 in the vicinity of TJ structures of the duodenum following activation of the Toll-like receptor 2 signalling pathway by *L. plantarum* WCFS1 [11].

Although the direct effects of carbohydrate substrates, such as prebiotics, on the intestinal epithelium have been largely unexplored, a study by Wu et al. [13] demonstrated that prebiotics directly activate PKC, resulting in the induction of select TJs such as *OCLN* or *TJP1*, and as such can directly alter TJ expressions to affect epithelial barrier function. Additionally, prebiotics directly alter kinase activities (the kinome) of IECs to regulate host signalling pathways [85]. This suggests that carbohydrate substrates can directly act on the intestinal epithelium and elicit specific cell signalling responses and directly modulate intestinal homeostasis. Whether the combined effects of probiotic lactobacilli and CF act independently or synergistically on the same pathways for the enhancement of the intestinal barrier needs further exploration.

3.6. CF and Bacteria When Cultured Alone or in Combination Had Variable Effects on Mucins

Mucins are an important aspect of the protective capacity of the intestinal barrier. Probiotic bacteria either alone or in association with CF had contrasting effects on mucin gene and protein expression. Although the levels of mucin mRNA were modulated by some bacteria/CF combinations, this did not always translate to concomitant changes in the abundance of the respective mucin proteins.

Treatments were shown to have variable effects on mucin gene expression levels, although CF did not change the levels of any mucin gene investigated compared to untreated co-cultures (Figure 6A). Previously we reported that CF increased *MUC2* and *MUC5AC* gene expression levels in Caco-2:HT29–MTX (90:10) co-cultures [47] after 12 h incubation, whilst a study by Martinez-Augustin et al. [86] reported that levels of *MUC2* and *MUC4* expression was decreased in HT29–MTX cells after exposure to a goat's milk fraction enriched with oligosaccharides, suggesting increased exposure times of IECs to carbohydrates can have differential effects on mucin gene expression [86]. In contrast, co-cultures incubated with *L. rhamnosus* GG had increased levels of *MUC4*, *MUC2* and *MUC5AC* mRNA compared to untreated co-cultures. An increase in *MUC2* mRNA has previously been shown for the goblet cell line LS174T after 6 h incubation with *L. rhamnosus* GG [87]. This increase resulted from the activation of the EGFR/Akt pathway by the soluble protein p40 produced by *L. rhamnosus* GG, suggesting that this strain does not need to be adhered to the cells to stimulate mucin gene expression. Although Caco-2:HT29–MTX (90:10) co-cultures incubated with *L. rhamnosus* HN001 also had increased levels of all mucin mRNA investigated, only that of *MUC5AC* mRNA was significantly increased compared to untreated (Figure 6A). The expression levels of all mucin genes were similar between co-cultures incubated with *L. casei* Shirota and untreated, whilst incubation with *L. plantarum* 299v resulted in decreased levels of both *MUC2* and *MUC5AC* mRNA (Figure 6A). This result was in contrast to the study of Mack et al. [88] who showed that incubation of HT29 cells with *L. plantarum* 299v increased the expression of both *MUC2* and *MUC3* mRNA. This difference could be attributed to the use of cell co-cultures in this study as opposed to a monoculture of predominantly undifferentiated HT29 cells. Only the combination of *L. casei* Shirota/CF was associated with a decrease in the level of *MUC2* mRNA compared to untreated co-cultures (Figure 6B). This observation may be due to the combined effects of both CF and *L. casei* Shirota, because individually both treatments were noted to cause a decrease in *MUC2* mRNA although these decreases on their own were not significant. All other bacteria/CF combinations had similar levels of *MUC4*, *MUC2* and *MUC5AC* mRNA compared to untreated co-cultures (Figure 6B).

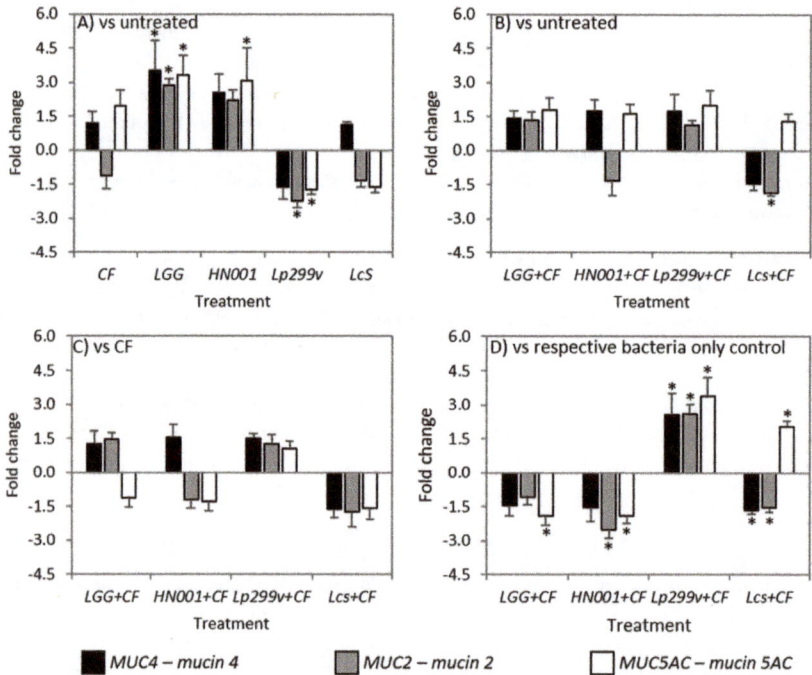

Figure 6. Fold change of *MUC4*, *MUC2*, and *MUC5AC* mRNA from Caco-2:HT29–MTX (90:10) co-cultures after 3 h incubation with (**A**) probiotic bacteria or a carbohydrate fraction (CF) relative to untreated co-cultures; (**B**) bacteria/CF combinations compared to untreated monolayers; (**C**) bacteria/CF combinations compared to monolayers incubated with CF; and (**D**) bacteria/CF combinations relative to bacteria only controls. Data are expressed as the mean fold change ($\pm$ SEM) of three replicates across three independent experiments; $n = 3$ A statistically significant difference in fold change at ± 1.5 is indicated by * ($P < 0.05$). LGG = *L. rhamnosus* GG; HN001 = *L. rhamnosus* HN001; Lp299v = *L. plantarum* 299v and LcS = *L. casei* Shirota.

Similar to that observed for TJ related gene expression, there was no difference in the levels of mucin mRNA between any bacteria/CF combinations and CF treated Caco-2:HT29–MTX (90:10) co-cultures (Figure 6C). However, it was of interest that the level of *MUC2* and *MUC5AC* mRNA between CF and the *L. plantarum* 299v/CF treated co-cultures were not different considering the decrease in the expression of these genes after incubation with *L. plantarum* 299v alone. This suggests that the CF when in combination with *L. plantarum* 299v abrogates the detrimental effect of this bacterial strain on the expression of these genes. Although the mechanisms through which CF when in combination with lactobacilli modulates mucin gene expression were not investigated in this study, previous reports have shown that neutral and acidic oligosaccharides from human milk activate EGFR [61], and that activation of EGFR and its downstream targets by probiotic lactobacilli stimulate mucin gene expression [87].

In comparison to co-cultures incubated with *L. rhamnosus* HN001, co-cultures incubated with the *L. rhamnosus* HN001/CF combination had decreased levels of both *MUC2* and *MUC5AC* mRNA. This result indicates that the CF abrogates the beneficial effect of *L. rhamnosus* HN001 in respect to *MUC5AC* mRNA and has an additive detrimental effect on the expression of *MUC2* mRNA (Figure 6D). The combination of *L. casei* Shirota/CF was associated with decreased levels of both *MUC4* and *MUC2* mRNA compared to *L. casei* Shirota alone (Figure 6D), the decrease of *MUC2* which could be attributed to an additive effect of the bacteria and the CF, whilst the decrease of *MUC4* could be viewed as a combined effect. In contrast the levels of *MUC5AC* mRNA were increased for *L. casei* Shirota/CF compared to its bacteria control. Additionally, the levels of all the mucin genes investigated were increased in co-cultures incubated with the *L. plantarum* 299v/CF combination compared to co-cultures incubated with *L. plantarum* 299v alone (Figure 6D), the result of which was not unexpected because *L. plantarum* 299v alone was shown to reduce the expression of all mucin mRNA when compared to untreated co-cultures.

The abundance of MUC2 mucin protein was similar for all monolayers after incubation with any bacteria/CF treatment. In contrast, all bacteria/CF preparations were shown to increase the abundance of MUC5AC compared to untreated co-cultures, except those treated with *L. rhamnosus* HN001. Additionally, monolayers treated with the *L. rhamnosus* HN001/CF combination had an increased relative abundance of MUC5AC protein compared to its respective bacteria control (Figure 7). There was no difference in the abundance of MUC5AC protein between co-cultures incubated with CF and any of the bacteria/CF combinations, but there was a significant increase in the abundance of this protein in CF treated co-cultures compared to untreated (Figure 7). Only Caco-2:HT29–MTX (90:10) co-cultures treated with the combination of *L. plantarum* 299v/CF had an increased MUC4 abundance compared to both untreated and respective bacteria alone co-cultures. However, there was no increase in the relative abundance of MUC4 in co-cultures treated with CF compared to untreated co-cultures (Figure 7). The abundance of MUC4 was similar for all other treatment groups. Wan et al. [89] suggested that the disparity between the changes in the levels of mucin genes and respective mucin proteins levels, such as occurred for the *L. rhamnosus* HN001/CF combination may be attributable to "methods used for quantifying mRNA transcripts levels are more sensitive than those for protein identification and quantification".

An increase in mucin abundance following incubation with probiotic lactobacilli when compared to untreated co-cultures could potentially enhance their ability to colonise the intestinal tract [39]. However, there was no association between changes in the abundance of specific mucin proteins which resulted in the modulation of bacterial adherence. Such interactions do exist between the lactic acid bacteria, *Lactococcus lactis* subsp. *lactis* BGKP1 and MUC3 and MUC5AC proteins, which aids in the adherence of this bacterial species to the mucus layer [90].

Only the *L. plantarum* 299v/CF combination was associated with an increased abundance of MUC4 mucin protein compared to its respective bacterial control (Figure 7). Membrane-bound mucins such as MUC4, are major components of the glycocalyx, and in addition to their role in providing a physical barrier, are also involved in a wide range of interactions in the luminal environment [91] (such as intracellular signalling events [8]), and play an important role in foetal development, epithelial renewal and differentiation, and epithelial integrity [92,93].

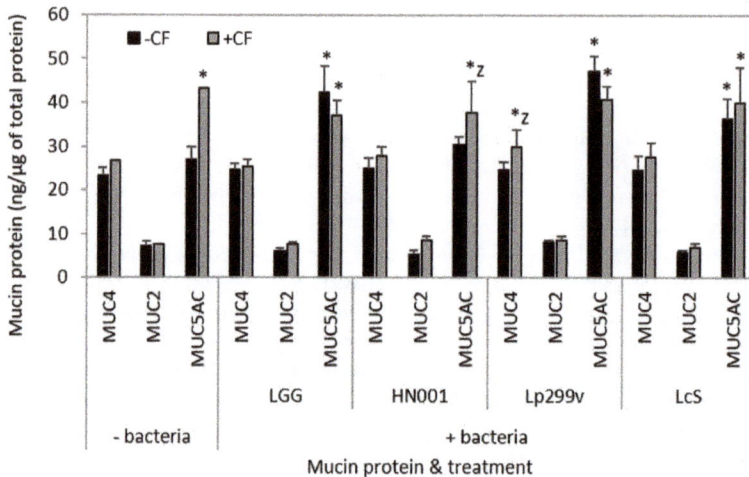

Figure 7. The abundance of MUC4, MUC2 and MUC5AC mucin protein from Caco-2:HT29–MTX (90:10) co-cultures after 3 h incubation with bacteria or a carbohydrate fraction (CF) from caprine milk either alone or in combination. Results are expressed as the mean abundance (±SEM); $n = 3$. * =significantly different ($P < 0.05$) compared to untreated co-cultures, and z = significantly different ($P < 0.05$) compared to co-cultures incubated with the respective bacteria only. UNT = untreated; LGG = *L. rhamnosus* GG; HN001 = *L. rhamnosus* HN001; Lp299v = *L. plantarum* 299v; and LcS = *L. casei* Shirota.

Binding of bacteria to the extracellular domain of membrane mucins can result in cleavage of the mucin. Such cleavage could be an activation signal to the intracellular domain and activation of mucin-specific signalling pathways that alter inflammatory responses, epithelial cell adhesion, and differentiation of epithelial cells [94]. Although the relationship between bacterial binding, cleavage of mucins and activation of the intracellular domain has not been fully elucidated, membrane-bound mucins may act as signalling receptors that sense the external environment and activate intracellular signal transduction pathways essential for barrier maintenance and damage repair [94]. Additionally, the secretion of mucins from goblet cells can be regulated by the host sensing intestinal microbes or their metabolites such as SCFAs or cytokines [95].

4. Conclusions

This work demonstrates that probiotic bacteria, when used in combination with CF, are able to increase the barrier integrity to a greater extent than the bacteria or the CF alone, in a Caco-2: HT29–MTX (90:10) co-culture model of the small intestinal epithelium. The precise mechanism through which barrier integrity was increased could not clearly be linked to changes in IEC metabolism associated with CF utilisation, or enhanced mucin gene or protein expression. However, both barrier integrity (TEER) and transcription levels of occludin were enhanced during incubation of co-cultures with bacteria and CF. Global analysis of mRNA and proteins from co-cultures incubated with CF or bacteria alone, and compared to mRNA from co-cultures incubated with CF and bacteria may provide important information on contrasting inter, and intra-cellular signalling cascades and IEC immunomodulation influenced by probiotic bacteria and/or dietary carbohydrates.

Author Contributions: Conceptualisation, A.M.B., N.C.R., A.L.C., and W.C.M.; Methodology, A.M.B.; Formal Analysis, A.M.B.; Investigation, A.M.B, and A.L.C.; Writing—Original Draft Preparation, A.M.B.; Writing—Review & Editing, N.C.R, A.L.C., and W.C.M.; Supervision, A.L.C.; Project Administration, W.C.M.; Funding Acquisition, N.C.R., A.L.C, and W.C.M.

Funding: Riddet Institute Centre of Research Excellence (CoRE) and AgResearch Core funding for the AB PhD scholarship and research costs.

Acknowledgments: Alicia M. Barnett acknowledges the Riddet Institute Centre of Research Excellence (CoRE) and AgResearch Core funding for the PhD scholarship and research cost. The authors would like to thank Mark McCann for technical help with qPCR; Rachel Anderson and Dulantha Ulluwishewa for manuscript reviewing.

Conflicts of Interest: The authors declare no conflict of interest.

References

1. Pereira, P.C. Milk nutritional composition and its role in human health. *Nutrition* **2014**, *30*, 619–627. [CrossRef] [PubMed]

2. Muehlhoff, E.; Bennett, A.; MacMahon, D. *Milk and Dairy Products in Human Nutrition*; Food and Agriculture Organization of the United Nations: Rome, Italy, 2013.

3. Martinez-Ferez, A.; Rudloff, S.; Guadix, A.; Henkel, C.A.; Pohlentz, G.; Boza, J.J.; Guadix, E.M.; Kunz, C. Goats' milk as a natural source of lactose-derived oligosaccharides: Isolation by membrane technology. *Int. Dairy J.* **2006**, *16*, 173–181. [CrossRef]

4. Donovan, S.M. Role of human milk components in gastrointestinal development: Current knowledge and future NEEDS. *J. Pediatr.* **2006**, *149*, S49–S61. [CrossRef]

5. Veereman-Wauters, G. Neonatal gut development and postnatal adaptation. *Eur. J. Pediatr.* **1996**, *155*, 627–632. [CrossRef] [PubMed]

6. Halpern, M.D.; Denning, P.W. The role of intestinal epithelial barrier function in the development of NEC. *Tissue Barriers* **2015**, *3*, e1000707. [CrossRef] [PubMed]

7. Gouyer, V.; Wiede, A.; Buisine, M.-P.; Dekeyser, S.; Moreau, O.; Lesuffleur, T.; Hoffmann, W.; Huet, G. Specific secretion of gel-forming mucins and TFF peptides in HT-29 cells of mucin-secreting phenotype. *BBA Mol. Cell Res.* **2001**, *1539*, 71–84. [CrossRef]

8. Hasnain, S.Z.; Evans, C.M.; Roy, M.; Gallagher, A.L.; Kindrachuk, K.N.; Barron, L.; Dickey, B.F.; Wilson, M.S.; Wynn, T.A.; Grencis, R.K.; et al. Muc5ac: A critical component mediating the rejection of enteric nematodes. *J. Exp. Med.* **2011**, *208*, 893–900. [CrossRef] [PubMed]

9. McGuckin, M.A.; Eri, R.; Simms, L.A.; Florin, T.H.; Radford-Smith, G. Intestinal barrier dysfunction in inflammatory bowel diseases. *Inflamm. Bowel Dis.* **2009**, *15*, 100–113. [CrossRef] [PubMed]

10. Ulluwishewa, D.; Anderson, R.C.; Young, W.; McNabb, W.C.; van Baarlen, P.; Moughan, P.J.; Wells, J.M.; Roy, N.C. Live *Faecalibacterium prausnitzii* in an apical anaerobic model of the intestinal epithelial barrier. *Cell. Microbiol.* **2015**, *17*, 226–240. [CrossRef] [PubMed]

11. Karczewski, J.; Troost, F.J.; Konings, I.; Dekker, J.; Kleerebezem, M.; Brummer, R.-J.M.; Wells, J.M. Regulation of human epithelial tight junction proteins by *Lactobacillus plantarum* in vivo and protective effects on the epithelial barrier. *Am. J. Physiol. Gastrointest. Liver Physiol.* **2010**, *298*, G851–G859. [CrossRef] [PubMed]

12. De Santis, S.; Cavalcanti, E.; Mastronardi, M.; Jirillo, E.; Chieppa, M. Nutritional Keys for Intestinal Barrier Modulation. *Front. Immunol.* **2015**, *6*, 612. [CrossRef] [PubMed]

13. Wu, R.Y.; Abdullah, M.; Määttänen, P.; Pilar, A.V.C.; Scruten, E.; Johnson-Henry, K.C.; Napper, S.; O'Brien, C.; Jones, N.L.; Sherman, P.M. Protein kinase C δ signaling is required for dietary prebiotic-induced strengthening of intestinal epithelial barrier function. *Sci. Rep.* **2017**, *7*, 40820. [CrossRef] [PubMed]

14. Chin, A.M.; Hill, D.R.; Aurora, M.; Spence, J.R. Morphogenesis and maturation of the embryonic and postnatal intestine. *Semin. Cell Dev. Biol.* **2017**, *66*, 81–93. [CrossRef] [PubMed]

15. Aagaard, K.; Ma, J.; Antony, K.M.; Ganu, R.; Petrosino, J.; Versalovic, J. The Placenta Harbors a Unique Microbiome. *Sci. Transl. Med.* **2014**, *6*, 237ra65. [CrossRef] [PubMed]

16. Dominguez-Bello, M.G.; Costello, E.K.; Contreras, M.; Magris, M.; Hidalgo, G.; Fierer, N.; Knight, R. Delivery mode shapes the acquisition and structure of the initial microbiota across multiple body habitats in newborns. *Proc. Natl. Acad. Sci. USA* **2010**, *107*, 11971–11975. [CrossRef] [PubMed]

17. Pacheco, A.R.; Barile, D.; Underwood, M.A.; Mills, D.A. The Impact of the Milk Glycobiome on the Neonate Gut Microbiota. *Annu. Rev. Anim. Biosci.* **2015**, *3*, 419–445. [CrossRef] [PubMed]

18. Kleessen, B.; Hartmann, L.; Blaut, M. Fructans in the diet cause alterations of intestinal mucosal architecture, released mucins and mucosa-associated bifidobacteria in gnotobiotic rats. *Br. J. Nutr.* **2003**, *89*, 597–606. [CrossRef] [PubMed]

19. Van den Abbeele, P.; Gérard, P.; Rabot, S.; Bruneau, A.; El Aidy, S.; Derrien, M.; Kleerebezem, M.; Zoetendal, E.G.; Smidt, H.; Verstraete, W.; et al. Arabinoxylans and inulin differentially modulate the mucosal and luminal gut microbiota and mucin-degradation in humanized rats. *Environ. Microbiol.* **2011**, *13*, 2667–2680. [CrossRef] [PubMed]

20. Leforestier, G.; Blais, A.; Blachier, F.; Marsset-Baglieri, A.; Davila-Gay, A.-M.; Perrin, E.; Tomé, D. Effects of galacto-oligosaccharide ingestion on the mucosa-associated mucins and sucrase activity in the small intestine of mice. *Eur. J. Clin. Nutr.* **2009**, *48*, 457–464. [CrossRef] [PubMed]

21. Walker, W.A. The importance of appropriate initial bacterial colonization of the intestine in newborn, child, and adult health. *Pediatr. Res.* **2017**, *82*, 387. [CrossRef] [PubMed]

22. Raynal-Ljutovac, K.; Lagriffoul, G.; Paccard, P.; Guillet, I.; Chilliard, Y. Composition of goat and sheep milk products: An update. *Small Rumin. Res.* **2008**, *79*, 57–72. [CrossRef]

23. Macfarlane, S.; Macfarlane, G.T. Composition and Metabolic Activities of Bacterial Biofilms Colonizing Food Residues in the Human Gut. *Appl. Environ. Microbiol.* **2006**, *72*, 6204–6211. [CrossRef] [PubMed]

24. Kavanaugh, D.W.; O'Callaghan, J.; Buttó, L.F.; Slattery, H.; Lane, J.; Clyne, M.; Kane, M.; Joshi, L.; Hickey, R.M. Exposure of *Bifidobacterium longum* subsp. *infantis* to Milk Oligosaccharides Increases Adhesion to Epithelial Cells and Induces a Substantial Transcriptional Response. *PLoS ONE* **2013**, *8*, e67224. [CrossRef] [PubMed]

25. Kadlec, R.; Jakubec, M. The effect of prebiotics on adherence of probiotics. *J. Dairy Sci.* **2014**, *97*, 1983–1990. [CrossRef] [PubMed]

26. Collins, M.D.; Gibson, G.R. Probiotics, prebiotics, and synbiotics: Approaches for modulating the microbial ecology of the gut. *Am. J. Clin. Nutr.* **1999**, *69*, 1052S–1057S. [CrossRef] [PubMed]

27. Donaldson, G.P.; Lee, S.M.; Mazmanian, S.K. Gut biogeography of the bacterial microbiota. *Nat. Rev. Microbiol.* **2016**, *14*, 20–32. [CrossRef] [PubMed]

28. Derrien, M.; van Hylckama Vlieg, J.E.T. Fate, activity, and impact of ingested bacteria within the human gut microbiota. *Trends Microbiol.* **2015**, *23*, 354–366. [CrossRef] [PubMed]

29. Hove, H.; Noergaard, H.; Mortensen, P.B. Lactic acid bacteria and the human gastrointestinal tract. *Eur. J. Clin. Nutr.* **1999**, *53*, 339–350. [CrossRef] [PubMed]

30. Johansson, M.L.; Molin, G.; Jeppsson, B.; Nobaek, S.; Ahrné, S.; Bengmark, S. Administration of different *Lactobacillus* strains in fermented oatmeal soup: In vivo colonization of human intestinal mucosa and effect on the indigenous flora. *Appl. Environ. Microbiol.* **1993**, *59*, 15–20. [PubMed]

31. Robins-Browne, R.M.; Levine, M.M. The fate of ingested lactobacilli in the proximal small intestine. *Am. J. Clin. Nutr.* **1981**, *34*, 514–519. [CrossRef] [PubMed]

32. Blackwood, B.P.; Yuan, C.Y.; Wood, D.R.; Nicolas, J.D.; Grothaus, J.S.; Hunter, C.J. Probiotic Lactobacillus Species Strengthen Intestinal Barrier Function and Tight Junction Integrity in Experimental Necrotizing Enterocolitis. *J. Probiotics Health* **2017**, *5*, 159. [CrossRef] [PubMed]

33. Anderson, R.C.; Cookson, A.L.; McNabb, W.C.; Park, Z.; McCann, M.J.; Kelly, W.J.; Roy, N.C. *Lactobacillus plantarum* MB452 enhances the function of the intestinal barrier by increasing the expression levels of genes involved in tight junction formation. *BMC Microbiol.* **2010**, *10*, 316. [CrossRef] [PubMed]

34. Anderson, R.C.; Cookson, A.L.; McNabb, W.C.; Kelly, W.J.; Roy, N.C. *Lactobacillus plantarum* DSM 2648 is a potential probiotic that enhances intestinal barrier function. *FEMS Microbiol. Lett.* **2010**, *309*, 184–192. [CrossRef] [PubMed]

35. Sultana, R.; McBain, A.J.; O'Neill, C.A. Strain-Dependent Augmentation of Tight-Junction Barrier Function in Human Primary Epidermal Keratinocytes by *Lactobacillus* and *Bifidobacterium* Lysates. *Appl. Environ. Microbiol.* **2013**, *79*, 4887–4894. [CrossRef] [PubMed]

36. Seth, A.; Yan, F.; Polk, D.B.; Rao, R.K. Probiotics ameliorate the hydrogen peroxide-induced epithelial barrier disruption by a PKC- and MAP kinase-dependent mechanism. *Am. J. Physiol. Gastrointest. Liver Physiol.* **2008**, *294*, G1060–G1069. [CrossRef] [PubMed]

37. Madsen, K.; Cornish, A.; Soper, P.; McKaigney, C.; Jijon, H.; Yachimec, C.; Doyle, J.; Jewell, L.; De Simone, C. Probiotic Bacteria Enhance Murine and Human Intestinal Epithelial Barrier Function. *Gastroenterology* **2001**, *121*, 580–591. [CrossRef] [PubMed]

38. Resta-Lenert, S.; Barrett, K.E. Live probiotics protect intestinal epithelial cells from the effects of infection with enteroinvasive *Escherichia coli* (EIEC). *Gut* **2003**, *52*, 988–997. [CrossRef] [PubMed]

39. Caballero-Franco, C.; Keller, K.; De Simone, C.; Chadee, K. The VSL#3 probiotic formula induces mucin gene expression and secretion in colonic epithelial cells. *Am. J. Physiol. Gastrointest. Liver Physiol.* **2007**, *292*, G315–G322. [PubMed]

40. Coconnier, M.H.; Klaenhammer, T.R.; Kerneis, S.; Bernet, M.F.; Servin, A.L. Protein-mediated adhesion of *Lactobacillus acidophilus* BG2FO4 on human enterocyte and mucus-secreting cell lines in culture. *Appl. Environ. Microbiol.* **1992**, *58*, 2034–2039. [PubMed]

41. Laparra, J.M.; Sanz, Y. Comparison of in vitro models to study bacterial adhesion to the intestinal epithelium. *Lett. Appl. Microbiol.* **2009**, *49*, 695–701. [CrossRef] [PubMed]

42. Bernet, M.F.; Brassart, D.; Neeser, J.R.; Servin, A.L. Adhesion of human bifidobacterial strains to cultured human intestinal epithelial cells and inhibition of enteropathogen-cell interactions. *Appl. Environ. Microbiol.* **1993**, *59*, 4121–4128. [PubMed]

43. Chichlowski, M.; De Lartigue, G.; German, J.B.; Raybould, H.E.; Mills, D.A. Bifidobacteria Isolated From Infants and Cultured on Human Milk Oligosaccharides Affect Intestinal Epithelial Function. *J. Pediatr. Gastroenterol. Nutr.* **2012**, *55*, 321–327. [CrossRef] [PubMed]

44. Wickramasinghe, S.; Pacheco, A.R.; Lemay, D.G.; Mills, D.A. Bifidobacteria grown on human milk oligosaccharides downregulate the expression of inflammation-related genes in Caco-2 cells. *BMC Microbiol.* **2015**, *15*, 172. [CrossRef] [PubMed]

45. Hilgendorf, C.; Spahn-Langguth, H.; Regårdh, C.G.; Lipka, E.; Amidon Gordon, L.; Langguth, P. Caco-2 versus caco-2/HT29-MTX co-cultured cell lines: Permeabilities via diffusion, inside- and outside-directed carrier-mediated transport. *J. Pharm. Sci.* **2000**, *89*, 63–75. [CrossRef]

46. Thum, C.; Cookson, A.; McNabb, W.C.; Roy, N.C.; Otter, D. Composition and enrichment of caprine milk oligosaccharides from New Zealand Saanen goat cheese whey. *J. Food Compos. Anal.* **2015**, *42*, 30–37. [CrossRef]

47. Barnett, A.M.; Roy, N.C.; McNabb, W.C.; Cookson, A.L. Effect of a Semi-Purified Oligosaccharide-Enriched Fraction from Caprine Milk on Barrier Integrity and Mucin Production of Co-Culture Models of the Small and Large Intestinal Epithelium. *Nutrients* **2016**, *8*, 267. [CrossRef] [PubMed]

48. Lesuffleur, T.; Barbat, A.; Dussaulx, E.; Zweibaum, A. Growth Adaptation to Methotrexate of HT-29 Human Colon Carcinoma Cells Is Associated with Their Ability to Differentiate into Columnar Absorptive and Mucus-secreting Cells. *Cancer Res.* **1990**, *50*, 6334–6343. [PubMed]

49. Lesuffleur, T.; Barbat, A.; Luccioni, C.; Beaumatin, J.; Clair, M.; Kornowski, A.; Dussaulx, E.; Dutrillaux, B.; Zweibaum, A. Dihydrofolate reductase gene amplification-associated shift of differentiation in methotrexate-adapted HT-29 cells. *J. Cell Biol.* **1991**, *115*, 1409–1418. [CrossRef] [PubMed]

50. Martínez-Maqueda, D.; Miralles, B.; De Pascual-Teresa, S.; Reverón, I.; Muñoz, R.; Recio, I. Food-Derived Peptides Stimulate Mucin Secretion and Gene Expression in Intestinal Cells. *J. Agric. Food Chem.* **2012**, *60*, 8600–8605. [CrossRef] [PubMed]

51. Konsoula, R.; Barile, F.A. Correlation of in vitro cytotoxicity with paracellular permeability in Caco-2 cells. *Toxicol. In Vitro* **2005**, *19*, 675–684. [CrossRef] [PubMed]

52. Tajima, A.; Iwase, T.; Shinji, H.; Seki, K.; Mizunoe, Y. Inhibition of Endothelial Interleukin-8 Production and Neutrophil Transmigration by Staphylococcus aureus Beta-Hemolysin. *Infect. Immun.* **2009**, *77*, 327–334. [CrossRef] [PubMed]

53. de Kok, J.B.; Roelofs, R.W.; Giesendorf, B.A.; Pennings, J.L.; Waas, E.T.; Feuth, T.; Swinkels, D.W.; Span, P.N. Normalization of gene expression measurements in tumor tissues: Comparison of 13 endogenous control genes. *Lab. Investig.* **2004**, *85*, 154–159. [CrossRef] [PubMed]

54. Lebrero-Fernández, C.; Wenzel, U.A.; Akeus, P.; Wang, Y.; Strid, H.; Simrén, M.; Gustavsson, B.; Börjesson, L.G.; Cardell, S.L.; Öhman, L.; et al. Altered expression of Butyrophilin (BTN) and BTN-like (BTNL) genes in intestinal inflammation and colon cancer. *Immun. Inflamm. Dis.* **2016**, *4*, 191–200. [CrossRef] [PubMed]

55. McCann, M.J.; Rowland, I.R.; Roy, N.C. Anti-proliferative effects of physiological concentrations of enterolactone in models of prostate tumourigenesis. *Mol. Nutr. Food Res.* **2013**, *57*, 212–224. [CrossRef] [PubMed]

56. Schwab, C.; Gänzle, M. Lactic acid bacteria fermentation of human milk oligosaccharide components, human milk oligosaccharides and galactooligosaccharides. *FEMS Microbiol. Lett.* **2011**, *315*, 141–148. [CrossRef] [PubMed]

57. Kuntz, S.; Rudloff, S.; Kunz, C. Oligosaccharides from human milk influence growth-related characteristics of intestinally transformed and non-transformed intestinal cells. *Br. J. Nutr.* **2008**, *99*, 462–471. [CrossRef] [PubMed]

58. Hester, S.N.; Donovan, S.M. Individual and combined effects of nucleotides and human milk oligosaccharides on proliferation, apoptosis and necrosis in a human fetal intestinal cell line. *Food Nutr. Sci.* **2012**, *3*, 1567–1576. [CrossRef]

59. Purup, S.; Vestergaard, M.; Pedersen, L.O.; Sejrsen, K. Biological activity of bovine milk on proliferation of human intestinal cells. *J. Dairy Res.* **2006**, *74*, 58–65. [CrossRef] [PubMed]

60. Takeda, T.; Sakata, M.; Minekawa, R.; Yamamoto, T.; Hayashi, M.; Tasaka, K.; Murata, Y. Human milk induces fetal small intestinal cell proliferation involvement of a different tyrosine kinase signaling pathway from epidermal growth factor receptor. *J. Endocrinol.* **2004**, *181*, 449–457. [CrossRef] [PubMed]

61. Kuntz, S.; Kunz, C.; Rudloff, S. Oligosaccharides from human milk induce growth arrest via G2/M by influencing growth-related cell cycle genes in intestinal epithelial cells. *Br. J. Nutr.* **2009**, *101*, 1306–1315. [CrossRef] [PubMed]

62. Ouwehand, A.C.; Tuomola, E.M.; Tölkkö, S.; Salminen, S. Assessment of adhesion properties of novel probiotic strains to human intestinal mucus. *Int. J. Food Microbiol.* **2001**, *64*, 119–126. [CrossRef]

63. Shoaf, K.; Mulvey, G.L.; Armstrong, G.D.; Hutkins, R.W. Prebiotic galactooligosaccharides reduce adherence of enteropathogenic *Escherichia coli* to tissue culture cells. *Infect. Immun.* **2006**, *74*, 6920–6928. [CrossRef] [PubMed]

64. Zivkovic, A.M.; German, J.B.; Lebrilla, C.B.; Mills, D.A. Human milk glycobiome and its impact on the infant gastrointestinal microbiota. *Proc. Natl. Acad. Sci. USA* **2011**, *108*, 4653–4658. [CrossRef] [PubMed]

65. Van den Abbeele, P.; Grootaert, C.; Possemiers, S.; Verstraete, W.; Verbeken, K.; Van de Wiele, T. In vitro model to study the modulation of the mucin-adhered bacterial community. *Appl. Microbiol. Biotechnol.* **2009**, *83*, 349–359. [CrossRef] [PubMed]

66. Kankainen, M.; Paulin, L.; Tynkkynen, S.; von Ossowski, I.; Reunanen, J.; Partanen, P.; Satokari, R.; Vesterlund, S.; Hendrickx, A.P.A.; Lebeer, S.; et al. Comparative genomic analysis of *Lactobacillus rhamnosus* GG reveals pili containing a human- mucus binding protein. *Proc. Natl. Acad. Sci. USA* **2009**, *106*, 17193–17198. [CrossRef] [PubMed]

67. MacKenzie, D.A.; Jeffers, F.; Parker, M.L.; Vibert-Vallet, A.; Bongaerts, R.J.; Roos, S.; Walter, J.; Juge, N. Strain-specific diversity of mucus-binding proteins in the adhesion and aggregation properties of *Lactobacillus reuteri*. *Microbiology* **2010**, *156*, 3368–3378. [CrossRef] [PubMed]

68. Lebeer, S.; Verhoeven, T.L.A.; Francius, G.; Schoofs, G.; Lambrichts, I.; Dufrêne, Y.; Vanderleyden, J.; De Keersmaecker, S.C.J. Identification of a Gene Cluster for the Biosynthesis of a Long, Galactose-Rich Exopolysaccharide in *Lactobacillus rhamnosus* GG and Functional Analysis of the Priming Glycosyltransferase. *Appl. Environ. Microbiol.* **2009**, *75*, 3554–3563. [CrossRef] [PubMed]

69. Suzuki, C.; Aoki-Yoshida, A.; Aoki, R.; Sasaki, K.; Takayama, Y.; Mizumachi, K. The distinct effects of orally administered *Lactobacillus rhamnosus* GG and *Lactococcus lactis* subsp. *lactis* C59 on gene expression in the murine small intestine. *PLoS ONE* **2017**, *12*, e0188985. [CrossRef] [PubMed]

70. Adlerberth, I.; Ahrne, S.; Johansson, M.L.; Molin, G.; Hanson, L.A.; Wold, A.E. A mannose-specific adherence mechanism in *Lactobacillus plantarum* conferring binding to the human colonic cell line HT-29. *Appl. Environ. Microbiol.* **1996**, *62*, 2244–2251. [PubMed]

71. Pretzer, G.; Snel, J.; Molenaar, D.; Wiersma, A.; Bron, P.A.; Lambert, J.; de Vos, W.M.; van der Meer, R.; Smits, M.A.; Kleerebezem, M. Biodiversity-Based Identification and Functional Characterization of the Mannose-Specific Adhesin of Lactobacillus plantarum. *J. Bacteriol.* **2005**, *187*, 6128–6136. [CrossRef] [PubMed]

72. Cook, R.; Harris, R.; Reid, G. Effect of culture media and growth phase on the morphology of lactobacilli and on their ability to adhere to epithelial cells. *Curr. Microbiol.* **1988**, *17*, 159–166. [CrossRef]

73. Deepika, G.; Karunakaran, E.; Hurley, C.; Biggs, C.; Charalampopoulos, D. Influence of fermentation conditions on the surface properties and adhesion of *Lactobacillus rhamnosus* GG. *Microb. Cell Fact.* **2012**, *11*, 1–12. [CrossRef] [PubMed]

74. Yang, F.; Wang, A.; Zeng, X.; Hou, C.; Liu, H.; Qiao, S. *Lactobacillus reuteri* I5007 modulates tight junction protein expression in IPEC-J2 cells with LPS stimulation and in newborn piglets under normal conditions. *BMC Microbiol.* **2015**, *15*, 32. [CrossRef] [PubMed]

75. Commane, D.M.; Shortt, C.T.; Silvi, S.; Cresci, A.; Hughes, R.M.; Rowland, I.R. Effects of Fermentation Products of Pro- and Prebiotics on Trans-Epithelial Electrical Resistance in an In Vitro Model of the Colon. *Nutr. Cancer* **2005**, *51*, 102–109. [CrossRef] [PubMed]

76. Le Leu, R.K.; Hu, Y.; Brown, I.L.; Woodman, R.J.; Young, G.P. Synbiotic intervention of *Bifidobacterium lactis* and resistant starch protects against colorectal cancer development in rats. *Carcinogenesis* **2010**, *31*, 246–251. [CrossRef] [PubMed]

77. Orlando, A.; Linsalata, M.; Notarnicola, M.; Tutino, V.; Russo, F. *Lactobacillus* GG restoration of the gliadin induced epithelial barrier disruption: The role of cellular polyamines. *BMC Microbiol.* **2014**, *14*, 19. [CrossRef] [PubMed]

78. Yan, F.; Liu, L.; Cao, H.; Moore, D.J.; Washington, M.K.; Wang, B.; Peek, R.M.; Acra, S.A.; Polk, D.B. Neonatal Colonization of Mice with LGG Promotes Intestinal Development and Decreases Susceptibility to Colitis in Adulthood. *Mucosal Immunol.* **2017**, *10*, 117–127. [CrossRef] [PubMed]

79. Robinson, K.; Deng, Z.; Hou, Y.; Zhang, G. Regulation of the Intestinal Barrier Function by Host Defense Peptides. *Front. Vet. Sci.* **2015**, *2*, 57. [CrossRef] [PubMed]

80. Patel, R.M.; Myers, L.S.; Kurundkar, A.R.; Maheshwari, A.; Nusrat, A.; Lin, P.W. Probiotic Bacteria Induce Maturation of Intestinal Claudin 3 Expression and Barrier Function. *Am. J. Pathol.* **2012**, *180*, 626–635. [CrossRef] [PubMed]

81. Yan, F.; Cao, H.; Cover, T.L.; Whitehead, R.; Washington, M.K.; Polk, D.B. Soluble Proteins Produced by Probiotic Bacteria Regulate Intestinal Epithelial Cell Survival and Growth. *Gastroenterology* **2007**, *132*, 562–575. [CrossRef] [PubMed]

82. Dai, C.; Zhao, D.-H.; Jiang, M. VSL#3 probiotics regulate the intestinal epithelial barrier in vivo and in vitro via the p38 and ERK signaling pathways. *Int. J. Mol. Med.* **2012**, *29*, 202–208. [PubMed]

83. Otte, J.-M.; Podolsky, D.K. Functional modulation of enterocytes by gram-positive and gram-negative microorganisms. *Am. J. Physiol. Gastrointest. Liver Physiol.* **2004**, *286*, G613–G626. [CrossRef] [PubMed]

84. Klingberg, T.D.; Pedersen, M.H.; Cencic, A.; Budde, B.B. Application of measurements of transepithelial electrical resistance of intestinal epithelial cell monolayers to evaluate probiotic activity. *J. Appl. Environ. Microbiol.* **2005**, *71*, 7528–7530. [CrossRef] [PubMed]

85. Wu, R.Y.; Määttänen, P.; Napper, S.; Scruten, E.; Li, B.; Koike, Y.; Johnson-Henry, K.C.; Pierro, A.; Rossi, L.; Botts, S.R.; et al. Non-digestible oligosaccharides directly regulate host kinome to modulate host inflammatory responses without alterations in the gut microbiota. *Microbiome* **2017**, *5*, 135. [CrossRef] [PubMed]

86. Martinez-Augustin, O.; Puerta, V.; Marti, A.; Baro, L.; Lo, E.; Suarez, M. Goat's milk oligosaccharides modulate mucin and trefoil factors production in the mucus producing intestinal cell line HT29/MTX. *Clin. Nutr.* **2003**, *22*, S42. [CrossRef]

87. Wang, L.; Cao, H.; Liu, L.; Wang, B.; Walker, W.A.; Acra, S.A.; Yan, F. Activation of Epidermal Growth Factor Receptor Mediates Mucin Production Stimulated by p40, a Lactobacillus rhamnosus GG-derived Protein. *J. Biol. Chem.* **2014**, *289*, 20234–20244. [CrossRef] [PubMed]

88. Mack, D.R.; Ahrne, S.; Hyde, L.; Wei, S.; Hollingsworth, M.A. Extracellular MUC3 mucin secretion follows adherence of Lactobacillus strains to intestinal epithelial cells in vitro. *Gut* **2003**, *52*, 827–833. [CrossRef] [PubMed]

89. Wan, L.-Y.M.; Allen, K.J.; Turner, P.C.; El-Nezami, H. Modulation of Mucin mRNA (MUC5AC and MUC5B) Expression and Protein Production and Secretion in Caco-2/HT29-MTX Co-cultures Following Exposure to Individual and Combined Fusarium Mycotoxins. *Toxicol. Sci.* **2014**, *139*, 83–98. [CrossRef] [PubMed]

90. Lukic, J.; Strahinic, I.; Jovcic, B.; Filipic, B.; Topisirovic, L.A.; Kojic, M.; Begovic, J. Different Roles for Lactococcal Aggregation Factor and Mucin Binding Protein in Adhesion to Gastrointestinal Mucosa. *Appl. Environ. Microbiol.* **2012**, *78*, 7993–8000. [CrossRef] [PubMed]

91. Corfield, A. Eukaryotic protein glycosylation: A primer for histochemists and cell biologists. *Histochem. Cell. Biol.* **2017**, *147*, 119–147. [CrossRef] [PubMed]

92. Liu, Y.; Yin, X.M.; Xia, R.W.; Huo, Y.J.; Zhu, G.Q.; Wu, S.L.; Bao, W.B. Association between the *MUC4* g.243A > G polymorphism and immune and production traits in large white pigs. *Turk. J. Vet. Anim. Sci.* **2015**, *39*, 141–146. [CrossRef]

93. Moniaux, N.; Escande, F.; Porchet, N.; Aubert, J.P.; Surinder, K.B. Structural Organisation and Classification of the Human Mucin Genes. *Front. Biosci.* **2001**, *6*, 1192–1206. [CrossRef]

94. van Putten, J.P.M.; Strijbis, K. Transmembrane mucins: Signaling receptors at the intersection of inflammation and cancer. *J. Innate Immun.* **2017**, *9*, 281–299. [CrossRef] [PubMed]

95. Okumura, R.; Takeda, K. Roles of intestinal epithelial cells in the maintenance of gut homeostasis. *Exp. Mol. Med.* **2017**, *49*, e338. [CrossRef] [PubMed]

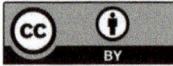

![nutrients logo]

nutrients

MDPI

Article

Importance of Health Aspects in Polish Consumer Choices of Dairy Products

Marta Sajdakowska *, Jerzy Gębski, Krystyna Gutkowska and Sylwia Żakowska-Biemans

Department of Organization and Consumption Economics, Faculty of Human Nutrition and Consumer Sciences, Warsaw University of Life Sciences (SGGW-WULS), 159C Nowoursynowska Street, 02-787 Warsaw, Poland; jerzy_gebski@sggw.pl (J.G.); krystyna_gutkowska@sggw.pl (K.G.); sylwia_zakowska_biemans@sggw.pl (S.Ż.-B.)
* Correspondence: marta_sajdakowska@sggw.pl; Tel.: +48-225-937-145

Received: 29 June 2018; Accepted: 30 July 2018; Published: 2 August 2018

Abstract: In general, dairy products are well regarded for their nutritional value. Consumer perception of dairy products is influenced by many interrelated factors but healthiness remains one of the key attributes and values for consumers. Furthermore, contemporary consumers increasingly seek out dairy products with additional health benefits and, therefore, it is essential to explore which attributes are important drivers of food choices and how producers can better respond to shifting consumer values and needs in each dairy product category. Therefore, the aims of the study were: (a) to identify consumer segments based on the importance they attached to selected attributes of dairy products, (b) to explore differences between the identified segments in their perceptions of health-related attributes of dairy products, (c) to determine if health-related aspects influenced consumers decisions to buy high-quality dairy products, and (d) to identify if consumers were open to novelties in dairy products. The data were collected within a CAPI (Computer Assisted Personal Interview) survey on a representative sample of 983 adult Polish consumers. The non-hierarchical K-means clustering method was used to identify four clusters of consumers, namely: Enthusiastic, Involved, Ultra-involved and Neutral. Enthusiastic consumers attach more importance to the influence of dairy products on immunity and are more willing to agree with the opinion that dairy products are a source of mineral nutrients as well as vitamins. Ultra-involved and Involved consumers pay less attention to some health aspects of dairy products compared to other clusters; however, the Ultra-involved are more quality-oriented than are the Involved. Neutral consumers are more open to accept changes on the dairy product market and are relatively more inclined to choose new dairy products. However, these consumers have scored lower on those aspects related to the healthiness of dairy products and, in order to target them effectively, it is essential to develop well-tailored communication strategies highlighting the health benefits of dairy products. These results relate to the Polish market and are important for the development of new dairy products and for targeting public nutrition as well as for directing marketing communication. The results may provide important insights for those who develop educational strategies and campaigns.

Keywords: consumer; dairy products; health aspects

---

1. Introduction

Dairy products are characterized by an appropriate nutritional value which contributes positively to human health [1–3]. Dairy products also play a key role in the prevalence and/or treatment of some diseases; examples include obesity [4–6], hypertension [7,8], type 2 diabetes [5,9,10], and cardiovascular disease [5,11–13]. Some kinds of dairy products are valued for their favorable effect on the digestive system [14,15]. Moreover, the consumption of dairy products is associated with lower body weight and/or body fat [16–18]. In general, the consumption of dairy products provides various health benefits [2]; however, some study results also show that, besides consumption-related benefits for example flavoring milk with added sugar may promote milk intake, this consumption may not be without adverse effects in terms of caloric intake and possibly obesity for children and adolescents [19]. Results of other studies also show that the possibility that milk intake is simply a marker of diets with good nutritional quality cannot be excluded, and this aspect needs further research [20].

The food sector faces an increasingly competitive and more globalized market and more demanding consumers who exhibit greater concern about quality and health benefits with respect to products [21]. Among the different product sectors, the dairy sector is the one that has undergone the greatest change, with the introduction of new products claiming healthy characteristics [22]. Polish consumers are increasingly interested in healthiness and the safety of food [23,24], and health is perceived as the most important value [25,26]. Consumer opinions on health are crucial, particularly when it comes to benefits and risks to health and disease prevention [27,28]. In addition, the effect on health is important in consumers' choice behavior concerning dairy products [29].

Therefore, the aims of the current study were: (a) to identify consumer segments based on the importance they attached to selected attributes of dairy products, (b) to explore differences between the identified segments in their perceptions of health-related attributes of dairy products, (c) to determine if health-related aspects influenced consumers decision to buy high quality dairy products, and (d) to identify if consumers were open to novelties in dairy products.

2. Materials and Methods

2.1. Data Collection Process

Quantitative data were collected in 2013 within the project "BIOFOOD-Innovative, Functional Products of Animal Origin" aimed at increasing innovation in the Polish agro-food sector through the development of products of animal origin providing functional and nutritional benefits. This paper presents some of the findings from a larger multidisciplinary study identifying drivers of and obstacles to innovation in products of animal origin [30], including consumer perception and acceptance of innovative food products [31].

The sample in our study (N = 983) was drawn from the Social Security addresses database and was representative for the national population in terms of age, gender and the region that consumers lived in. The survey was conducted in each of the 16 voivodships in Poland. After drawing the starting addresses, the random route method was used in the selection of the sample [32,33]. A number of sampling points were drawn with probability proportional to population size, for total coverage of the country, and to population density. In order to do so, the sampling points were drawn systematically from each of the "administrative regional units", after stratification by individual unit and type of area. They thus represent the whole of Poland as well as the distribution of the resident population. In each of the selected sampling points, a starting address was drawn at random. Further addresses were selected by standard "random route" procedures from the initial address. In each household, a respondent was drawn, at random (following the "closest birthday rule").

The interviews were conducted face-to-face at respondents' homes by a professional market research agency in accordance with the ESOMAR (European Society for Opinion and Marketing Research) code of conduct using the CAPI (Computer Assisted Personal Interview) technique. All respondents were aged 21+. Only those respondents who met the recruitment criteria, i.e., made their own or cooperative food purchases and declared dairy product consumption, participated in the study.

2.2. Description of Questionnaire

The questionnaire used in the study was structured in two main blocks and covered aspects such as consumer perception of food quality and consumer perception of health aspects of dairy products. In order to identify consumer segments, a question related to the importance of different attributes of dairy products in consumer food choices was used for the factor and then cluster analysis ("Please specify to what extent the factors listed below encourage you to consume dairy products"). A 7–point scale was used, where 1–meant "definitely does not encourage to consume dairy products", and 7–"definitely encourages you to consume dairy products". Analysis of statements' reliability in a given question was performed using Cronbach Coefficient Alpha. The obtained value of Cronbach Coefficient Alpha = 0.803 confirmed the right choice of questions for factor analysis (Principal Component Analysis–PCA). To profile segments, three further questions were used regarding opinions on dairy products. One of these referred to opinions on selected attributes of products. The next question identified opinions on high-quality products, including health aspects. In the following question, a scale designed for the needs of other studies on products of animal origin was used [34], including statements from other scales used in available literature on the subject [35,36]. The question was worded as follows: "People have different opinions on food. Please specify to what extent you agree or disagree with the statements on dairy products listed below". For these 3 questions, a 7–point scale was used, where 1–meant "I strongly agree", and 7–"I strongly disagree". Analyses were conducted using the SAS 9.4 statistical package (SAS Institute, Cary, NC, USA).

3. Results

Consumer segmentation was preceded by a factor analysis using PCA with a varimax rotation of 14 statements. Based on eigenvalues (eigenvalues higher than 1), a 3–factor solution describing the phenomenon analyzed was suggested (Table 1). The factors obtained via PCA analysis explained 54.54% of total variation. Qualification for particular factors was based on the minimum value of factor loadings estimated at 0.4. Factor adequacy for the requirements of factor analysis, as studied by the Kaiser-Mayer-Olkin measure (KMO). The KMO value indicating collective correlation of variables was 0.89, which clearly confirmed the logic behind using the variable reduction method. Identified factors presented in Table 1 were used for cluster analysis (segmentation).

Table 1. Principal components analysis (PCA) of consumers' use of dairy product consumption factors; varimax rotated factor loadings percentage of explained variance (N = 983, Poland).

Food Characteristics	Factor 1 Hedonic Aspects	Factor 2 Health Aspects	Factor 3 Health Concerns
Easy to prepare	0.754		
A quick snack which can be eaten between meals	0.711		
Taste	0.696		
Wide product range	0.691		
Variety to the menu	0.661		
Habits	0.579		
Mineral and vitamin content	0.538		
Medical/dietary recommendations		0.797	
Appropriate animal breeding		0.675	
Health reasons		0.617	
Low level of processing		0.549	
Presence of preservatives			0.804
Presence of flavors			0.704
Fat content			0.447
The variance explained/% explained variance	34.79	10.66	9.09

The division of consumers into segments was conducted in two stages. Firstly, a cluster analysis using hierarchical methods was performed. In the second stage of consumer segmentation, a cluster analysis was used based on non-hierarchical method K-means with initial cluster seeds obtained through the hierarchical method. The non-hierarchical K-means clustering method led to the identification of four clusters: Enthusiastic, Ultra-Involved, Involved, and Neutral. In general, the names of the clusters related to consumers' perceptions of dairy products and reflected their mean scores; the highest for the Enthusiastic, average for the Ultra-Involved, relatively lower for the

Involved and the lowest for the Neutral. The profiles of the resulting segments were determined using chi square cross-tabulation and ANOVA (Analysis of Variance) with post-hoc Waller-Duncan K-ratio *t* Test comparison of mean scores. The socio-demographic characteristics, including gender, age, education, place of residence, number of members in the household, number of children in the household, the subjective evaluation of health and income satisfaction, are presented in Table 2. The results of cluster analysis, together with the size of each cluster, are reported in Tables 2–5. The data analysis presented in Table 2 indicates that, in the sample tested, there were statistically significant differences observed in terms of all the clusters identified. In the total sample, a slight majority of respondents were women. In terms of the age of the total sample, it can be seen that the largest age group was 45–54, people aged 65–75 were the least numerous. Over 40% of the surveyed declared the lowest education level, and people with university education were the least numerous group. Over 1/3 of the respondents declared living in rural areas, while every 10th respondent indicated living in big cities with over 500 thousand inhabitants. Almost 75% respondents lived in households comprising 2–4 persons, and over half of the people surveyed declared having children. A subjective evaluation of income satisfaction showed that almost 40% of the surveyed people lived frugally and had enough money to buy what they needed and over 1/3 lived very frugally to save money for major purchases. About half of the surveyed people evaluated their health as good, more than 20% as very good, and almost one quarter of respondents selected a neutral answer (i.e., "neither good nor bad").

Cluster 1 (Enthusiastic–29.09%) was dominated by women and people aged 45–54, 55–64 as well as 35–44. Over 2/5 respondents were those with the lowest level of education, over 1/3 declared secondary education, and one fifth of respondents had a university education. The most numerous group were inhabitants of rural areas. A subjective evaluation of health showed that half of the respondents described their health as good and almost 20% as very good. A subjective evaluation of income satisfaction showed that the majority of the surveyed people lived frugally and had enough money or lived very frugally to save money for major purchases. Two- and three-person households were the most numerous in segment 2. Families with children constituted over half of this segment.

Cluster 2 (Ultra-involved–18.82%) was dominated by men, people aged 45–64 and by people with secondary or lower education levels, one fifth of respondents, similar to cluster 2, declared a university education; the biggest group of respondents came from rural areas. More than half of the people in this segment assessed their health as good and almost 30% as very good. A subjective evaluation of income satisfaction showed that over 2/5 of the surveyed people lived frugally and had enough money to buy what they needed. Compared with other segments, the largest share of people who have children was noted in segment 3.

Cluster 3 (Involved–27.56%) was dominated by people with lower education levels (primary, lower secondary and vocational) living in rural areas, small towns (up to 100 thousand inhabitants) and medium-sized cities (200–500 thousand inhabitants). In this segment, almost half of the people were those respondents who assessed their health as good, more than 25% assessed it as very good. Over 1/3 of this segment was constituted by people from two-person households. In this segment there was the lowest share of people with children, compared with other segments.

In cluster 4 (Neutral–24.41%) half of the people were respondents with the lowest levels of education (primary, lower secondary and vocational). In this segment, over 1/4 of those surveyed were people living in rural areas, and almost 60% of the people came from towns of over 20 thousand inhabitants (the aggregate of percentages for towns of 20 thousand–100 thousand, 100 thousand–500 thousand and of more than 500 thousand). More than 50% of the surveyed people from this segment assessed their health as good, and one tenth of respondents assessed it as very good. A subjective evaluation of income satisfaction showed that more than 2/5 of the surveyed people lived very frugally to save money for major purchases, and almost 1/3 lived frugally and had enough money to buy what they needed. The most represented households in this segment were 2-and 3-person ones. Moreover, an average share of people with children was noted among the Neutral group (Table 2).

Table 2. Socio-demographic characteristics of the consumers surveyed (*N* = 983, Poland).

Variables	Total Sample (%)	Cluster 1 Enthusiastic *N* = 286	Cluster 2 Ultra-Involved *N* = 185	Cluster 3 Involved *N* = 271	Cluster 4 Neutral *N* = 240	*p*-Value for χ^2 Test
Gender						0.0185
Women	50.97	58.04	44.32	50.92	47.72	
Men	49.03	41.96	55.68	49.08	52.28	
Age (years)						0.0182
21–27	16.3	11.19	22.16	17.34	16.6	
28–34	15.9	13.64	17.3	15.5	17.84	
35–44	18.3	17.83	20.54	16.61	19.09	
45–54	20.2	22.73	21.62	18.82	17.84	
55–64	18.4	19.58	12.43	22.14	17.43	
65–75	10.89	15.03	5.95	9.59	11.2	
Education						0.011
Vocational	46.80	44.41	41.08	50.18	53.53	
Secondary	37.81	36.36	39.46	36.53	37.34	
Higher	15.39	19.23	19.46	13.28	9.13	
Place of residence						<0.0001
Rural area	35.62	37.41	52.97	29.52	26.81	
Cities up to 20,000	13.51	13.99	9.73	14.76	14.47	
Cities above 20,000 to 100,000	19.96	18.53	16.22	20.3	24.26	
Cities above 100,000 to 500,000	19.75	19.23	14.05	24.72	19.15	
Cities above 500,000	11.16	10.84	7.03	10.7	15.32	
Number of persons in the household						0.0056
1	13.10	11.87	11.36	12.25	16.96	
2	27.71	28.06	21.59	31.62	27.68	
3	25.56	27.34	25.57	21.34	28.13	
4	21.70	21.22	21.02	22.92	21.43	
5 and more	11.92	11.51	20.45	11.86	5.8	
Children (Yes)	52.74	53.50	63.46	45.87	50.81	0.0087
Subjective assessment of financial situation						0.0155
Sufficient budget without necessity to economize	8.33	7.04	13.1	6.53	8.3	
We live frugally and have enough money to buy what we need	38.8	39.63	44.05	42.04	30.57	
We live very frugally to save money for major purchases	35.8	34.44	28.57	34.29	44.1	
We have enough money for the cheapest food or clothes and less	17.10	18.89	14.29	17.14	17.03	
Health assessment						0.0008
Very good	21.28	19.23	29.19	25.46	12.92	
Good	50.81	50.0	51.35	49.08	53.33	
Neither good nor bad	23.93	25.52	18.92	20.66	29.58	
Bad	3.56	4.9	0	4.06	4.17	
Very bad	0.41	0.35	0.54	0.74	0	

3.1. Consumer Perception of Health-Related Attributes of Dairy Products

Regarding opinions on perception of dairy products, respondents declared the highest level of agreement with the statement that dairy products are a rich source of protein and that dairy products, particularly yogurts, kefirs and butter milk, have a beneficial influence on immunity. In all the statements analyzed (Table 3), statistically significant (*p* < 0.05) differences were noted between mean scores in particular clusters. An additional post-hoc test (Waller-Duncan K-ratio *t* Test) compared mean values of opinions between pairs of clusters.

Table 3. Profile of the segments in terms of different perceptions of dairy products (*N* = 983, Poland).

Statements	Mean	Cluster 1 Enthusiastic N = 286	Cluster 2 Ultra-Involved N = 185	Cluster 3 Involved N = 271	Cluster 4 Neutral N = 240	*p*-Value
Dairy products are a rich source of protein	6.13	6.61 [a]	6.52 [a]	6.05 [b]	5.35 [c]	<0.0001
Dairy products, particularly yogurts, kefirs and butter milk, have a beneficial influence on immunity	5.85	6.33 [a]	6.09 [b]	5.68 [c]	5.28 [d]	<0.0001
Dairy products are a rich source of minerals	5.76	6.28 [a]	6.04 [b]	5.54 [c]	5.18 [d]	<0.0001
Dairy products are a rich source of vitamins	5.73	6.17 [a]	5.95 [b]	5.58 [c]	5.19 [d]	<0.0001
Healthy nutrients in dairy products have a beneficial influence on the digestive system	5.61	6.13 [a]	5.94 [a]	5.28 [b]	5.10 [b]	<0.0001
Dairy products with reduced fat content are the best for health	4.74	5.14 [a]	4.53 [b,c]	4.32 [c]	4.84 [a,b]	<0.0001

[a,b,c,d] Means with the same letter are not significantly different; ANOVA (Analysis of Variance) post-hoc Waller-Duncan K-ratio *t* Test.

When compared to other segments, the Enthusiastic attached the most importance to the influence of dairy products on immunity (dairy products, particularly yogurts, kefirs and butter milk have a beneficial influence on immunity). They have agreed to a greater extent with the opinion that dairy products are a rich source of minerals as well as vitamins, and that products with reduced fat content are the best for one's health. The Ultra-involved, to a greater extent than two other segments (i.e., Involved and Neutral), agreed with the statement that dairy products have a beneficial influence on immunity, that they are a source of minerals and vitamins and that healthy nutrients in dairy products have a beneficial influence on the digestive system.

The Involved, more often than the Neutral, agreed with the opinion that dairy products are a rich source of protein and have a beneficial influence on immunity and that dairy products are a rich source of minerals as well as vitamins. Moreover, the Neutral, more often than the Involved, agreed with the opinion that dairy products with reduced fat content are the best for one's health.

In all the analyzed statements on health aspects of dairy products, statistically significant (*p* < 0.05) differences were noted between mean scores in particular clusters.

3.2. Quality Attributes of Dairy Products as Drivers of Food Purchasing Decisions

The degree of agreement with the statement on the importance of dairy product quality in the choice of food shows its significant role in consumers' decisions, whereby the Enthusiastic agreed with it to the highest extent and Neutrals to the least extent (Table 4).

Table 4. Profiles of the segments in terms of different perceptions of high quality dairy products (*N* = 983, Poland).

Statements	Mean	Cluster 1 Enthusiastic N = 286	Cluster 2 Ultra-Involved N = 185	Cluster 3 Involved N = 271	Cluster 4 Neutral N = 240	*p*-Value
Quality matters to me while choosing dairy products	5.71	6.22 [a]	5.98 [b]	5.48 [c]	5.14 [d]	<0.0001
I buy high-quality dairy products because they have a beneficial influence on my children's health	4.59	4.95 [a]	4.63 [a]	3.96 [b]	4.78 [a]	<0.0001
I buy high-quality dairy products because they have a beneficial influence on my body shape	4.08	4.39 [a,b]	4.07 [b]	3.32 [c]	4.51 [a]	<0.0001
I buy high-quality dairy products only for those family members who have health issues	3.18	3.12 [b]	2.57 [c]	2.82 [b,c]	4.07 [a]	<0.0001

[a,b,c,d] Means with the same letter are not significantly different; ANOVA post-hoc Waller-Duncan K-ratio *t* Test.

Compared with other clusters, the Involved to a lesser extent expressed their agreement with the statement that they bought high-quality dairy products due to their beneficial influence on children's health or that they bought high-quality dairy products due to their beneficial influence on their body shape. The Neutral, more often than the respondents from other clusters, agreed with the opinion that they bought high-quality dairy products only for those family members who had health issues.

3.3. Consumers' Willingness to Accept Innovation in Dairy Products

In order to identify respondents' opinions on their willingness to buy dairy products and to accept changes on the food market regarding dairy products, those surveyed were asked about the level of their agreement with statements describing selected opinions on the willingness to buy dairy products and to accept some changes on the dairy product market. In all the analyzed statements on openness to new milk-based products, statistically significant differences were noted between mean scores in particular clusters (Table 5). An additional post-hoc test (Waller-Duncan K-ratio *t* Test) compared mean values of opinions between pairs of clusters.

The highest degree of agreement amongst respondents was noted for the statement: "If I do not know what is in a food, I will not try it", "I am very particular about the foods I will eat". Analysis of the responses in individual clusters showed that, compared with other consumers, the Neutral expressed the highest level of agreement with the majority of suggested statements concerning openness to new products, which may indicate that they exhibit greater pro-innovative attitudes. The Enthusiastic, to a greater extent than the Ultra-involved, declared that they usually know more than others about the latest products, they seek information on new dairy products appearing on the market and that they have concerns about eating dairy products they have not tried before. Compared with consumers from other clusters, the Involved declared a lower level of agreement with the majority of statements, which indicates the lowest level of openness to changes (innovation) on the dairy product market. Regarding concerns about eating products which have not been tried before, the Involved declared a relatively high level of agreement, a similar level to the Neutral respondents (Table 5).

Table 5. Profiles of the segments in terms of different perceptions referring to openness to buy new products and changes in the market of dairy products ($N = 983$, Poland).

Statements	Mean	Cluster 1 Enthusiastic $N = 286$	Cluster 2 Ultra-Involved $N = 185$	Cluster 3 Involved $N = 271$	Cluster 4 Neutral $N = 240$	*p*-Value
I like to buy new and different products	3.85	3.86 [b]	3.90 [b]	3.33 [c]	4.38 [a]	<0.0001
New products excite me	4.00	4.17 [a,b]	3.92 [b]	3.54 [c]	4.37 [a]	<0.0001
I try new products before my friends and neighbors	2.80	2.69 [b]	2.46 [b]	2.12 [c]	3.93 [a]	<0.0001
I know more than others about the latest new products	2.83	2.71 [b]	2.34 [c]	2.13 [c]	4.03 [a]	<0.0001
I look for information about what new food appears on the market	2.79	2.67 [b]	2.35 [c]	2.22 [c]	3.93 [a]	<0.0001
I am usually amongst the first to try new products	3.22	3.11 [b]	3.03 [b]	2.58 [c]	4.17 [a]	<0.0001
I am constantly sampling new and different foods	3.36	3.25 [b]	3.11 [b,c]	2.88 [c]	4.20 [a]	<0.0001
I do not trust new foods	3.79	3.69 [b,c]	3.79 [b]	3.40 [c]	4.30 [a]	<0.0001
If I do not know what is in a food, I will not try it	4.55	4.81 [b]	4.34 [b]	4.52 [a,b]	4.43 [a,b]	0.0461
I like foods from different countries	3.29	3.3 [b]	3.22 [b]	2.57 [c]	4.09 [a]	<0.0001
Ethnic food looks too weird to eat (e.g., Asian cuisine)	3.72	3.56 [b]	3.5 [b]	3.42 [c]	4.31 [a]	<0.0001
At dinner parties, I will try a new food	3.64	3.81 [b]	3.51 [b]	2.99 [c]	4.25 [a]	<0.0001
I am afraid to eat things I have never eaten before	3.90	3.69 [b]	3.34 [c]	4.15 [a]	4.31 [a]	<0.0001
I am very particular about the foods I will eat	4.48	4.68 [a]	4.57 [a,b]	4.23 [b]	4.45 [a,b]	0.0331
I will eat almost anything	4.10	3.99 [b]	4.39 [a]	3.72 [b]	4.43 [a]	0.0003
I like to try ethnic restaurants (e.g., Asian cuisine)	2.92	2.56 [b]	2.75 [b]	2.58 [b]	3.85 [a]	<0.0001

[a,b,c] Means with the same letter are not significantly different; ANOVA post-hoc Waller-Duncan K-ratio *t* Test.

4. Discussion

Our findings show that, compared with other consumers, the Enthusiastic assessed dairy products the most favorably due to their influence on immunity and their mineral and vitamin content. This group demonstrated the highest levels of agreement with the statement that dairy products with reduced fat content are the best for one's health. The segment of the Enthusiastic comprised a higher share of women and mature respondents that exhibit higher health concerns and better knowledge on health-related aspects of food.

Female consumers show high acceptance for some functional dairy products, such as yogurt enriched with calcium, fiber and probiotics. Acceptance of functional dairy products increases amongst consumers with higher diet/health-related knowledge, as well as with age [37]. When it comes to fat content, for the choice of calorie reduced dairy products the highest priorities were: a low fat content, healthiness and good taste [38]. Moreover, low-fat dairy products, when consumed regularly as part of a balanced diet, may have a number of beneficial outcomes for neurocognitive health during ageing [39]. Furthermore, the main reason for choosing functional fermented dairy products is prevention of diseases, followed by the positive impact of low-fat content on body weight [40].

Agreement with the opinion that dairy products are a rich source of protein observed in our study was equally significant for the Enthusiastic and Ultra-involved. In general, milk proteins are precursors of bioactive peptides, so dairy products (e.g., fermented products) may be regarded as functional foods and targeted for imparting several biologically beneficial attributes [41]. Moreover, from the consumers' point of view, products enriched with proteins could be beneficial for the elderly [42] as well as for people on special dietary regimes and those with certain health issues [43]. Results of other studies show that, for example, the use of protein-enriched drinking yogurt, consumed as part of regular meals, can be a promising and feasible solution to increase the protein intake of ill patients [44].

The results of our study showed that quality is the most important factor in choosing dairy products for the Enthusiastic, and the least important for the Neutral. It must, however, be added that consumers perceive the notion of 'quality' in a complex way. From the consumers' perspective, there are many aspects which can describe the quality of a food product, i.e., intrinsic qualities (e.g., taste), as well as external factors (e.g., origin or labeling) [45,46]. Moreover, from the consumers' point of view, the factors of dairy product quality include health and process-related quality that are credence dimensions. The above-mentioned quality components must be clearly communicated to a consumer to establish trust in them [47]. In our own studies respondents exhibited concerns about dairy products which they had not previously consumed, which is supported by high levels of agreement with the statements: "If I do not know what is in a food, I will not try it" and "I am very particular about the foods I will eat". These opinions may also confirm the willingness to seek information, for example, about the composition of products in this category, which has also been noted in other studies [29,48].

Our research revealed that consumers' choice of high-quality dairy products for their influence on children's health was the most important factor for the following segments: Enthusiastic, Ultra-involved and Neutral. In the case of the first two segments, it is connected with the biggest share of families with children in these segments, which is confirmed in other studies [49]. As shown in the literature of the subject, dairy products contain many of the nutrients which are responsible, amongst other things, for the proper growth of children [50]. When it comes to yogurts [51], their frequent consumption, for example amongst American children, is associated with better diet quality, lower levels of fasting insulin, reduced insulin resistance scores and improved insulin sensitivity scores.

Our own findings show that agreement with the opinions about buying high-quality dairy products for those family members who have health issues is the highest amongst Neutral respondents. The literature on the subject concerning health aspect of dairy products emphasizes that various types of dairy products have different importance levels for health, which is shown by the so-called risk markers of cardiovascular disease [52]. In addition, for health reasons it is advisable to consume dairy products with low fat content rather than products with high fat content [53]. The intake of milk and yogurts should be increased and the intake of cheese should be decreased [54]. However, a growing interest of consumers in the development of new functional foods and their introduction into healthy diets has been observed [15]. Functional dairy products will still play a significant role in a healthy diet [55].

Compared with other segments, the Neutral placed greater importance on the influence of body shape aspect, which can indicate that this group, to a greater extent, may be motivated by hedonic values and, therefore, exhibit greater concern for their appearance, which has also been noted in other studies [56].

As noted earlier, our own studies showed that the Neutral, compared with other consumers, were the least concerned about selected attributes of dairy products, such as their protein content, influence on immunity or presence of vitamins and minerals. However, the attributes discussed were rated relatively highly in the opinion of people in this segment, which could indicate that they matter during the decision-making process. Moreover, the Neutral, compared with other segments, showed the greatest acceptance for changes on the dairy food market and were relatively more willing to declare choosing new products. Consequently, this segment can be a potential group of people interested in new products on the market, including health-promoting food products. Moreover, other studies [57] have shown that health-promoting food products are important for consumers and the importance of the health aspect as the criterion for food choice is growing [34]. However, the Neutral segment does not possess characteristic socio-demographic attributes typical of innovative consumers. Other studies have shown that younger consumers declare higher acceptance for the suggested changes in products of animal origin [34,58,59]. The acceptance for changes also concerns, to a greater extent, better educated people [34,58,59] and those of higher income [34,60]. However, the Neutral segment is dominated by those living in cities, including the biggest cities, i.e., with over 500 thousand inhabitants. Findings from other authors [59–61] have shown that this group exhibits the greatest acceptance for changes to food including changes to products of animal origin [34,58]. Furthermore, big cities offer consumers more choice of products, which has been reported by other authors [62], who claim that small towns offer consumers a significantly narrower range of available goods.

5. Conclusions

Growing interest in health-related attributes of food has given rise to a new range of foods and products on the market that, as well as providing nourishment, improve health by increasing well-being and reducing the risk of certain diseases. Our research has revealed that consumers appreciate health-promoting attributes of dairy products declaring their use for a specific purpose and target group, i.e., for children or family members with health issues. Neutral respondents exhibited greater acceptance of changes in the dairy food market, which could indicate that this will be the group of people particularly interested in new products. However, they scored lower on those aspects related to the healthiness of dairy products and to target them effectively it is essential to develop well-tailored communication strategies highlighting the health benefits of dairy products.

Our results need to be repeated under different socio-cultural conditions and/or in other countries.

These results are of relevance for professionals involved in public nutrition issues as well as for marketers aiming at development of well-tailored communication strategies. The results may provide important insights for those who develop educational strategies and campaigns.

Author Contributions: M.S. developed the concept of the study. J.G. analyzed the data and contributed to its interpretation. M.S. interpreted the data and wrote the original draft. M.S. and S.Ž.-B. were involved in writing—review & editing. K.G. was responsible for funding acquisition and supervision. All Authors were involved in critically revising the manuscript, and have given their approval to the manuscript submitted.

Acknowledgments: The survey was a part of the "BIOFOOD—Innovative, Functional Products of Animal Origin", Project No. POIG.01.01.02-014-090/09 that was co-financed by the European Union from the European Regional Development Fund within the Innovative Economy Operational Programme 2007–2013; Research financed by Polish Ministry of Science and Higher Education within funds of Faculty of Human Nutrition and Consumer Sciences, Warsaw University of Life Sciences (WULS), for scientific research.

Conflicts of Interest: The authors declare no conflict of interest.

References

1. Dror, D.K.; Allen, L.H. Dairy product intake in children and adolescents in developed countries: Trends, nutritional contribution, and a review of association with health outcomes. *Nutr. Rev.* **2014**, *72*, 68–81. [CrossRef] [PubMed]
2. Hess, J.M.; Jonnalagadda, S.S.; Slavin, J.L. Dairy Foods: Current Evidence of their Effects on Bone, Cardiometabolic, Cognitive, and Digestive Health. *Compr. Rev. Food Sci. Food Saf.* **2016**, *15*, 251–268. [CrossRef]
3. Jones, V.S.; Drake, M.A.; Harding, R.; Kuhn-Sherlock, B. Consumer perception of soy and dairy products: a cross cultural study. *J. Sens. Stud.* **2008**, *23*, 65–79. [CrossRef]
4. Barrea, L.; Di Somma, C.; Macchia, P.E.; Falco, A.; Savanelli, M.C.; Orio, F.; Colao, A.; Savastano, S. Influence of nutrition on somatotropic axis: Milk consumption in adult individuals with moderate-severe obesity. *Clin. Nutr.* **2017**, *36*, 293–301. [CrossRef] [PubMed]
5. Thorning, T.K.; Raben, A.; Tholstrup, T.; Soedamah-Muthu, S.S.; Givens, I.; Astrup, A. Milk and dairy products: Good or bad for human health? An assessment of the totality of scientific evidence. *Food Nutr. Res.* **2016**, *60*, 32527. [CrossRef] [PubMed]
6. Wądołowska, L.; Ulewicz, N.; Sobas, K.; Wuenstel, J.W.; Slowinska, M.A.; Niedzwiedzka, E.; Czlapka-Matyasik, M. Dairy-Related Dietary Patterns, Dietary Calcium, Body Weight and Composition: A Study of Obesity in Polish Mothers and Daughters, the MODAF Project. *Nutrients* **2018**, *10*, 90. [CrossRef] [PubMed]
7. Gopinath, B.; Flood, V.M.; Burlutsky, G.; Louie, J.C.Y.; Baur, L.A.; Mitchell, P. Dairy food consumption, blood pressure and retinal microcirculation in adolescents. *Nutr. Metab. Cardiovasc. Dis.* **2014**, *24*, 1221–1227. [CrossRef] [PubMed]
8. Yuan, W.L.; Kakinami, L.; Gray-Donald, K.; Czernichow, S.; Lambert, M.; Paradis, G. Influence of dairy product consumption on Children's blood Pressure: Results from the quality cohort. *J. Acad. Nutr. Diet.* **2013**, *113*, 936–941. [CrossRef] [PubMed]
9. Gille, D.; Schmid, A.; Walther, B.; Vergères, G. Fermented Food and Non-Communicable Chronic Diseases: A Review. *Nutrients* **2018**, *10*, 448. [CrossRef] [PubMed]
10. Moslehi, N.; Shab-Bidar, S.; Mirmiran, P.; Sadeghi, M.; Azizi, F. Associations between dairy products consumption and risk of type 2 diabetes: Tehran lipid and glucose study. *Int. J. Food Sci. Nutr.* **2015**, *66*, 692–699. [CrossRef] [PubMed]
11. Lordan, R.; Tsoupras, A.; Mitra, B.; Zabetakis, I. Dairy Fats and Cardiovascular Disease: Do We Really Need to Be Concerned? *Foods* **2018**, *7*, 29. [CrossRef] [PubMed]
12. Markey, O.; Vasilopoulou, D.; Givens, D.I.; Lovegrove, J.A. Dairy and cardiovascular health: Friend or foe? *Nutr. Bull.* **2014**, *39*, 161–171. [CrossRef] [PubMed]
13. Ribeiro, A.G.; Mill, J.G.; Cade, N.V.; Velasquez-Melendez, G.; Matos, S.M.A.; Molina, M.C.B. Associations of Dairy Intake with Arterial Stiffness in Brazilian Adults: The Brazilian Longitudinal Study of Adult Health (ELSA-Brasil). *Nutrients* **2018**, *10*, 701. [CrossRef] [PubMed]
14. Guyonnet, D.; Schlumberger, A.; Mhamdi, L.; Jakob, S.; Chassany, O. Fermented milk containing Bifidobacterium lactis DN-173 010 improves gastrointestinal well-being and digestive symptoms in women reporting minor digestive symptoms: A randomised, double-blind, parallel, controlled study. *Br. J. Nutr.* **2009**, *102*, 1654–1662. [CrossRef] [PubMed]
15. Kandylis, P.; Pissaridi, K.; Bekatorou, A.; Kanellaki, M.; Koutinas, A.A. Dairy and non-dairy probiotic beverages. *Curr. Opin. Food Sci.* **2016**, *7*, 58–63. [CrossRef]
16. Abargouei, A.S.; Janghorbani, M.; Salehi-Marzijarani, M.; Esmaillzadeh, A. Effect of dairy consumption on weight and body composition in adults: A systematic review and meta-analysis of randomized controlled clinical trials. *Int. J. Obes.* **2012**, *36*, 1485–1493. [CrossRef] [PubMed]
17. Chen, M.; Pan, A.; Malik, V.S.; Hu, F.B. Effects of dairy intake on body weight and fat: A meta-analysis of randomized controlled trials. *Am. J. Clin. Nurs.* **2012**, *96*, 735–747. [CrossRef] [PubMed]
18. Louie, J.C.Y.; Flood, V.M.; Hector, D.J.; Rangan, A.M.; Gill, T.P. Dairy consumption and overweight and obesity: A systematic review of prospective cohort studies. *Obes. Rev.* **2011**, *12*, e582–e592. [CrossRef] [PubMed]

19. Patel, A.I.; Moghadam, S.D.; Freedman, M.; Hazari, A.; Fang, M.L.; Allen, I.E. The association of flavored milk consumption with milk and energy intake, and obesity: A systematic review. *Prev. Med.* **2018**, *111*, 151–162. [CrossRef] [PubMed]

20. Lamarche, B.; Givens, D.I.; Soedamah-Muthu, S.; Krauss, R.M.; Jakobsen, M.U.; Bischoff-Ferrari, H.A.; Pan, A.; Després, J.P. Does Milk Consumption Contribute to Cardiometabolic Health and Overall Diet Quality? *Can. J. Cardiol.* **2016**, *32*, 1026–1032. [CrossRef] [PubMed]

21. Barrena, R.; Garcia, T.; Sanchez, M. Analysis of personal and cultural values as key determinants of novel food acceptance. Application to an ethnic product. *Appetite* **2015**, *87*, 205–214. [CrossRef] [PubMed]

22. Bayarri, S.; Carbonell, I.; Barrios, E.X.; Costell, E. Acceptability of Yogurt and Yogurt-like Products: Influence of Product Information and Consumer Characteristics and Preferences. *J. Sens. Stud.* **2010**, *25*, 171–189. [CrossRef]

23. Ozimek, I.; Żakowska-Biemans, S. Determinants of Polish consumers' food choices and their implication for the national food industry. *Br. Food J.* **2011**, *113*, 138–154. [CrossRef]

24. Żakowska-Biemans, S. Polish consumer food choices and beliefs about organic food. *Br. Food J.* **2011**, *113*, 122–137. [CrossRef]

25. Dąbrowska, A.; Gutkowska, K.; Janoś-Kresło, M.; Ozimek, I. *Serwicyzacja Konsumpcji w Polskich Gospodarstwach Domowych: Uwarunkowania i Tendencje*; Difin: Warszawa, Poland, 2010. (In Polish)

26. Gutkowska, K.; Jankowski, P.; Sajdakowska, M.; Żakowska-Biemans, S.; Kowalczuk, I. Kryteria różnicujące zachowania konsumentów wobec produktów żywnościowych na przykładzie mięsa i przetworów mięsnych. *Żywność Nauka Technol. Jakość* **2014**, *96*, 85–100. (In Polish)

27. Jeżewska-Zychowicz, M. Impact of beliefs and attitudes on young consumers' willingness to use functional food. *Pol. J. Food Nutr. Sci.* **2009**, *59*, 183–187.

28. Verbeke, W.; Frewer, L.J.; Scholderer, J.; de Brabander, H.F. Why consumers behave as they do with respect to food safety and risk information. *Anal. Chim. Acta* **2006**, *586*, 2–7. [CrossRef] [PubMed]

29. Rahnama, H.; Rajabpour, S. Factors for consumer choice of dairy products in Iran. *Appetite* **2017**, *111*, 46–55. [CrossRef] [PubMed]

30. BIOŻYWNOŚĆ—Innowacyjne, Funkcjonalne Produkty Pochodzenia Zwierzęcego. Available online: http://www.biozywnosc.edu.pl/ (accessed on 31 July 2018). (In Polish)

31. Żakowska-Biemans, S.; Tekień, A. Free Range, Organic? Polish Consumers Preferences Regarding Information on Farming System and Nutritional Enhancement of Eggs: A Discrete Choice Based Experiment. *Sustainability* **2017**, *9*, 1999. [CrossRef]

32. Bauer, J.J. Selection errors of random route samples. *Sociol. Methods Res.* **2014**, *43*, 519–544. [CrossRef]

33. Kent, R. *Marketing Research in Action. Sampling Cases*; Kent, R., Ed.; Routledge: London, UK, 1993; p. 53.

34. Sajdakowska, M.; Jankowski, P.; Gutkowska, K.; Guzek, D.; Żakowska-Biemans, S.; Ozimek, I. Consumer acceptance of innovations in food: A survey among Polish consumers. *J. Consum. Behav.* **2018**, *17*, 253–267. [CrossRef]

35. Pliner, P.; Hobden, K. Development of a scale to measure the trait of food neophobia in humans. *Appetite* **1992**, *19*, 105–120. [CrossRef]

36. Roehrich, G. Consumer innovativeness: Concepts and measurements. *J. Bus. Res.* **2004**, *57*, 671–677. [CrossRef]

37. Bimbo, F.; Bonanno, A.; Nocella, G.; Viscecchia, R.; Nardone, G.; De Devitiis, B.; Carlucci, D. Consumers' acceptance and preferences for nutrition-modified and functional dairy products: A systematic review. *Appetite* **2017**, *113*, 141–154. [CrossRef] [PubMed]

38. Johansen, S.B.; Næs, T.; Hersleth, M. Motivation for choice and healthiness perception of calorie-reduced dairy products. A cross-cultural study. *Appetite* **2011**, *56*, 15–24. [CrossRef] [PubMed]

39. Camfield, D.A.; Owen, L.; Scholey, A.B.; Pipingas, A.; Stough, C. Dairy constituents and neurocognitive health in ageing. *Br. J. Nutr.* **2011**, *106*, 159–174. [CrossRef] [PubMed]

40. Cerjak, M.; Tomić, M. Buying Motives and Trust of Young Consumers for Functional Fermented Dairy Products: Evidence from Croatian Students. *J. Int. Food Agribus. Mark.* **2015**, *27*, 177–187. [CrossRef]

41. Choi, J.; Sabikhi, L.; Hassan, A.; Anand, S. Bioactive peptides in dairy products. *Int. J. Dairy Technol.* **2012**, *65*, 1–12. [CrossRef]

42. van der Zanden, L.D.T.; van Kleef, E.; de Wijk, E.R.; van Trijp, H.C.M. Knowledge, perceptions and preferences of elderly regarding protein-enriched functional food. *Appetite* **2014**, *80*, 16–22. [CrossRef] [PubMed]

43. Banovic, M.; Arvola, A.; Pennanen, K.; Duta, D.E.; Brückner-Gühmann, M.; Lähteenmäki, L.; Grunert, K.G. Foods with increased protein content: A qualitative study on European consumer preferences and perceptions. *Appetite* **2018**, *125*, 233–243. [CrossRef] [PubMed]

44. Stelten, S.; Dekker, I.M.; Ronday, E.M.; Thijs, A.; Boelsma, E.; Peppelenbos, H.W.; de van der Schueren, M.A.E. Protein-enriched 'regular products' and their effect on protein intake in acute hospitalized older adults; a randomized controlled trial. *Clin. Nutr.* **2015**, *34*, 409–414. [CrossRef] [PubMed]

45. Bernués, A.; Olaizola, A.; Corcoran, K. Extrinsic attributes of red meat as indicators of quality in Europe. An application for market segmentation. *Food Qual. Pref.* **2003**, *14*, 265–276. [CrossRef]

46. Grunert, K.G. Current issues in the understanding of consumer food choice. *Trends Food Sci. Technol.* **2002**, *13*, 275–285. [CrossRef]

47. Grunert, K.G.; Bech-Larsen, T.; Bredahl, L. Three issues in consumer quality perception and acceptance of dairy products. *Int. Dairy J.* **2000**, *10*, 575–584. [CrossRef]

48. Visschers, V.H.M.; Hartmann, C.; Leins-Hess, R.; Dohle, S.; Siegrist, M. A consumer segmentation of nutrition information use and its relation to food consumption behaviour. *Food Policy* **2013**, *42*, 71–80. [CrossRef]

49. Roos, E.; Lehto, R.; Ray, C. Parental family food choice motives and children's food intake. *Food Qual. Pref.* **2012**, *24*, 85–91. [CrossRef]

50. Jung, M.E.; Bourne, J.E.; Buchholz, A.; Martin Ginis, K.A. Strategies for public health initiatives targeting dairy consumption in young children: A qualitative formative investigation of parent perceptions. *Publ. Health Nutr.* **2017**, *20*, 2893–2908. [CrossRef] [PubMed]

51. Zhu, Y.; Wang, H.; Hollis, J.H.; Jacques, P.F. The associations between yogurt consumption, diet quality, and metabolic profiles in children in the USA. *Eur. J. Nutr.* **2015**, *54*, 543–550. [CrossRef] [PubMed]

52. Steijns, J.M. Dairy products and health: Focus on their constituents or on the matrix? *Int. Dairy J.* **2008**, *18*, 425–435. [CrossRef]

53. Abedini, M.; Falahi, E.; Roosta, S. Dairy product consumption and the metabolic syndrome. *Diabetes Metab. Syndr. Clin. Res. Rev.* **2015**, *9*, 34–37. [CrossRef] [PubMed]

54. Clerfeuille, E.; Maillot, M.; Verger, E.O.; Lluch, A.; Darmon, N.; Rolf-Pedersen, N. Dairy Products: How They Fit in Nutritionally Adequate Diets. *J. Acad. Nutr. Diet.* **2013**, *113*, 950–956. [CrossRef] [PubMed]

55. de Toledo Guimaraes, J.; Silva, E.K.; de Almeida Meireles, M.A.; Gomes da Cruz, A. Non-thermal emerging technologies and their effects on the functional properties of dairy products. *Curr. Opin. Food Sci.* **2018**, *22*, 62–66. [CrossRef]

56. Kowalczuk, I.; Gutkowska, K.; Sajdakowska, M.; Żakowska-Biemans, S.; Kozłowska, A.; Olewnik-Mikołajewska, A. Innowacyjny konsument żywności pochodzenia zwierzęcego. *Żywność Nauka Technol. Jakość* **2013**, *5*, 177–194. (In Polish)

57. McCarthy, B.; Liu, B.H.; Chen, T. Innovations in the agro-food system: Adoption of certified organic food and green food by Chinese consumers. *Br. Food J.* **2016**, *118*, 1334–1349. [CrossRef]

58. Gutkowska, K.; Sajdakowska, M.; Żakowska-Biemans, S.; Kowalczuk, I.; Kozłowska, A.; Olewnik-Mikołajewska, A. Poziom akceptacji zmian na rynku żywności pochodzenia zwierzęcego w opinii konsumentów. *Żywność Nauka Technol. Jakość* **2012**, *84*, 187–202. (In Polish)

59. Żakowska-Biemans, S. Czynniki różnicujące skłonność do zaakceptowania nowych produktów żywnościowych. *Handel Wewn.* **2016**, *363*, 384–398. (In Polish)

60. Kowalczuk, I.; Jeżewska-Zychowicz, M. Innowacyjność konsumentów na rynku żywności. *Stud. I Prace WNEiZ US* **2016**, *43*, 177–186. (In Polish) [CrossRef]

61. Kowalczuk, I. *Innowacyjna Żywność w Opinii Konsumentów i Producentów. Rozprawy Naukowe i Monografie. Treatises and Monographs*; Publications of WULS-SGGW; Wydawnictwo SGGW: Warszawa, Poland, 2011. (In Polish)

62. Handbury, J.; Weinstein, D.E. Goods Prices and Availability in Cities. *Rev. Econ. Stud.* **2015**, *82*, 258–296. [CrossRef]

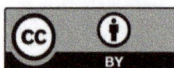

nutrients

MDPI

Review

Vitamin D Fortification of Fluid Milk Products and Their Contribution to Vitamin D Intake and Vitamin D Status in Observational Studies—A Review

Suvi T. Itkonen *, Maijaliisa Erkkola and Christel J. E. Lamberg-Allardt

Department of Food and Nutrition, P.O. Box 66, 00014 University of Helsinki, 00790 Helsinki, Finland;
maijaliisa.erkkola@helsinki.fi (M.E.); christel.lamberg-allardt@helsinki.fi (C.J.E.L.-A.)
* Correspondence: suvi.itkonen@helsinki.fi; Tel.: +358-44-356-1209

Received: 25 June 2018; Accepted: 7 August 2018; Published: 9 August 2018

Abstract: Fluid milk products are systematically, either mandatorily or voluntarily, fortified with vitamin D in some countries but their overall contribution to vitamin D intake and status worldwide is not fully understood. We searched the PubMed database to evaluate the contribution of vitamin D-fortified fluid milk products (regular milk and fermented products) to vitamin D intake and serum or plasma 25-hydroxyvitamin D (25(OH)D) status in observational studies during 1993–2017. Twenty studies provided data on 25(OH)D status (n = 19,744), and 22 provided data on vitamin D intake (n = 99,023). Studies showed positive associations between the consumption of vitamin D-fortified milk and 25(OH)D status in different population groups. In countries with a national vitamin D fortification policy covering various fluid milk products (Finland, Canada, United States), milk products contributed 28–63% to vitamin D intake, while in countries without a fortification policy, or when the fortification covered only some dairy products (Sweden, Norway), the contribution was much lower or negligible. To conclude, based on the reviewed observational studies, vitamin D-fortified fluid milk products contribute to vitamin D intake and 25(OH)D status. However, their impact on vitamin D intake at the population level depends on whether vitamin D fortification is systematic and policy-based.

Keywords: dairy; vitamin D; vitamin D-fortified milk; vitamin D intake; vitamin D fortification; 25-hydroxyvitamin D

1. Introduction

Vitamin D plays an important role in bone health, being necessary for calcium absorption [1]. Low vitamin D status in terms of low serum 25-hydroxyvitamin D (S-25(OH)D) concentration has also been linked to the increased risk of some common chronic diseases, such as type 2 diabetes or cardiovascular disease [2]. In Northern latitudes, especially in the wintertime, ultraviolet B (UVB) radiation is too low for dermal synthesis of vitamin D [3]. As there are only a few natural vitamin D-rich foods, such as fish, egg yolk, and some wild mushrooms [1], some countries, particularly populations at high latitudes, have initiated national policies of fortifying certain foods with vitamin D to prevent vitamin D deficiency. Usually these vitamin D-fortified products are low-fat milk, fat spreads, breakfast cereals, and certain baby foods [4,5]. To better cover different population groups with differing food habits, a wider vitamin D fortification of different products instead of concentrating on only a few staple foods has been suggested [5].

To our knowledge, a portion of milk products are systematically, either mandatorily or voluntarily, fortified with vitamin D only in Finland, Norway, Sweden, Canada, and United States (Table 1) [6–12]. In Finland, the recommended fortification level of all fluid milks except some organic products is currently 1 µg/100 g, but some products with a concentration of 2 µg/100 g are available on the market [6,7]. The fortification is voluntary, but all manufacturers unanimously follow the recommendations. In Norway, only one type of milk is recommended to be fortified with vitamin D at a concentration of 0.4 µg/100 g [8]. Sweden recently doubled the fortification levels of fluid milks to 1 µg/100 g and extended the mandatory fortification to cover all fluid milk products with <3% fat [9,10]. Health Canada has also proposed increasing the mandatory vitamin D fortification of fluid milks from around 1 µg/100 g to 2 µg/100 g as a consequence of the inadequate vitamin D intake among the population [11]. In the United States, fluid milks can be fortified with vitamin D by around 1 µg/100 g; the fortification is not mandate at the federal level, but most states mandate fortification [12]. In other countries, such as United Kingdom, Ireland, Spain, and Australia, the fortification is not systematic, but there is a varying number of vitamin D-fortified milk products available [13–17]. However, data on their proportion to the total amount of dairy products in different countries is not easily accessed due to fluctuations in the market. This causes a knowledge gap on the prevalence of vitamin D fortified fluid milks and their contribution to vitamin D intake worldwide.

In the latest updated systematic review and meta-analysis on the effects of vitamin D fortification in randomised controlled trials (RCT), 12 of the 16 included studies used different milk products, such as fluid milk or milk powder, as a carrier of vitamin D [18]. Four of these studies used vitamin D-fortified milk and two used vitamin D-fortified yoghurt drinks. All of the studies showed the efficacy of the studied milk products to increase the S-25(OH)D concentration or decrease the decline in S-25(OH)D status during the wintertime relative to the control group [19–24]. Further, in Finland, the vitamin D fortification of fluid milks has been shown to improve the S-25(OH)D status independently among regular milk users after extensive changes in the national vitamin D fortification policy in an 11-year follow-up study [25].

The aim of this review was to investigate the contribution of vitamin D-fortified fluid milk products (regular milk and fermented products, such as sour milk and yoghurt) (i) to vitamin D intake; and (ii) to vitamin D status (25(OH)D concentration in plasma or serum in observational studies with a special focus on differences possibly caused by different vitamin D fortification policies.

Table 1. Countries with a vitamin D fortification policy of fluid milk products.

Country	Vitamin D-Fortified Milk Products	Type of Fortification	Added Amount of Vitamin D	New Proposed Amounts of Vitamin D
Finland [6,7]	fluid milk products (milk, yoghurt, sourmilk) *	voluntary	1 μg/100 g	na
Norway [8]	extra low-fat milk (also lactose free)	voluntary	0.4 μg/100 g	na
Sweden [9,10]	low-fat milk (max 1.5% fat)	mandatory	0.38–0.50 μg/100 g	0.95–1.10 μg/100 g for milk <3% fat 0.75–1.10 μg/100 g for fermented milk <3% fat
Canada [11]	milk	mandatory	0.825–1.125 μg/100 g	2 μg/100 g
United States [12]	fluid milk (also acidified milk and cultured milk), yoghurt	voluntary ‡	1.05 μg/100 g for milk 2.225 μg/100 g for yoghurt §	na

* In regard to organic milk products, it is mandatory to add 1 μg/100 g vitamin D to homogenized fat-free milk (not allowed on other organic milk products). ‡ for milk products, only evaporated and non-fat dry milk are mandatorily fortified. § maximum amount; na = not applicable.

2. Materials and Methods

2.1. Data Sources and Search Strategy

The literature search was done in the PubMed database at the end of December 2017. The search terms were the following combination of keywords: "vitamin D" [MeSH Terms] OR "vitamin D" [All Fields] OR "ergocalciferols" [MeSH Terms] OR "ergocalciferols" [All Fields]) AND (dairy [All Fields] OR ("milk, human" [MeSH Terms] OR ("milk" [All Fields] AND "human" [All Fields]) OR "human milk" [All Fields] OR "milk" [All Fields] OR "milk" [MeSH Terms])) AND (fortification [All Fields] OR fortified [All Fields]". We limited the search to articles that had the search terms in their title, abstract or among keywords. The data search was restricted to the last 25 years from 1993 to 2017.

2.2. Eligibility and Study Selection

Two independent authors reviewed the titles and abstracts of all identified studies and selected observational studies that reported either vitamin D intake or 25(OH)D status in plasma or serum for full-text screening. Among the full-texts, the eligibility of the articles was screened using the following exclusion criteria: full-text in a language other than English, studies with disease outcomes, participants/patient groups with diagnosed diseases, participants aged less than one year, studies in which the contribution of *growing up milks* (special products marketed for 1 to 3-year-olds) could not be separated from that of other fluid milks, RCTs, and reviews. In addition, nationally representative study reports in local languages other than English were searched to cover vitamin D intake data from all countries with vitamin D fortification policy of fluid milks.

2.3. Data Extraction

The following information was extracted from eligible studies: first author's name, publication year, country, number and age range of subjects, dietary assessment method, total and/or dietary vitamin D intake (vitamin D intake studies), vitamin D intake from milk (vitamin D intake studies), contribution of milk to vitamin D intake (vitamin D intake studies), latitude (25(OH)D studies), season that blood was drawn (25(OH)D studies), 25(OH)D assay method and quality control of assay (25(OH)D studies), and 25(OH)D concentrations (25(OH)D studies). The results were stratified by the population groups as follows: "children and adolescents" (vitamin D and 25(OH)D studies), "pregnant women and mother-child pairs" (25(OH)D studies), and "adults, elderly, and all age groups" (vitamin D and 25(OH)D studies). In addition, the results were reported by country. In some cases, the results were stratified by supplement use or other factors, depending on the original study design. In 25(OH)D studies, the role of vitamin D-fortified milk on vitamin D status was examined as a determinant of vitamin D status or as a comparison of the 25(OH)D status between low or non-users of vitamin D-fortified milk and more frequent users. If the contribution of milk to total vitamin D intake was not provided, it was calculated from the reported total intake and vice versa. International units were converted to micrograms, and 25(OH)D concentrations in ng/ml were converted to nmol/L. In this study, we referred to the Institute of Medicine threshold for S-25(OH)D status, where ≤30 nmol/L is vitamin D deficient, 30–49.9 nmol/L is insufficient, and ≥50 nmol/L is sufficient [26].

3. Results

Figure 1 shows the literature search and study selection process. We found 337 articles that were published between 1993 and 2017, and their titles and abstracts were scanned. Fifty-one full-text review papers were selected. Of these, two were unavailable and the corresponding author could not be reached, and 15 were not relevant to the research questions. Thus, 34 papers were included in the review process. Of these, 20 provided data on the 25(OH)D status, and 20 provided data on vitamin D intake. Additionally, intake data in national surveys covering countries with a fluid milk vitamin D fortification policy that were not covered in the PubMed search (Norway, Sweden) were explored. One Norwegian [27] and one Swedish report [28] in local language were found and were included to provide data on vitamin D intake and the contribution of milk in those countries. Nationally representative data from other countries with a vitamin D fortification policy were already found in the literature search.

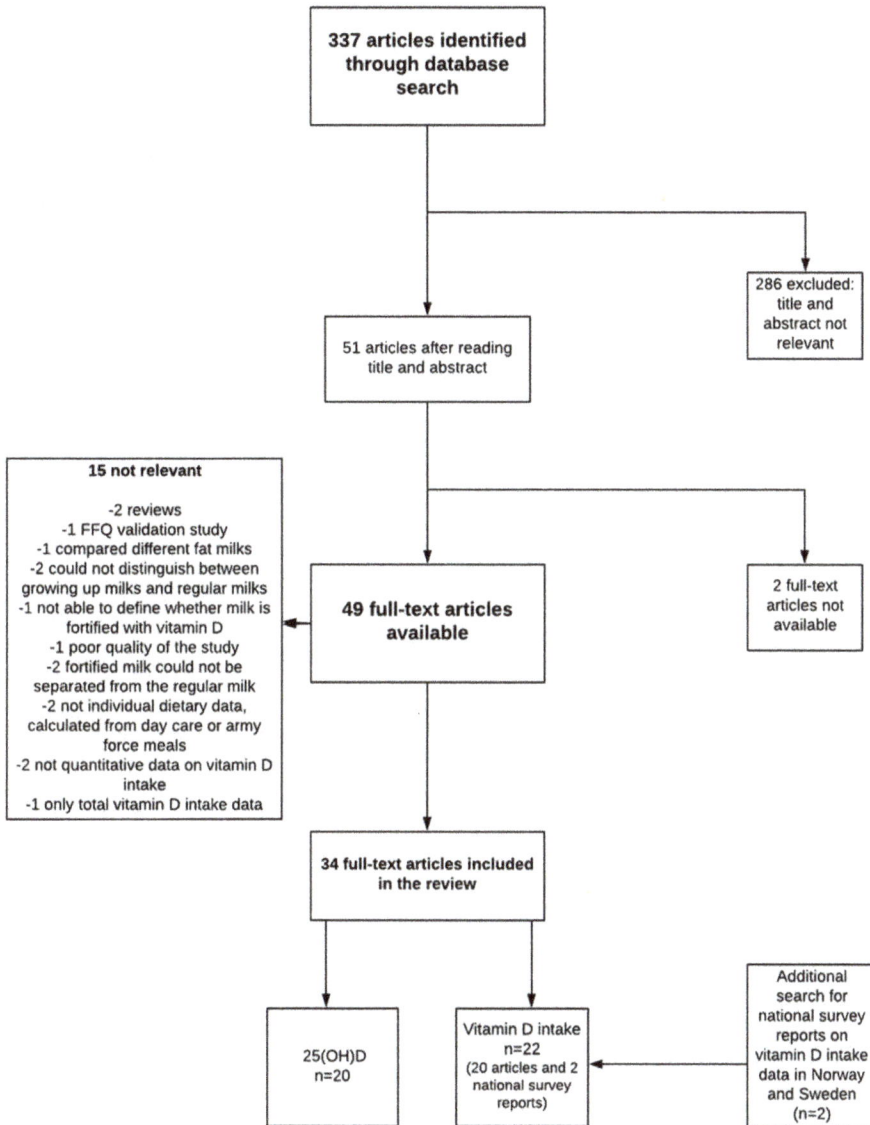

Figure 1. Literature search and study selection process.

3.1. Contribution of Vitamin D-Fortified Milk to Vitamin D Intakes

For this review, 22 observational studies reported data on the contribution of vitamin D-fortified milk to vitamin D intake including 99,023 subjects (Table 2). Data from the following countries were provided: United States (6 studies), Canada (4), Finland (4), Ireland (2), Australia (1), Norway (1), Spain (1), Sweden (1), and United Kingdom (1). Additionally, one study provided data from both the United

States and Canada. Various methods to assess vitamin D intake were used: food records (8 studies), 24 h recalls (7), food frequency questionnaires (FFQ) (4), one-week diet history (1), household food diary (1), and both FFQ and food records (1).

3.1.1. Children and Adolescents

In the studies of Irish and British children and adolescents, the total vitamin D intakes were 2.8–3.5 µg/day and dietary intakes were 1.6–2.6 µg/day [13–15]. Fortified milks provided 0.4 µg/day or less vitamin D [13–15]. It is notable that the consumption of vitamin D-fortified milk was not common; in the study of Black et al. [13], only 4–5% of subjects consumed vitamin D-fortified milk. In contrast, in countries with policy-based vitamin D fortification, i.e., in the United States, Canada, and Finland, the mean dietary vitamin D intakes in children were 4.4–5.9 µg/day, and 2.3–3.3 µg/day of that originated from milk products, covering more than half of the total dietary intake [29–32].

3.1.2. Adults and the Elderly, and Studies Including All Age Groups

In Spain and Australia, some of the fluid milks on the market are fortified with vitamin D and studies conducted in these countries among the adult population showed that the contribution of milk to total vitamin D intake was 15–18%, with total intakes being 3.5 and 4.4 µg/day, respectively [16,17]. In a Canadian population-based study among adults, the total vitamin D intake was shown to be 5.6 µg/day among females and 4.8 µg/day among males, and milk contributed 48% of the total vitamin D intake among females and 63% among males [33]. In other large American and Canadian population-based studies covering all age groups, 1.9–2.9 µg of vitamin D ingested per day originated from milk, while mean total vitamin D intakes ranged from 4.2 to 9.8 µg/day and dietary intakes from 3.9 to 7.0 µg/day, milk contributing 44–49% of the vitamin D intake [33–37]. In a smaller study carried out among the adult population in the United States as well in a Canadian study on Inuit and Inuvialuit women, vitamin D intakes were similar to those found in the larger studies; however, the contribution of milk to vitamin D intake was slightly lower, 31–43% [38,39]. In line with the newer studies, in two studies carried out among elderly people in the United States that were published in the 1990s, half of the vitamin D intake originated from milk [40,41]. The recent representative population-based study in Finland [25] showed that 34% of dietary vitamin D intake originated from vitamin D-fortified fluid milk products which is similar to the proportion observed in the latest National FINDIET Study—28–39%, varying between age and sex groups [42]. Dietary vitamin D intakes in the study of Jääskeläinen et al. were the highest among all of the studies included in this review: 14 µg/day among men and 12 µg/day among women [25]. Data on the contributions of milk to vitamin D intake in other Nordic European countries following the implementation of a national vitamin D fortification policy have also been provided. The latest Norwegian national dietary survey reported that extra-skimmed milk, the only vitamin D-fortified milk in Norway, provided 4% of dietary vitamin D intake, with the mean dietary vitamin D intake being 6 µg/day [27]. Despite the wider milk fortification policy in Sweden, only 12% of dietary vitamin D intake originated from milk products in the Swedish national survey, with the mean dietary vitamin D intake being 7 µg/day [28].

Table 2. Studies on the contribution of milk to total or dietary vitamin D intake.

Reference	Country	Study Population	Dietary Assessment Method	Total/Dietary Vitamin D Intake (µg/day)	SD (or SEM *)	Vitamin D Intake from (fortified) Fluid Milk or Related Products (µg/day)	SD	Contribution of (Fortified) Milk to Total or Dietary Vitamin D Intake (%)
Children and adolescents								
Black et al. (2014) [13]	Ireland	594 children, 5–12 years and 441 teenagers, 13–17 years	7-day (semi-) weighted food record	Total/dietary intake 5–8 years: 2.8/1.9 9–12 years: 2.8/2.2 13–17 years: 3.2/2.6	2.4/1.1 2.1/1.3 2.5/1.8	Fortified milk: 0.1 Milk and yoghurt: 0.3–0.4	na	Total intake Fortified milk: 2–3% Milk and yoghurt: 10–13%
Cole et al. (2010) [29]	United States	290 children, 1–5 years	3-day food record	Dietary intake: 4.4	3.0	Fortified milk: 2.7 †	na	Dietary intake Fortified milk: 62%
Cribb et al. (2015) [14]	United Kingdom	755 children, 1.5 years and 3.5 years	3-day food diary	Dietary intake 1.5 years: 1.6 3.5 years: 1.8	1.5 1.4	Yoghurt, cheese and milk 1.5 years: 0.035 µg/MJ/day 3.5 years: 0.023 µg/MJ/day	0.02 µg/MJ/day 0.02 µg/MJ/day	Dietary intake Yoghurt, cheese and milk 1.5 years: 9% 3.5 years: 6%
Hennessy et al. (2016) [15]	Ireland	500 children, 1–4 years	4-day weighted food diary	Total intake All subjects: 3.5 Fortified food consumers: 3.2	3.7 2.7	Fortified milk All subjects: 0.1 Fortified food consumers: 0.1	na	Total intake All subjects: 2% Fortified food consumers, supplement non-users: 13%
Mark et al. (2011) [30]	Canada	159 children, 8–11 years	3 × 24 h recalls	Total/dietary intake: 6.6/5.6	4.3/3.5	Milk: 3.3 †	na	Total/dietary intake Milk: 49/58%
Piirainen et al. (2007) [32]	Finland	36 children, 4 years	4-day food record	Total/dietary intake: 7.9/4.5	6.3–9.6/ 3.8–5.1 §	2.3	2.0–2.6 §	Total intake Milk: 54%
Soininen et al. (2016) [31]	Finland	374 children, 6–8 years	4-day food record	Total/dietary intake: 7.7/5.9	na/2.1	Fluid milk: 2.9 All milk products: 3.1	1.5 1.4	Total/dietary intake Fluid milk: 38/49% All milk products: 40/52%
Adults and the elderly								
Amcoff et al. (2012) [28]	Sweden	1797 adults, 18–80 years	4-day food diary	Dietary intake Women: 6.4 Men: 7.6	4.2/5.4	na	na	Dietary intake Milk products: 12%
Gonzalez-Rodríguez et al. (2013) [16]	Spain	418 adults, 18–60 years	24 h recall	Total/dietary intake: 3.5/3.2	4.0/3.8	Dairy products: 0.5 †	na	Total/dietary intake Dairy products: 15/17%

Table 2. Cont.

Reference	Country	Study Population	Dietary Assessment Method	Total/Dietary Vitamin D Intake (μg/day)	SD (or SEM *)	Vitamin D Intake from (fortified) Fluid Milk or Related Products (μg/day)	SD	Contribution of (Fortified) Milk to Total or Dietary Vitamin D Intake (%)
Holm Totland et al. (2012) [27]	Norway	1787 adults, 18–70 years	24 h recall	Total/dietary intake Women: 10/4.9 Men: 12/6.7	na/4.3 na/5.7	na	na	Dietary intake Vitamin D fortified extra-skimmed milk: 4%
Jayaratne et al. (2013) [17]	Australia	785 adults, ≥31 years	FFQ	Total intake: 4.4	4.0	Dairy and related products including margarine: 1.9 [†] Milk: 0.8 [†] Yoghurt: 0.3 [†]	na na na	Total intake Dairy and related products including margarine: 43% Milk: 18% Yoghurt: 6%
Jääskeläinen et al. (2017) [25]	Finland	3635 adults, ≥30 years	FFQ	Dietary intake Men: 14 Women: 12	14–15 [§] 11–12 [§]	na	na	Dietary intake Fluid milk products: 34%
Kinyamu et al. (1998) [41]	United States	376 elderly women, 65–77 years	7-day food record	Total intake Supplement non-users: 3.5 Supplement users: 13.4	2.2 2.0	Milk Supplement non-users: 2.0 Supplement users: 1.8	1.6 1.5	Total intake Milk: 51%
Kolahdooz et al. (2013) [38]	Canada	203 Inuit and Inuvialuit women, 19–44 years	FFQ	All subjects: 6.0 [‡] Traditional food eaters: 7.1 [‡] Non-traditional food eaters: 4.9 [‡]	6.3 5.3 3.2	Dairy group (milk, yoghurt, cheese and eggs) Traditional food eaters: 2.2 Non-traditional food eaters: 1.9	na na	Dairy group (milk, yoghurt, cheese and eggs) Traditional food eaters: 31% [‡] Non-traditional food eaters: 39% [‡]
Levy et al. (2015) [39]	United States	743 adults, 20–65 years	one week diet history	Total intake Winter season: 4.5 Summer season: 4.3	4.0 3.2	Dairy products Winter season: 1.9 Summer season: 1.9	2.5 3.8	Dietary intake Winter season: 43% Summer season: 41%
Moore et al. (2014) [37]	United States	9719 adults, ≥19 years	24 h recall	Total/dietary intake 8.6/4.4	0.3/0.1 *	Milk and milk drinks: 1.7 [†] Fortified milk and milk products: 1.9 [†]	na na	Total/dietary intake Milk and milk drinks: 20/39% Fortified milk and milk products: 22/44%
O'Dowd et al. (1993) [41]	United States	109 elderly, >60 years	FFQ or 3-day dietary record	Total/dietary intake All subjects: 9.5/ Supplement non-users: 7.3	5.1/2.5	Fortified milk All subjects: 4.7	1.9	Total intake Fortified milk: 50%

Table 2. *Cont.*

Reference	Country	Study Population	Dietary Assessment Method	Total/Dietary Vitamin D Intake (µg/day)	SD (or SEM *)	Vitamin D Intake from (fortified) Fluid Milk or Related Products (µg/day)	SD	Contribution of (Fortified) Milk to Total or Dietary Vitamin D Intake (%)
Poliquin et al. (2009) [33]	Canada	9425 adults, ≥25 years	interview-administered semi-quantitative FFQ	Total intake from milk and supplements Women: 5.6 Men: 4.8	5.9 5.5	Milk Women: 2.7 Men: 3.0	2.9 3.5	Total intake from milk and supplements Women: 48% Men: 63%
Raulio et al. (2017) [42]	Finland	1295 adults, 25–64 years	24 h recall	Total intake Women: all women: 17.5 Supplement non-users: 8.6 Supplement users: 24.7 Men: all men: 17.3 Supplement non-users: 11.2 Supplement users: 29.5	15.4 6.2 16.8 17.0 7.5 23.1	na	na	Dietary intake Milk: 28–39%, depending on age and sex
All ages								
Hill et al. (2012) [36]	United States and Canada	7837 US and 4025 Canadian citizens, ≥2 years	7- to 14-day household food diary	Total intake United States: 4.4 Canada: 4.2	0.03 * 0.5 *	Milk United States: 2.0 Canada: 1.9	na na	Total intake Milk: 44% in both countries
Moore et al. (2004) [34]	United States	18931 subjects, >1 years	24 h recall	Total/dietary intake: 5.3–9.8/3.9–7.0 depending on age and sex	na	na	na	Dietary intake Dairy products: 45–47%
Vatanparast et al. (2010) [35]	Canada	34789 subjects, >1 years	24 h recall	Dietary intake: 6.2	0.1 *	Milk products: 2.9	na	Dietary intake Milk products: 49%

FFQ, food frequency questionnaire; na, not applicable; * SE(M), standard error (of mean); † calculated from the proportion of milk contribution; ‡ unclear whether total or dietary vitamin D intake (3% supplement users); § 95% confidence interval.

143

3.2. Associations Between Consumption of Vitamin D-Fortified Milk and 25(OH)D Status

Twenty observational studies included in this review investigated associations between the consumption of vitamin D-fortified milk and 25(OH)D status (*n* = 19,744) (Table 3). Data from the following countries were provided: United States (5 studies), Canada (4), Finland (3), Sweden (2), Egypt (1), Ireland (1), Jordan (1), Norway (1), Spain (1), and Thailand (1). Various methods were used to assess 25(OH)D concentrations: different immunoassays (13 studies), LC-MS/MS (5) and competitive binding assays (2). Milk consumption was assessed by either a questionnaire (8 studies), FFQ (5), food records (4), 24 h recall (1), one-week diet history (1) or by both FFQ and food records (1).

3.2.1. Children and Adolescents

Among Egyptian children aged 9–11 years (*n* = 200), those who consumed vitamin D-fortified milk less than once a day had a significantly higher risk of vitamin D insufficiency (S-25(OH)D < 50 nmol/L) than those who consumed more milk [43]. In Jordan, children who consumed vitamin D-fortified fresh milk had higher S-25(OH)D concentrations than those who consumed unfortified milk (53 nmol/L vs. 43 nmol/L) (*n* = 93) [44]. These two studies did not provide data on the amounts of consumed milk. In Finland, higher consumption of vitamin D-fortified milk was associated with higher S-25(OH)D concentrations among children aged 6–8 years (*n* = 374) [31]. Children who drank at least 450 g/day of vitamin D-fortified milk had a 72–74% lower risk of having S-25(OH)D below 50 nmol/L than those who drank less than 300 g/day (adjusted for age and sex). However, another study on 10-year-old Finnish children (*n* = 171) found no association between vitamin D-fortified milk consumption frequency and S-25(OH)D status, but among those children with a history of cow's milk allergy (an indicator of milk avoidance), consumption of vitamin D-fortified milk as well as S-25(OH)D concentrations were lower than among their peers without allergy history [45]. Nevertheless, vitamin D supplement use was very common in this population (60% daily users), and thus was one important determinant of their vitamin D status [45].

A Canadian study in 1–6-year-old children (*n* = 2468) showed that children who drank only non-cow's milk (i.e. vegetable-based milk alternatives or goat's milk) were more than two-fold likely to have an S-25(OH)D concentration <50 nmol/L relative to children who drank cow's milk, which is mandatorily fortified in Canada (odds ratio 2.7, 95% CI 1.6–4.7) [46]. In another sample of Canadian children aged 8–11 years with a daily mean of 1.3 vitamin D-fortified milk servings (*n* = 159), one daily serving of milk contributed to a 2.9 nmol/L increase in plasma 25(OH)D concentration [30]. Further, among 2270 children aged 3–18 years in Canada, those consuming vitamin D-fortified milk daily were more likely to have sufficient S-25(OH)D concentration (≥50 nmol/L) than those who drank milk less frequently (odds ratio 2.4, 95% CI 1.7–3.3) [47,48]. A Spanish study in 9–13-year-old children (*n* = 102) showed that the number of daily dairy servings (mean 2.3 servings) was associated with the S-25(OH)D status [49]. Those who consumed ≥2.5 servings of milk daily had higher S-25(OH)D concentrations than those who did not (53 nmol/L vs. 46 nmol/L) [49]. In Sweden, fortified lean milk consumption (mean 230 g/day) correlated with S-25(OH)D status in a group of 13-year-old children (*n* = 165) [50]. Among 15–18-year-old adolescents in Norway (*n* = 890), the use of vitamin D-fortified milk was significantly associated with S-25(OH)D status in a multivariate model in boys, but not in girls [51]. Boys who were frequent milk consumers had higher S-25(OH)D concentrations than infrequent consumers, but this was not seen among girls, and no milk consumption data was provided [51].

3.2.2. Pregnant Women and Mother-Child Pairs

Two studies carried out in pregnant women in Thailand and Finland also showed an association between vitamin D-fortified milk and vitamin D status [52,53]. Among Thai women (*n* = 120), the consumption of multivitamin-fortified milk containing vitamin D was higher among those with vitamin D sufficiency (S-25(OH)D concentration > 50 nmol/L) in the third trimester than among those with insufficiency [52]. Consumption of multivitamin-fortified milk was associated with an increase in S-25(OH)D concentration between the first and third trimester. The mean multivitamin-fortified milk consumption was 1.0 daily serving in the first trimester and 1.4 servings in the third trimester. In a multivariate analysis, non-consumption of multivitamin-fortified milk was an independent predictor of vitamin D deficiency [52]. In a study carried out in 584 mother-child pairs in Finland, modifiers of umbilical cord blood (UCB) 25(OH)D status were studied [53]. The maternal dietary pattern "dairy and sandwich", including vitamin D-fortified milk and margarines, positively contributed to child UCB 25(OH)D status in mother-child pairs in whom an increase was seen in 25(OH)D concentration when comparing maternal 25(OH)D status in early pregnancy with UCB 25(OH)D status, but not in those in whom no increase was seen [53]. Among Jordanian women, no differences in S-25(OH)D concentration were seen among those who consumed vitamin D-fortified milk relative to those who consumed unfortified milk (26 nmol/L vs. 27 nmol/L) [44]. However, their vitamin D status was much worse than that of their children, whose vitamin D status was better if vitamin D-fortified milk was consumed [44].

3.2.3. Adults, the Elderly, and All Age Groups

Among adults aged 20–65 years in the United States (*n* = 743), the use of vitamin D-fortified milk was a significant predictor of S-25(OH)D status in the wintertime, but not in the summertime [39]. In an elderly American population aged >65 years (*n* = 376) [41], S-25(OH)D status correlated with milk calcium intake from vitamin D-fortified milk (an indicator of milk consumption). Among those who did not use vitamin D supplements, milk calcium was the main determinant of S-25(OH)D status; however, this was not the case among vitamin D supplement users. Among adult (≥18 years) Arab-American women (*n* = 87), vitamin D-fortified milk was not an independent determinant of S-25(OH)D status, but their milk consumption was minimal, and S-25(OH)D concentrations were extremely low [54]. In the Canadian National Survey consisting of a population aged 6–79 years (*n* = 5306), those who consumed vitamin D-fortified milk once a day or more had higher S-25(OH)D concentrations than those with consumption of less than once a day [55]. People who consumed milk more than once a day had a mean S-25(OH)D concentration of 75 nmol/L, while the corresponding mean among those who consumed milk less than once a day was 63 nmol/L. In a Swedish study on elderly women aged >60 years (*n* = 116), consumption of vitamin D-fortified reduced-fat dairy correlated with S-25(OH)D status, and the intake of two daily portions of fortified milk (300 g) was associated with a 6.2 nmol/L increment in S-25(OH)D concentration in a multiple linear regression model [56]. Further, in an Irish study of three large cohorts of elderly subjects (*n* = 1233, *n* = 1895, *n* = 1316), vitamin D-fortified milk consumption predicted a higher S-25(OH)D concentration in two of the three cohorts [57].

Table 3. Studies in which the contribution of vitamin D-fortified milk to serum or plasma 25-hydroxyvitamin D status was evaluated.

Reference	Country (Latitude)	Season Blood Drawn	Study Population	25(OH)D Assay Method (Quality Control of Assay: Certificate; CV% <15%)	Dietary Assessment Method	Serum or Plasma 25(OH)D nmol/L Mean (or Median *)	SD (or IQR † or 95% CI ‡ or SE §)
Children and adolescents							
Abu Shady et al. (2016) [43]	Egypt (31° N)	April, May	200 children, 9–11 years	Quantitative enzyme immunoassay (na; na)	Questionnaire	41	14
Barman et al. (2015) [50]	Sweden (63° N)	All	165 children, 13 years	LC-MS/MS (na; na)	FFQ	51	14
Cole et al. (2010) [29]	United States (33° N)	All	290 children, 1–5 years	LC-MS/MS (na; na)	3-day food record	65	19
Lee et al. (2014) [46]	Canada (43° N)	All	2468 children, 1–6 years	Diasorin LIAISON (na; yes except inter CV% 17.4% at high concentrations)	Questionnaire	80 *	66–99 †
Mark et al. (2011) [30]	Canada (45° N)	All	159 children, 8–11 years	IDS radioimmunoassay (na; yes)	3 × 24 h recalls	Winter/spring: 50 Summer/autumn: 58	10 15
Munasinghe et al. (2017) [47,48]	Canada (various latitudes)	All	2270 children, 3–18 years	Diasorin LIAISON (na; yes)	FFQ	62	56–69 ‡
Rodríguez–Rodríguez et al. (2011) [49]	Spain (40° N)	February	102 children, 9–13 years	Chemiluminescence (na; na)	3-day weighted food diary	50	16
Rosendahl et al. (2017) [45]	Finland (60° N)	January–June	171 children, 10 years	Roche Diagnostics immunochemiluminescence (na; na)	FFQ	73	22
Soininen et al. (2016) [31]	Finland (62° N)	All but July	374 children, 6–8 years	Diasorin LIAISON (na; yes)	4-day food record	69	24
Öberg et al. (2014) [51]	Norway (69° N)	September–April	890 children, 15–18 years	LC-MS/MS (DEQAS; yes)	Questionnaire	Boys: 41 Girls: 54	21 23
Pregnant women and mother-child pairs							
Charatcharoenwitthaya et al. (2013) [52]	Thailand (14° N)	Winter season: 72%, rainy season: 28%	120 pregnant women, 18–40 years	LC-MS/MS MassCrom (na; yes)	Interviewed questionnaire	1st trimester: 61 2nd trimester: 84 3rd trimester: 90	17 20 22
Gharaibeh et al. (2009) [44]	Jordan (31° N)	June and July	93 children (4–5 years) and mothers (mean age 34 years) dyads	IDS ELISA (na; na)	Questionnaire	Mothers: 26 Children: 56	10 20

Table 3. *Cont.*

Reference	Country (Latitude)	Season Blood Drawn	Study Population	25(OH)D Assay Method (Quality Control of Assay: Certificate; CV% <15%)	Dietary Assessment Method	Serum or Plasma 25(OH)D nmol/L Mean (or Median *)	SD (or IQR †, or 95% CI ‡ or SE §)
Hauta-alus et al. (2017) [53]	Finland (60° N)	All	584 newborns and mothers (18–43 years)	IDS-iSYS (DEQAS; yes)	FFQ	Mothers: 89 / Cord blood: 88	19 / 22
Adults and the elderly							
Burgaz et al. (2007) [56]	Sweden (60° N)	January–March	116 elderly women, 61–86 years	IDS EIA (na; yes)	FFQ	69	23
Hobbs et al. (2009) [54]	United States (42° N)	April	87 women, ≥18 years	Diasorin LLAISON (na; na)	Questionnaire	Unveiled subjects: 21 * / Veiled supplement users: 17 * / Veiled supplement non-users: 10 *	14–34 † / 10–29 † / 5–17 †
Kinyamu et al. (1998) [41]	United States (41° N)	All	376 elderly women, 65–77 years	Competitive binding assay (na; yes)	7-day food record	Supplement non-users: 74 / Supplement users: 88	23 / 28
Levy et al. (2015) [39]	United States (various latitudes)	February–April and August–October	743 adults, 20–65 years	Diasorin LLAISON (College of American Pathology; na)	One week diet history	Summer: 101 / Winter: 93	42 / 39
McCarroll et al. (2015) [57]	Ireland (52° N)	All	3 cohorts (1233, 1895, 1316) of elderly subjects, >60 years	LC-MS (DEQAS; yes)	Questionnaire	Supplement non-users: 46/61/68 / Supplement users: 67/83/74	24/32/23 / 27/27/30
ODowd et al. (1993) [40]	United States (41° N)	January–May	109 elderly, >60 years	Competitive binding assay (na; yes)	FFQ or 3-day dietary record	All subjects: 45 / Supplement non-users: 40 / Supplement users: 65	2 § / 2 § / 3 §
All ages							
Langlois et al. (2010) [55]	Canada (various latitudes)	All	5306 subjects, 6–79 years	Diasorin Liaison (DEQAS; yes)	Interviewed questionnaire	All subjects 68 / April-October 70 / November–March 64	65–70 ‡ / 66–74 ‡ / 60–68 ‡

CI, confidence interval; CV coefficient of variation; DEQAS, Vitamin D External Quality Assessment Scheme; EIA enzyme immunoassay; ELISA enzyme linked immunosorbent assay; FFQ, food frequency questionnaire; IQR interquartile range; LC-MS/MS liquid chromatography-tandem mass spectrometry; SE standard error; 25(OH)D, 25-hydroxyvitamin D. * Median; † IQR; ‡ 95% CI; § SE.

4. Discussion

Based on these observational studies on vitamin D intake and vitamin D-fortified milk consumption, it seems that in countries with wide vitamin D fortification policies (Finland, Canada, United States), the total vitamin D intake as well as the contribution of milk to total vitamin D intake is higher than in the countries without fortification policies (Ireland, United Kingdom, Spain, Australia). It is notable that in Norway and Sweden, where some of the fluid milks are fortified with vitamin D amounts lower than in Finland, Canada, or United States, the contribution of fluid milk to vitamin D intake was shown to be as low as 4% and 12%, respectively, compared with around 50% in the other fortification policy countries.

Concerning the vitamin D status, we observed that the consumption of vitamin D-fortified milk was positively associated with 25(OH)D status in almost all studies included in this review within heterogeneous population groups, independent of country-specific vitamin D-fortification policies. Even though the consumed amounts of milk varied, the associations between milk and 25(OH)D status were seen also at fairly low consumption levels. Further, the association was seen in different population groups: children (with the exception of 10-year old Finns), teenagers (except in Norwegian girls), adults (except in Arab-American women), pregnant women, and the elderly. This mostly positive association between vitamin D-fortified milk consumption and vitamin D status was supported by a recent standardized representative population-based study in Finland, where the vitamin D fortification policy of fluid milks, in particular, was shown to be successful in improving vitamin D status in the Finnish population [25]. It would be useful to have systematic follow-up data from the other countries with vitamin D fortification policies, as the present evidence is based mainly on the Finnish follow-up study. Vatanparast et al. [35] stated that despite vitamin D fortification being mandatory in Canada, the vitamin D intakes are inadequate and recently, Canada implemented new guidelines to increase the fortification levels [11]. Sweden has also extended their vitamin D fortification policy [10]; thus, in the following years there is an opportunity to evaluate the effects of vitamin D fortification at the population level also in those countries.

4.1. Limitations of the Study

The studies included in this review were carried out in populations of differing size, age, and gender in numerous countries and at a range of latitudes with different levels of UVB exposure. Different assay methods for 25(OH)D analysis have been used, increasing the heterogeneity of the studies [58], and not all studies have provided quality control data. LC-MS/MS, which is considered the golden standard and reference method in 25(OH)D assays [58], was used in 25% of the reviewed studies. However, as our aim was to investigate the associations between the consumption of vitamin D fortified milk and 25(OH)D status, the differences among the assays probably do not mitigate the power of the overall conclusions, as the trends in 25(OH)D concentrations usually remain similar independent of the analysis method used [59]. Of greater importance is that most studies considered the variability of 25(OH)D concentrations between seasons and took the samples at a time when UVB availability is low or over a short time period or adjusted the data for the season [39,56]. Also, the dietary assessment methods used in the studies varied and the validity of the methods was not described in all papers. Some used validated FFQs [25,47] and some only used questionnaires on milk consumption [43,46]. Moreover, the portion sizes used were not defined in all studies. The consumed amounts of milk and the vitamin D contents differed, as did the confounding factors used in statistical analyses. The representativeness of the samples was not described in most of the studies, but representative data from national health surveys in the United States, Canada, Sweden, Norway, and Finland were included when describing the contributions of fluid milk to vitamin D intake [25,27,28,33–35,37]. We only searched data from PubMed, and some studies might have been missed in our limited literature search. However, these are probably studies that have not taken a stand on vitamin D fortification of fluid milks as such, and therefore, have not emphasized it in the abstracts or in the keywords. Nevertheless, publication bias may have occurred, as some studies that found no association between vitamin D-fortified milk and vitamin D status may not have been published.

4.2. Future Perspectives in Vitamin D Fortification

Vitamin D fortification of foodstuffs has proven to be a suitable vehicle to increase vitamin D intake at the population level [5], and the present review shows that vitamin D-fortified fluid milk products contribute to both vitamin D intake and 25(OH)D status. Cashman and Kiely [5], however, stated that the fortification of fluid milks may not be enough. Thus, country-specific staple foods should be chosen as optimal vitamin D carriers based on the results of simulation studies. Also, the biofortification of foodstuffs should be considered [5]. In many countries without a current fortification policy, the option of systematic vitamin D fortification of food is under consideration, and simulation studies have been carried out in recent years. A study using Swedish, British, and Dutch data, for instance, showed that increased fortification of fluid milk to the level currently used in Finland (1 μg/100 g) and fortification of margarines to 15 μg/100 g would substantially increase vitamin D intake [60]. Another study based on British data [61] revealed that the best option would be the fortification of wheat flour with vitamin D, this being a more efficient option to increase S-25(OH)D concentration than milk alone or combined fortification of milk and wheat flour. In Germany, the effects of fortification on the seasonal variation of S-25(OH)D concentrations were simulated, but milk was not considered to be a good carrier of vitamin D [62]. Simulation studies in Irish and British children showed that the fortification of cow's milk would improve vitamin D intake [14,63]. Further, an Australian simulation demonstrated that with vitamin D fortification of all milk and breakfast cereals, vitamin D intake would increase almost two-fold [17]. These studies reflect the interest in widening the fortification policies. However, the results of the above-described simulation studies show that fortification of milk products may not be the most effective option in all countries.

5. Conclusions

The reviewed studies indicated that in countries with a national vitamin D fortification policy for fluid milks at a level of around 1 μg/100 g, such as Finland, United States, and Canada, milk products contribute substantially to vitamin D intake, while in countries without a fortification policy or with only a few milk products being mandatorily fortified, the contribution is low. Studies carried out at different latitudes among different population groups have also shown that the consumption of vitamin D-fortified milk is associated with a higher 25(OH)D concentration. Based on the reviewed observational studies, vitamin D fortification of milk is an effective vehicle in improving vitamin D intake and 25(OH)D status in populations with adequate average milk consumption. However, other food sources, natural or fortified, as well as national recommendations on the use of vitamin D supplements should not be overlooked when planning national nutrition policies to ensure adequate vitamin D intake.

Author Contributions: Conceptualization: S.T.I., M.E. and C.J.E.L.-A.; Methods: S.T.I. and C.J.E.L.-A.; Data search: S.T.I.; Study Selection: S.T.I. and C.J.E.L.-A.; Data Extraction: S.T.I.; Writing—Original Draft Preparation: S.T.I.; Writing—Review & Editing: S.T.I., M.E. and C.J.E.L.-A.; Project Administration: S.T.I.; Funding Acquisition: S.T.I.

Funding: This research was funded by [Foundation for Nutrition Research].

Conflicts of Interest: The authors declare no conflict of interest. The funders had no role in the design of the study; in the collection, analyses, or interpretation of data; in the writing of the manuscript, and in the decision to publish the results.

References

1. Lamberg-Allardt, C.; Brustad, M.; Meyer, H.E.; Steingrimsdottir, L. Vitamin D—A systematic literature review for the 5th edition of the Nordic Nutrition Recommendations. *Food Nutr. Res.* **2013**, *57*, 22671. [CrossRef] [PubMed]

2.   Theodoratou, E.; Tzoulaki, I.; Zgaga, L.; Ioannidis, J.P. Vitamin D and multiple health outcomes: Umbrella review of systematic reviews and meta-analyses of observational studies and randomized trials. *BMJ* **2014**, *348*, 2035. [CrossRef] [PubMed]

3.   O'Neill, C.M.; Kazantzidis, A.; Ryan, M.J.; Barber, N.; Sempos, C.T.; Durazo-Arvizu, R.A.; Jorde, R.; Grimnes, G.; Eiriksdottir, G.; Gudnason, V.; et al. Seasonal changes in vitamin D-effective UVB-availability in Europe and associations with population serum 25-hydroxyvitamin D. *Nutrients* **2016**, *8*, 533–538. [CrossRef] [PubMed]

4.   European Union. Commission Directive 2006/141/EC on infant formulae and follow-on formulae and amending Directive 1999/21/EC. *Off. J. Eur Union* **2006**, *401*, 15.

5.   Cashman, K.D.; Kiely, M. Tackling inadequate vitamin D intakes within the population: Fortification of dairy products with vitamin D may not be enough. *Endocrine* **2016**, *251*, 38–46. [CrossRef] [PubMed]

6.   National Nutrition Council. Report of vitamin D Working Group (Valtion Ravitsemusneuvottelukunta D-Vitamiinityöryhmän Raportti In Finnish). 2010. Available online: https://www.evira.fi/globalassets/vrn/pdf/d-vitamiiniraportti2010.pdf (accessed on 1 January 2018).

7.   Ministry of Agriculture and Forestry of Finland. Maa-ja metsätalousministeriön asetus rasvattoman homogenoidun maidon D-vitaminoinnista. Available online: http://www.finlex.fi/fi/laki/alkup/2016/20160754 (accessed on 1 March 2018).

8.   Nasjonalt råd for Ernaering. Tiltak for å Sikre en God Vitamin D-Status I Befolkningen. 2006. Available online: https://helsedirektoratet.no/Documents/Om%20oss/R%C3%A5d%20og%20utvalg/Nasjonalt%20r%C3%A5d%20for%20ern%C3%A6ring/Tiltak%20for%20%C3%A5%20sikre%20en%20god%20vitamin%20D-status%20i%20befolkningen%20IS-1408.pdf (accessed on 1 January 2018).

9.   Livsmedelsverket. Livsmedelverkets Föreskrifter (SLVFS 1983:2) om Berikning av Vissa Livsmedel (Food Agency's Order about Fortification of Foodstuffs). Available online: https://www.livsmedelsverket.se/globalassets/om-oss/lagstiftning/berikn---kosttillsk---livsm-spec-gr-fsmp/slvfs-1983-02-kons.pdf (accessed on 1 January 2018).

10.   Livsmedelsverket. Livsmedelverkets föreskrifter (LIVSFS 2018:5) om berikning av vissa livsmedel (Food Agency's order about fortification of foodstuffs). Available online: https://www.livsmedelsverket.se/globalassets/om-oss/lagstiftning/berikn---kosttillsk---livsm-spec-gr-fsmp/livsfs-2018-5_web.pdf (accessed on 1 June 2018).

11.   Department of Health. Regulations Amending Certain Regulations Made Under the Food and Drugs Act (Nutrition Symbols, Other Labelling Provisions Partially Hydrogenated Oils and Vitamin D.). *Can. Gazette.* **2018**, *152*, 6. Available online: http://gazette.gc.ca/rp-pr/p1/2018/2018-02-10/pdf/g1-15206.pdf (accessed on 1 June 2018).

12.   Calvo, M.S.; Whiting, S.J. Vitamin D Fortification in North America: Current Status and Future Considerations. In *The Handbook of Food Fortification from Concepts to Public Health Applications*; Preedy, R.V., Srirajaskanthan, R., Patel, V., Eds.; Springer Science + Business Media: New York, NY, USA, 2013; Volume 2, pp. 259–271.

13.   Black, L.J.; Walton, J.; Flynn, A.; Kiely, M. Adequacy of vitamin D intakes in children and teenagers from the base diet, fortified foods and supplements. *Public Health Nutr.* **2014**, *17*, 721–731. [CrossRef] [PubMed]

14.   Cribb, V.L.; Northstone, K.; Hopkins, D.; Emmett, P.M. Sources of vitamin D and calcium in the diets of preschool children in the UK and the theoretical effect of food fortification. *J. Hum. Nutr. Diet.* **2015**, *28*, 583–592. [CrossRef] [PubMed]

15.   Hennessy, Á.; Browne, F.; Kiely, M.; Walton, J.; Flynn, A. The role of fortified foods and nutritional supplements in increasing vitamin D intake in Irish preschool children. *Eur. J. Nutr.* **2017**, *56*, 1219–1231. [CrossRef] [PubMed]

16.   González-Rodríguez, L.G.; Estaire, P.; Peñas-Ruiz, C.; Ortega, R.M.; UCM Research Group VALORNUT (920030). Vitamin D intake and dietary sources in a representative sample of Spanish adults. *J. Hum. Nutr. Diet.* **2013**, *26*, 64–72. [CrossRef]

17.   Jayaratne, N.; Hughes, M.C.; Ibiebele, T.I.; Van den Akker, S.; Van der Pols, J.C. Vitamin D intake in Australian adults and the modeled effects of milk and breakfast cereal fortification. *Nutrition* **2013**, *29*, 1048–1053. [CrossRef] [PubMed]

18.   Black, L.J.; Seamans, K.M.; Cashman, K.D.; Kiely, M. An updated systematic review and meta-analysis of the efficacy of vitamin D food fortification. *J. Nutr.* **2012**, *142*, 1102–1108. [CrossRef] [PubMed]

19. McKenna, M.J.; Freaney, R.; Byrne, P.; McBrinn, Y.; Murray, B.; Kelly, M.; Donne, B.; O'Brien, M. Safety and efficacy of increasing wintertime vitamin D and calcium intake by milk fortification. *QJM* **1995**, *88*, 895–898. [PubMed]

20. Keane, E.M.; Healy, M.; O'Moore, R.; Coakley, D.; Walsh, J.B. Vitamin D-fortified liquid milk: Benefits for the elderly community-based population. *Calcif. Tissue Int.* **1998**, *62*, 300–302. [CrossRef] [PubMed]

21. Daly, R.M.; Brown, M.; Bass, S.; Kukuljan, S.; Nowson, C. Calcium- and vitamin D3-fortified milk reduces bone loss at clinically relevant skeletal sites in older men: A 2-year randomized controlled trial. *J. Bone Miner. Res.* **2006**, *21*, 397–405. [CrossRef] [PubMed]

22. Kukuljan, S.; Nowson, C.; Bass, S.; Sanders, K.; Nicholson, G.C.; Seibel, M.J.; Salmon, J.; Daly, R.M. Effects of a multi-component exercise program and calcium-vitamin-D3-fortified milk on bone mineral density in older men: A randomised controlled trial. *Osteoporos. Int.* **2009**, *20*, 1241–1251. [CrossRef] [PubMed]

23. Nikooyeh, B.; Neyestani, T.R.; Farvid, M.; Alavi-Majd, H.; Houshiarrad, A.; Kalayi, A.; Shariatzadeh, N.; Gharavi, A.; Heravifard, S.; Tayebinejad, N.; et al. Daily consumption of vitamin D– or vitamin D + calcium-fortified yogurt drink improved glycemic control in patients with type 2 diabetes: A randomized clinical trial. *Am. J. Clin. Nutr.* **2011**, *93*, 764–771. [CrossRef] [PubMed]

24. Shab-Bidar, S.; Neyestani, T.R.; Djazayery, A.; Eshraghian, M.R.; Houshiarrad, A.; Gharavi, A.; Kalayi, A.; Shariatzadeh, N.; Zahedirad, M.; Khalaji, N.; et al. Regular consumption of vitamin D-fortified yogurt drink (Doogh) improved endothelial biomarkers in subjects with type 2 diabetes: A randomized double-blind clinical trial. *BMC Med.* **2011**, *9*, 125. [CrossRef] [PubMed]

25. Jääskeläinen, T.; Itkonen, S.T.; Lundqvist, A.; Erkkola, M.; Koskela, T.; Lakkala, K.; Dowling, K.G.; Hull, G.; Kröger, H.; Karppinen, J.; et al. The positive impact of general food fortification policy on vitamin D status in a representative adult Finnish population: Evidence from an 11-year follow-up based on standardized 25-hydroxyvitamin D. data. *Am. J. Clin. Nutr.* **2017**, *105*, 1512–1520. [CrossRef] [PubMed]

26. Institute of Medicine Food and Nutrition Board. *Dietary Reference Intakes for Adequacy: Calcium and Vitamin D*; The National Academies Press: Washington, DC, USA, 2011.

27. Holm Totland, T.; Kjerpeseth Melnaes, B.; Lundberg-Hallén, N.; Helland-Kigen, K.M.; Lund-Blix, N.A.; Borch Myhre, J.; Wetting Johansen, A.M.; Bjørge Løken, E.; Frost Andersen, L. A representative Study on Nutrient Intakes among 18–70 Year-Old Men and Women in Norway). Available online: https://helsedirektoratet.no/Lists/Publikasjoner/Attachments/301/Norkost-3-en-landsomfattende-kostholdsundersokelse-blant-menn-og-kvinner-i-norge-i-alderen-18-70-ar-2010-11-IS-2000.pdf (accessed on 1 June 2018).

28. Amcoff, E.; Edberg, A.; Enghardt Barbieri, H.; Lindroos, A.K.; Nälsén, C.; Pearson, M.; Warensjö Lemming, E. Livsmedels-och näringsintag bland vuxna i Sverige. Available online: https://www.livsmedelsverket.se/globalassets/publikationsdatabas/rapporter/2011/riksmaten_2010_20111.pdf?id=3588 (accessed on 1 June 2018).

29. Cole, C.R.; Grant, F.K.; Tangpricha, V.; Swaby-Ellis, E.D.; Smith, J.L.; Jacques, A.; Chen, H.; Schleicher, R.L.; Ziegler, T.R. 25-hydroxyvitamin D status of healthy, low-income, minority children in Atlanta, Georgia. *Pediatrics* **2010**, *125*, 633–639. [CrossRef] [PubMed]

30. Mark, S.; Lambert, M.; Delvin, E.E.; O'Loughlin, J.; Tremblay, A.; Gray-Donald, K. Higher vitamin D intake is needed to achieve serum 25(OH)D levels greater than 50 nmol/L in Québec youth at high risk of obesity. *Eur J. Clin Nutr* **2011**, *65*, 486–492. [CrossRef] [PubMed]

31. Soininen, S.; Eloranta, A.M.; Lindi, V.; Venäläinen, T.; Zaproudina, N.; Mahonen, A.; Lakka, T.A. Determinants of serum 25-hydroxyvitamin D concentration in Finnish children: The Physical Activity and Nutrition in Children (PANIC) study. *Br. J. Nutr.* **2016**, *115*, 1080–1091. [CrossRef] [PubMed]

32. Piirainen, T.; Laitinen, K.; Isolauri, E. Impact of national fortification of fluid milks and margarines with vitamin D on dietary intake and serum 25-hydroxyvitamin D concentration in 4-year-old children. *Eur. J. Clin. Nutr.* **2007**, *61*, 123–128. [CrossRef] [PubMed]

33. Poliquin, S.; Joseph, L.; Gray-Donald, K. Calcium and vitamin D intakes in an adult Canadian population. *Can. J. Diet. Pract. Res.* **2009**, *70*, 21–27. [CrossRef] [PubMed]

34. Moore, C.; Murphy, M.M.; Keast, D.R.; Holick, M.F. Vitamin D intake in the United States. *J. Am. Diet. Assoc.* **2004**, *104*, 980–983. [CrossRef] [PubMed]

35. Vatanparast, H.; Calvo, M.S.; Green, T.J.; Whiting, S.J. Despite mandatory fortification of staple foods, vitamin D intakes of Canadian children and adults are inadequate. *J. Steroid. Biochem. Mol. Biol.* **2010**, *121*, 301–303. [CrossRef] [PubMed]

36. Hill, K.M.; Jonnalagadda, S.S.; Albertson, A.M.; Joshi, N.A.; Weaver, C.M. Top food sources contributing to vitamin D intake and the association of ready-to-eat cereal and breakfast consumption habits to vitamin D intake in Canadians and United States Americans. *J. Food. Sci.* **2012**, *77*, H170–175. [CrossRef] [PubMed]

37. Moore, C.E.; Radcliffe, J.D.; Liu, Y. Vitamin D intakes of adults differ by income, gender and race/ethnicity in the USA, 2007 to 2010. *Public Health Nutr.* **2014**, *17*, 756–763. [CrossRef] [PubMed]

38. Kolahdooz, F.; Barr, A.; Roache, C.; Sheehy, T.; Corriveau, A.; Sharma, S. Dietary adequacy of vitamin D and calcium among Inuit and Inuvialuit women of child-bearing age in Arctic Canada: A growing concern. *PLoS ONE* **2013**, *8*, e78987. [CrossRef] [PubMed]

39. Levy, M.A.; McKinnon, T.; Barker, T.; Dern, A.; Helland, T.; Robertson, J.; Cuomo, J.; Wood, T.; Dixon, B.M. Predictors of vitamin D status in subjects that consume a vitamin D supplement. *Eur. J. Clin. Nutr.* **2015**, *69*, 84–89. [CrossRef] [PubMed]

40. O'Dowd, K.J.; Clemens, T.L.; Kelsey, J.L.; Lindsay, R. Exogenous calciferol (vitamin D) and vitamin D endocrine status among elderly nursing home residents in the New York City area. *J. Am. Geriatr. Soc.* **1993**, *41*, 414–421. [CrossRef] [PubMed]

41. Kinyamu, H.K.; Gallagher, J.C.; Rafferty, K.A.; Balhorn, K.E. Dietary calcium and vitamin D intake in elderly women: Effect on serum parathyroid hormone and vitamin D. metabolites. *Am. J. Clin. Nutr.* **1998**, *67*, 342–348. [CrossRef] [PubMed]

42. Raulio, S.; Erlund, I.; Männistö, S.; Sarlio-Lähteenkorva, S.; Sundvall, J.; Tapanainen, H.; Vartiainen, E.; Virtanen, S.M. Successful nutrition policy: Improvement of vitamin D intake and status in Finnish adults over the last decade. *Eur. J. Public Health* **2017**, *27*, 268–273. [CrossRef] [PubMed]

43. Abu Shady, M.M.; Youssef, M.M.; Salah El-Din, E.M.; Abdel Samie, O.M.; Megahed, H.S.; Salem, S.M.; Mohsen, M.A.; Abdel Aziz, A.; El-Toukhy, S. Predictors of serum 25-hydroxyvitamin D concentrations among a sample of Egyptian schoolchildren. *Sci. World J.* **2016**, *2016*, 8175768. [CrossRef] [PubMed]

44. Gharaibeh, M.A.; Stoecker, B.J. Assessment of serum 25(OH)D concentration in women of childbearing age and their preschool children in Northern Jordan during summer. *Eur. J. Clin. Nutr.* **2009**, *63*, 1320–1326. [CrossRef] [PubMed]

45. Rosendahl, J.; Fogelholm, M.; Pelkonen, A.; Mäkelä, M.J.; Mäkitie, O.; Erkkola, M. A history of cow's milk allergy is associated with lower vitamin D status in schoolchildren. *Horm. Res. Paediatr.* **2017**, *88*, 244–250. [CrossRef] [PubMed]

46. Lee, G.J.; Birken, C.S.; Parkin, P.C.; Lebovic, G.; Chen, Y.; L'Abbé, M.R.; Maguire, J.L. TARGet Kids! Collaboration. Consumption of non-cow's milk beverages and serum vitamin D levels in early childhood. *CMAJ* **2014**, *186*, 1287–1293. [CrossRef] [PubMed]

47. Munasinghe, L.L.; Yuan, Y.; Willows, N.D.; Faught, E.L.; Ekwaru, J.P.; Veugelers, P.J. Vitamin D deficiency and sufficiency among Canadian children residing at high latitude following the revision of the RDA of vitamin D intake in 2010. *Br. J. Nutr.* **2017**, *117*, 457–465. [CrossRef] [PubMed]

48. Munasinghe, L.L.; Yuan, Y.; Willows, N.D.; Faught, E.L.; Ekwaru, J.P.; Veugelers, P.J. Vitamin D deficiency and sufficiency among Canadian children residing at high latitude following the revision of the RDA of vitamin D intake in 2010—CORRIGENDUM. *Br. J. Nutr.* **2017**, *117*, 1052–1054. [CrossRef] [PubMed]

49. Rodríguez-Rodríguez, E.; Aparicio, A.; López-Sobaler, A.M.; Ortega, R.M. Vitamin D status in a group of Spanish schoolchildren. *Minerva Pediatr.* **2011**, *63*, 11–18. [PubMed]

50. Barman, M.; Jonsson, K.; Hesselmar, B.; Sandin, A.; Sandberg, A.S.; Wold, A.E. No association between allergy and current 25-hydroxy vitamin D in serum or vitamin D intake. *Acta Paediatr.* **2015**, *104*, 405–413. [CrossRef] [PubMed]

51. Öberg, J.; Jorde, R.; Almås, B.; Emaus, N.; Grimnes, G. Vitamin D deficiency and lifestyle risk factors in a Norwegian adolescent population. *Scand. J. Public Health* **2014**, *42*, 593–602. [CrossRef] [PubMed]

52. Charatcharoenwitthaya, N.; Nanthakomon, T.; Somprasit, C.; Chanthasenanont, A.; Chailurkit, L.O.; Pattaraarchachai, J.; Ongphiphadhanakul, B. Maternal vitamin D status, its associated factors and the course of pregnancy in Thai women. *Clin. Endocrinol. (Oxf.)* **2013**, *78*, 126–133. [CrossRef] [PubMed]

53. Hauta-Alus, H.H.; Holmlund-Suila, E.M.; Rita, H.J.; Enlund-Cerullo, M.; Rosendahl, J.; Valkama, S.M.; Helve, O.M.; Hytinantti, T.K.; Surcel, H.M.; Mäkitie, O.M.; et al. Season, dietary factors, and physical activity modify 25-hydroxyvitamin D concentration during pregnancy. *Eur. J. Nutr.* **2018**, *57*, 1369–1379. [CrossRef] [PubMed]

54. Hobbs, R.D.; Habib, Z.; Alromaihi, D.; Idi, L.; Parikh, N.; Blocki, F.; Rao, D.S. Severe vitamin D deficiency in Arab-American women living in Dearborn, Michigan. *Endocr. Pract.* **2009**, *15*, 35–40. [CrossRef] [PubMed]

55. Langlois, K.; Greene-Finestone, L.; Little, J.; Hidiroglou, N.; Whiting, S. Vitamin D status of Canadians as measured in the 2007 to 2009 Canadian Health Measures Survey. *Health Rep.* **2010**, *21*, 47–55. [PubMed]

56. Burgaz, A.; Akesson, A.; Oster, A.; Michaëlsson, K.; Wolk, A. Associations of diet, supplement use, and ultraviolet B radiation exposure with vitamin D status in Swedish women during winter. *Am. J. Clin. Nutr.* **2007**, *86*, 1399–1404. [CrossRef] [PubMed]

57. McCarroll, K.; Beirne, A.; Casey, M.; McNulty, H.; Ward, M.; Hoey, L.; Molloy, A.; Laird, E.; Healy, M.; Strain, J.J.; et al. Determinants of 25-hydroxyvitamin D in older Irish adults. *Age Ageing* **2015**, *44*, 847–853. [CrossRef] [PubMed]

58. Carter, G.D. 25-hydroxyvitamin D: A difficult analyte. *Clin. Chem.* **2012**, *58*, 486–488. [CrossRef] [PubMed]

59. Binkley, N.; Carter, G.D. Toward clarity in clinical vitamin D status assessment: 25(OH)D assay standardization. *Endocrinol. Metab. Clin. N. Am.* **2017**, *46*, 885–899. [CrossRef] [PubMed]

60. Harika, R.K.; Dötsch-Klerk, M.; Zock, P.L.; Eilander, A. Compliance with Dietary Guidelines and Increased Fortification Can Double Vitamin D Intake: A. Simulation Study. *Ann. Nutr. Metab.* **2016**, *69*, 246–255. [CrossRef] [PubMed]

61. Allen, R.E.; Dangour, A.D.; Tedstone, A.E.; Chalabi, Z. Does fortification of staple foods improve vitamin D intakes and status of groups at risk of deficiency? A United Kingdom modeling study. *Am. J. Clin. Nutr.* **2015**, *102*, 338–344. [CrossRef] [PubMed]

62. Brown, J.; Sandmann, A.; Ignatius, A.; Amling, M.; Barvencik, F. New perspectives on vitamin D food fortification based on a modeling of 25(OH)D concentrations. *Nutr. J.* **2013**, *12*, 151. [CrossRef] [PubMed]

63. Kehoe, L.; Walton, J.; McNulty, B.A.; Nugent, A.P.; Flynn, A. Dietary strategies for achieving adequate vitamin D and iron intakes in young children in Ireland. *J. Hum. Nutr. Diet.* **2017**, *30*, 405–416. [CrossRef] [PubMed]

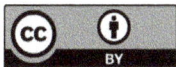

nutrients

MDPI

Article

Bioavailability of Vitamin B_{12} from Dairy Products Using a Pig Model

Danyel Bueno Dalto, Isabelle Audet, Christiane L. Girard and Jean-Jacques Matte *

Sherbrooke Research and Development Centre, Agriculture and Agri-Food Canada, Sherbrooke, QC J1M 0C8, Canada; danyel.buenodalto@agr.gc.ca (D.B.D.); isabelle.audet@agr.gc.ca (I.A.); christiane.girard@agr.gc.ca (C.L.G.)
* Correspondence: jacques.matte@agr.gc.ca; Tel.: +1-819-564-5507

Received: 20 June 2018; Accepted: 18 August 2018; Published: 21 August 2018

Abstract: The present study compares the bioavailability of vitamin B_{12} (B_{12}) of dairy products or synthetic B_{12}, using the pig as an experimental model for humans. Eleven pigs were used in a cross-over design to assess the net portal drained viscera (PDV) flux of blood plasma B_{12} after ingestion of tofu (TF; devoid of B_{12}), Swiss cheese (SC), Cheddar cheese (CC), yogurt (YG), and synthetic B_{12} (TB_{12}; TF supplemented with cyanocobalamin), providing a total of 25 µg of B_{12} each. PDV blood plasma flow for SC and CC were higher than for TF and TB_{12} ($p \leq 0.04$) whereas YG was higher than TF ($p = 0.05$). Porto-arterial difference of blood plasma B_{12} concentrations were higher for CC and TB_{12} than for TF and YG ($p \leq 0.04$) but not different from SC ($p \geq 0.15$). Net PDV flux of B_{12} was only different from zero for CC. However, the net PDV flux of B_{12} for CC was not different from SC or TB_{12}. Cumulative net PDV flux of B_{12} for SC, TB_{12}, and CC were 2.9, 4.4, and 8.3 µg 23 h post-meal, corresponding to a bioavailability of 11.6%, 17.5%, and 33.0%, respectively. In conclusion, CC had the best bioavailability of B_{12} among the tested dairy products or compared to synthetic B_{12}.

Keywords: bioavailability; dairy; pig model; vitamin B_{12}

---

1. Introduction

Animal products and by-products are the only natural source of vitamin B_{12} (B_{12}) in human diets. Considering that B_{12} is synthesized exclusively by bacteria and archaebacteria (when cobalt is not limiting), ruminant animals (e.g., cows) obtain the vitamin from synthesis by their ruminal microflora. The vitamin is further absorbed and stored in their body, which explain why the tissues and milk of these animals are especially rich in B_{12}.

Among animal-derived products, milk stands out as an excellent source of B_{12}. Milk intake was reported to be better correlated with B_{12} status than eggs, red meat, poultry, fish and seafood consumption [1,2]. Using a food-frequency questionnaire, Vogiatzoglou et al. [3] showed that at similar intakes, dairy products have a greater impact on plasma concentrations of B_{12} than the above mentioned products, suggesting a better bioavailability of this vitamin from dairy products. Using a direct measurement, Matte et al. [4] reported greater bioavailability of B_{12} from milk than from the synthetic form (cyanocobalamin) present in most supplements. Considering that similar forms of B_{12} (adenosylcobalamin, hydroxocobalamin, and methylcobalamin) are found in cow's milk and dairy products [5], they would be expected to have similar B_{12}-related nutritional characteristics. However, because of distinct manufacturing processes, the various dairy products are nutritionally different among them or compared to milk. For example, whereas only 60–70% of the original content of B_{12} from milk remains in the curd for Cheddar cheese [6], Swiss cheese increases its original B_{12} content due to the indispensable use of *Propionibacterium shermanii* bacteria, which is known to synthesise this vitamin [7]. For yogurt, the addition of starter cultures does not affect B_{12} concentrations but fermentation of heat-treated milk resulted in losses of 25% [8]. Therefore, it is possible that these different processes impact some nutritional aspects related to this vitamin, such as its bioavailability.

The present study compares the net flux of B_{12} across portal-drained viscera (PDV) after ingestion of different dairy products or cyanocobalamin (synthetic B_{12}) using, as Matte et al. [4], the pig as an experimental model for humans. It aims to determine if, as previously observed for milk, the provision of B_{12} brought by dairy products is better absorbed through the gastrointestinal tract than that of the synthetic form used in vitamin supplements.

2. Methods

The experimental procedures followed the guidelines of the Canadian Council on Animal Care [9] and were approved by the Institutional Animal Care Committee (#490) of the Sherbrooke Research and Development Centre (Sherbrooke, QC, Canada). All animals were cared for according to the recommended code of practice of the National Farm Animal Care Council [10].

3. Initial Analysis and Selection of Dairy Products

Because of the wide variety of dairy products available on the market, those commonly consumed worldwide were initially chosen (cheese and yogurt). Considering the huge variation in B_{12} content among these products, different types and brands of cheese and yogurt were selected and analyzed for their content in B_{12}. Based on these analyses, Swiss cheese (SC; 32 ng B_{12}/g; Agropur, Longueil, QC, Canada), Cheddar cheese (CC; 15 ng B_{12}/g; Laiterie de Coaticook, Coaticook, QC, Canada), and plain natural yogurt (YG; 4 ng B_{12}/g; Liberté, St-Hubert, QC, Canada) were chosen. Tofu (TF; Horium, Montreal, QC, Canada) was chosen as a negative control diet because foodstuffs from plant origin are naturally devoid of B_{12} [11]. TF was also used as a carrier for the synthetic form of B_{12}, cyanocobalamin (TB$_{12}$; positive control).

In order to minimize variations in B_{12} levels among products throughout the experiment, one single batch of each product was purchased. The concentration of B_{12} in each product was determined (Table 1) before being frozen at $-20\,^\circ$C. One single solution of cyanocobalamin (V-2876, Sigma-Aldrich, St Louis, MO, USA) was prepared, analyzed for its B_{12} content (0.125 mg B_{12}/mL) and frozen at $-20\,^\circ$C in individual portions.

Table 1. Composition of the experimental products (as-fed basis) and their calculated provision of dry matter, protein, fat, salt, and vitamin B_{12} [1].

Item	Tofu	Swiss Cheese	Cheddar Cheese	Yogurt [2]
	Composition			
Dry matter, %	34.60	62.40	52.90	12.70 (23.7)
Protein, g/g	0.17	0.27	0.23	0.06 (0.11)
Fat, g/g	0.05	0.27	0.33	0.02 (0.04)
Sodium, mg/g	0.10	5.33	5.00	0.49 (0.91)
Vitamin B_{12}, ng/g	0.12	31.88	14.87	3.77 (6.79)
	Calculated provision per meal			
Dry matter, g	692.0	833.0	883.0	865.1
Protein, g	340.0	380.6	384.1	401.5
Fat, g	100.0	260.6	551.1	146.0
Sodium, g	0.2	4.26	8.35	3.32
Vitamin B_{12}, ng	0.2	25.1	24.8	24.8

[1] The amount of each experimental product fed was: tofu = 2000 g, Swiss cheese = 780 g, Cheddar cheese = 1670 g, yogurt = 3650 g. [2] Values within brackets refer to the preparation of fresh + lyophilized yogurt.

4. Preliminary Animal Trial

Considering that pigs are not normally fed this type of foodstuffs, a preliminary animal trial was necessary to assess the maximum consumption of each dairy product in order to standardize B_{12} ingestion among treatments.

Twenty Yorkshire-Landrace x Duroc pigs were selected at 44.4 ± 4.8 kg of body weight (BW) and 70–77 days of age. They were penned individually (1 m × 1.8 m) and randomly allocated to one of 4 treatments: (1) increasing amounts of TF; (2) increasing amounts of SC; (3) increasing amounts of CC; and (4) increasing amounts of YG. Animals were allowed one single daily meal. When the consumption of the tested products did not provide the equivalent of 1200 g of dry matter, the meal was complemented with a conventional growing-phase feed after the 1 h feeding trial. Evaluations of maximum ingestion capacity, meal duration, and intestinal health (presence of diarrhea) were performed. The trial ended when a similar average consumption was achieved during two consecutive days. This happened at day 7 for TF, day 8 for SC and CC, and day 10 for YG. In average, pigs were able to eat 2.3 kg of TF, 1.8 kg of SC, 1.8 kg of CC, and 7.2 kg of YG within 1 h. No diarrhea was observed during this preliminary trial.

5. Description of Treatments

Based on the results of the B_{12} analyses and the preliminary trial, the experimental dose of B_{12} to be administered to animals was fixed at 25 µg. This amount was found to be sufficient to produce a detectable response of post-prandial portal net fluxes in a previous experiment [12]. It also corresponds to the current daily allowance given to market pigs of this age [13]. Therefore, the total volume of each product to be used was 1670 g of CC, 780 g of SC, 3650 g of YG, 2000 g of TF and 2000 g of TB_{12} (a dice of TF was infused with 200 µL of the cyanocobalamin solution at 0.125 mg B_{12}/mL). For SC, considering that 780 g represents less than 70% of a normal pig feed intake, 1 kg of TF was added to the treatment (offered after SC was completely consumed). For YG, based on the above described analysis and trial, it would not be possible to reach the fixed dose of 25 µg by using fresh YG. Therefore, a part of experimental YG was lyophilized (dosed B_{12} concentration was 27.16 ng/g) to be further incorporated into fresh YG just before feeding to animals. Pre-trial analyses of B_{12} concentration were performed in mixes of fresh + lyophilized YG to ensure an accurate concentration.

6. Experimental Animals and Palatability Test

Forty four pigs were selected (based on BW and average daily gain) two weeks before surgery and fed ad libitum a conventional growing-phase diet. Diet composition was 87.43% of dry matter, 3243 Kcal of metabolizable energy, 16.4% of crude protein, 3.29% of fat, 2.69% of crude fiber, 0.83% of calcium, and 0.54% of phosphorus. In order to identify pigs with the greatest predisposition to ingest the studied products, a palatability test was performed. Without any fasting period, pigs were offered each product as follows: Day 1 and 2: 400 and 500 g of TF; day 3 and 4: 400 and 500 g of SC; day 5 and 6: 400 and 500 g of CC; day 7 and 8: 750 and 1500 g of YG. The amount of product left in the feeder after 1h was weighted and used to calculate intake. Twenty-six pigs with the highest average intake for all or most of the products were pre-selected for surgery.

7. Surgery

Average BW at surgery was 47.7 ± 7.5 kg. The surgical procedure has been described by Hooda et al. [14]. Briefly, a catheter was inserted in the portal vein at approximately 2.5 cm before its entry into the liver and an ultrasonic flow probe (Transonic Systems, Inc., Ithaca, NY, USA) was installed around the portal vein 1.0 cm distal to the catheter. Another catheter was inserted through the carotid artery up to the junction between the carotid and subclavian arteries.

Improvements were made on the original pre-, intra-, and post-surgical procedures. Instead of completely withdrawing feed 16h prior to surgery, pigs had access to a total of 400 g of feed overnight. After surgery, pigs had access to 750 g of plain yogurt immediately after waking-up in order to stimulate food consumption. For animals that did not eat during the first morning after surgery, another 750 g of plain yogurt was offered. These procedures reduced fasting time and attenuated the risk of post-operatory gastric ulcerations without any impact on intra- or post-operatory procedures. The portal catheter, originally inserted in direction of the blood flow after installing a V-shaped suture heading the liver, was inserted against the blood flow with the V-shaped suture heading in the opposite direction to the liver. This procedure has reduced the obstruction of catheters by fibrin as compared to previous studies of this laboratory using this technique. The flow probe, which was originally installed after a major dissection of the portal vein, was installed with a minor dissection laterally to the vein. In most cases, the removal of a lymph node that is attached between the vein and the pancreas was necessary. This procedure has reduced surgical time, the risk of rupture of the vein and the occurrence of post-operatory intestinal adhesions without any disturbance of flow probe's signal.

After these improvements, a total of 15 surgeries were performed; 2 animals were eliminated because of post-operatory intestinal adhesions and 2 animals had their portal catheters blocked.

8. Post-Operatory Procedures and Experimental Days

After surgery, animals were penned individually (1 m × 1.8 m) and fed the conventional growing-phase diet described above in a single daily meal, according to their BW (1.0 kg/day until 50 kg BW; 1.2 kg/day from 50–60 kg BW; and 1.5 kg/day after 60 kg BW). Seven to 10 days after surgery, when animals have fully recovered (appetite and normal growth rate), they were gradually adapted (3–5 days) to the metabolic cage (with free access to water). On days -3 and -2 prior to each experimental day (day 0), pigs were adapted to consume an increasing amount of the respective experimental product (1.0 and 2.0 kg for TF; 0.5 and 1.0 kg for SC, 1.0 and 2.0 kg for CC; 1.7 and 3.5 kg for YG). On day -1, no adaptation was performed. On experimental days (one per week), animals were placed in metabolic cages and fed tofu (absent in B_{12}) or one of the experimental products providing a total of 25 µg of B_{12}. Treatments (TF, SC, CC, YG, and TB_{12}) were distributed according to a duplicate 5 × 5 Latin Square design.

Blood samples (4 mL) were collected simultaneously from the two catheters 5 min before the experimental meal and every 60 min post-meal during 23 h Portal blood flow was recorded continuously during 23 h using a flowmeter (Transonic® 400-series; Ithaca, NY, USA) and the PowerLab System (AD Instruments, Colorado Springs, CO, USA). Between experimental days, animals were moved back to their respective pens and fed the basal diet described above.

9. Sample Handling and Analyses

Immediately after sampling, arterial and PDV blood were transferred from syringes into EDTA-treated tubes (Vacutainer, Becton Dickinson, Franklin Lakes, NJ, USA). Packed cell volume (PCV) was measured in duplicate on fresh PDV blood by micro-centrifugation. Aliquots of arterial and PDV blood were frozen for hemoglobin determination according to the method of Drabkin [15]. Arterial and PDV plasma were collected after centrifugation of blood at 1800 × g for 10 min at 4 °C and frozen at −20 °C for further analysis. Arterial and PDV plasma concentrations of B_{12} were measured in duplicate by radioassay (SimulTRAC-S Radioasssay kit, Vitamin B_{12} (^{57}Co)/Folate (^{125}I), MP Biomedicals, Diagnostics Division, Orangeburg, NY, USA). For each sample, analyses of plasma B_{12} were made in duplicate. The upper limit for coefficients of variation between duplicate was fixed at ≤4%.

10. Calculations and Statistical Analysis

Two animals were not equipped with flow probes (technical reasons) whereas one animal lost flow probe functionality during one profile (YG) and another one during three profiles (SC, CC, and YG). For these animals, the estimation of PDV blood flow was performed using the average blood flows of all other pigs within the same treatment, at each sampling time. The estimated values for these periods were not included in the statistical analysis of PDV plasma flow but were used for the calculation of net PDV flux of B_{12}. Net flux of B_{12} across PDV was calculated as described by Girard et al. [16]. Positive net PDV flux indicates release of B_{12} from PDV, whereas negative net PDV flux indicates B_{12} uptake by the PDV. Statistical analyses of arterial concentrations of B_{12}, PCV on PDV blood, PDV plasma flows, porto-arterial difference, and net PDV flux of B_{12} were conducted on values for each sampling time.

All variables were analyzed using the MIXED procedure of SAS (SAS Institute Inc., Cary, NC, USA) [17] according to a cross-over design in which pigs, periods, and treatments were included in the model along with repeated measures in time (equally spaced). When the treatment effect was significant, multiple comparisons between treatments were performed using a *t*-test. Differences were considered significant at $p \leq 0.05$ and tendencies at $0.05 < p \leq 0.10$.

11. Results

Arterial concentrations of B_{12} were not affected by dietary treatments ($p = 0.18$; Table 2) but a time effect was observed in which values gradually decreased throughout the 23 h profile period (181.7 ± 7.3 to 162.1 ± 7.3 pg/mL; $p < 0.001$). Although an interaction treatment × time was observed ($p = 0.03$), no specific pattern could be associated to any particular treatment.

Packed cell volume in the portal blood was affected by dietary treatments ($p = 0.01$). Values for TF and TB_{12} (33.5 ± 0.4 and $33.8 \pm 0.5\%$) were or tended to be higher than SC, CC, and YG (31.9 ± 0.4, 32.5 ± 0.4, and $32.4 \pm 0.4\%$, respectively; $p \leq 0.07$). A time effect ($p < 0.001$) was observed in which PCV gradually decreased during the first 11 post-prandial hours (from 35.6 ± 0.7 to $31.5 \pm 0.7\%$) but remained stable thereafter until the end of the profile period (32.2 ± 0.7). No interaction treatment × time was observed ($p = 0.14$).

Portal-drained viscera plasma flow was affected by dietary treatments ($p = 0.01$). Values for SC and CC were higher ($p \leq 0.04$) than TF and TB_{12} whereas YG was higher than TF ($p = 0.05$; Table 2). A time effect ($p < 0.001$) was observed, with maximal values reached at the first post-prandial hour (1.30 ± 0.04 vs 1.09 ± 0.04 L/min for the pre-prandial PDV plasma flow) and this was followed by a gradual decrease until the end of the sampling period (1.14 ± 0.04 L/min). No treatment × time interaction was observed ($p = 0.19$) on this variable.

Table 2. Average B_{12} arterial concentration, PDV plasma flow, porto-arterial difference, and net PDV flux of vitamin B_{12} during 23 post-prandial hours according to dietary treatments.

Item	Tofu	Swiss Cheese	Cheddar Cheese	Yogurt	Tofu + B_{12}	*p* Value
Arterial B_{12}, ng/L	173.2 ± 14.2	177.2 ± 13.0	145.4 ± 143.0	187.7 ± 15.2	194.6 ± 16.4	0.18
PDV plasma flow, L/min [1]	$0.93^{\,c} \pm 0.08$	$1.31^{\,a} \pm 0.08$	$1.34^{\,a} \pm 0.08$	$1.19^{\,ab} \pm 0.09$	$1.06^{\,bc} \pm 0.08$	0.01
Porto-arterial difference, ng/L [1]	$-1.36^{\,b} \pm 1.56$	$1.58^{\,ab} \pm 1.46$	$4.68^{\,a} \pm 1.53$	$-0.21^{\,b} \pm 1.68$	$4.78^{\,a} \pm 1.81$	0.03
Net PDV flux of B_{12}, ng/min [2,3]	$-1.50^{\,c} \pm 1.84$	$2.10^{\,abc} \pm 1.73$	$5.99^{\,a} \pm 1.81$	$-0.31^{\,bc} \pm 1.98$	$3.17^{\,ab} \pm 2.14$	0.06

Different subscribed letters within a row indicate differences between treatments using *t* test ($p \leq 0.05$). PDV: portal drained viscera. [1] Values for tofu, Swiss cheese, and yogurt were not different from zero ($p \geq 0.29$). [2] Values for tofu, Swiss cheese, yogurt, and tofu + B_{12} were not different from zero ($p \geq 0.15$). [3] Because estimated values of PDV plasma flow were not included in the statistical analysis (due to missing data) of PDV plasma flow but were used for the calculation of arterial and PDV flux of B_{12}, net PDV flux of B_{12} does not reflect the multiplication of porto-arterial difference by PDV plasma flow.

Porto-arterial differences of plasma B_{12} concentrations were affected by dietary treatments ($p = 0.03$). Values differed from zero ($p \leq 0.01$) only for CC and TB_{12} and were higher than for TF and YG ($p \leq 0.04$) but not different from SC ($p \geq 0.15$; Table 2). No time effect or interaction treatment × time were observed ($p \geq 0.39$). Net PDV flux of B_{12} tended to be affected by dietary treatments ($p = 0.06$). Values differed from zero ($p \leq 0.01$) only for CC. Although the average net PDV fluxes of B_{12} (per min) for SC and TB_{12} were not statistically different from zero ($p \geq 0.15$), their cumulative net PDV flux for the whole 23 h post-meal were numerically positive at 2.9 and 4.4 µg, respectively, corresponding to a calculated bioavailability of 11.6 and 17.5%. Net PDV flux of B_{12}

(per min) for CC was higher than that of TF and YG ($p \leq 0.02$) but not different from SC and TB$_{12}$ ($p \geq 0.13$; Table 2). Cumulative net PDV flux of B$_{12}$ for CC during the whole post-prandial period of 23 h was 8.3 µg, corresponding to a calculated bioavailability of 33.0%.

12. Discussion

To the best of our knowledge, the present study using a net PDV flux approach to assess the amount of vitamin B$_{12}$ absorbed from dairy products through the gastrointestinal tract is unique in scientific literature. Pigs were used because this species is recognized as a reliable and valuable experimental model for studies in human nutrition [18]. More specifically for B$_{12}$, this is supported by previous results of this laboratory [12] reporting that several aspects of the nutritional metabolism of B$_{12}$ in pigs are similar to that in humans [19,20].

Although dietary treatment effects on PCV were unexpected, the values for all treatments were within the normal range. Therefore, the most likely explanation for the lower PCV in SC, CC, and YG compared to TF and TB$_{12}$ would be hemodilution of PDV blood. The calculated total provision of B$_{12}$, dry matter, and protein were standardized among treatments, however, levels of sodium were higher for SC, CC, and YG compared to TF (Table 1). Dietary salt intake is known to alter extracellular fluid volume [21]. Pigs in SC, CC, and YG treatments consumed between 16.6 and 41.8 times more salt than in TF, representing 125.8 to 316.3% of the daily amount of salt normally fed to 70–125 kg pigs, and this was ingested in one single meal. This high acute salt consumption might have caused a higher flow of extracellular fluid at the PDV level and increased the plasma fraction of portal blood. Incidentally, portal plasma flow of SC, CC, and YG were also greater than in TF. As for sodium, calculated total provisions of fat were not standardized between treatments and were higher for SC, CC, and YG compared to TF (Table 1). Fat has long been known to impact intestinal venous blood flow [22]. Indeed, Chou and Coatney [23], after evaluating the impact of various nutrients on postprandial intestinal hyperemia concluded that micellar fatty acids were the most effective in increasing intestinal blood flow. In this sense, SC, CC, and YG provided between 1.5 and 5.5 times more fat than TF.

The mean porto-arterial difference and net PDV flux of B$_{12}$ following a meal not supplemented with B$_{12}$ (TF) (Table 2) were not different from zero, as previously observed by Matte et al. [4,12]. These same authors reported conflicting results for cyanocobalamin (equivalent to TB$_{12}$ in the present study). Matte et al. [12] supplemented pigs with levels of 25 or 250 µg of cyanocobalamin in corn starch + casein-based diets and observed net B$_{12}$ flux different from zero whereas in Matte et al. [4] the net flux of that same synthetic form of B$_{12}$ did not differ from zero in diets incorporating B$_{12}$ solutions in plant-based feedstuff (44 and 71 µg B$_{12}$). Such inconsistent results may be related to the known effect of different food matrixes on B$_{12}$ absorption [24]. In dairy cows, Artegoitia et al. [25] reported a better absorption of B$_{12}$ after a post-ruminal infusion of a solution of cyanocobalamin + casein hydrolysate than after infusions of cyanocobalamin + whey protein or free cyanocobalamin solutions. Proteins are known to slow gastric emptying [26] and, although both casein and whey are proteins with high B$_{12}$-binding capacity [27], casein (hydrolyzed or not) has a gastric emptying time 33% slower than whey [28]. This may be caused by formation of curd-like structures by caseins once in the stomach whereas whey remains liquid. Therefore, it appears that the food matrix effect on the absorption of vitamin B$_{12}$ would be related to the rate of the vitamin release from this food matrix leaving the stomach. In this sense, a gradual gastric release of B$_{12}$ would enhance the duration and efficiency of its absorption whereas the presence of bulky transient arrival of B$_{12}$ at the site of absorption would result in a greater amount of unabsorbed B$_{12}$ in the intestinal lumen because B$_{12}$ receptors in the ileum are saturable [29]. This hypothesis is in line with the fact that increasing dietary levels of the vitamin, which is likely related to a greater gastric release, decreases the efficiency of B$_{12}$ absorption [30].

Mean porto-arterial difference and net PDV flux of B$_{12}$ for YG were not different from zero (Table 2). Considering its similarity with milk (high protein liquids) one would expect YG absorption to be comparable to that of milk (8–10%) [4]. Compared to milk, yogurt is richer in proteins (milk enriched with milk solids) which, in addition to various buffers produced during the fermentation process, provide a greater buffering capacity to this dairy product [31]. According to Jalan et al. [32], following ingestion of a standard 250 mL dose of yogurt or whole milk, 31 and 10 meq of gastric HCl would be required to reduce the pH of the meals to a pH of 2. In this sense, the present YG treatment (3650 g) would require 8.7 times more HCl than the milk treatment of Matte et al. [4] at 1300 g to reduce the pH of the meals to a pH of 2, which is critical for the release of B_{12} from its binding proteins in milk [33]. Additionally, according to Rioux and Turgeon [34], high viscous food matrixes may impair the digestion of nitrogenous compounds such as casein, the greater binder of B_{12} in milk [33]. In this sense, it has to be stated that the present YG treatment (fresh + lyophilized yogurt) was much more viscous than milk or even regular yogurt. Considering that the bioavailability of protein-bound B_{12} is dependent on the gastric degradation of B12-binding proteins, the above mentioned factors suggest that the release of cobalamin from these binding proteins, a crucial step in B_{12} intestinal absorption, was impaired.

For cheeses, mean porto-arterial difference and net PDV flux of B_{12} for SC did not differ from zero whereas CC did (Table 2). However, it has to be stated that net PDV flux of B_{12} for CC was not statistically different from that of SC. In fact, the cumulative net PDV flux of B_{12} for SC was numerically positive and corresponded to a calculated bioavailability of 11.6%. Although this value is lower than CC (33.0%), it is comparable to values reported by Matte et al. [12] for semi-purified diets supplemented with 25 µg of cyanocobalamin (9.7%) and Matte et al. [4] using milk preparations containing 44 or 71 µg of B_{12} (8–10%).

Although most steps of the manufacturing process of SC and CC are similar, differences in starter cultures, in particular the use of Propionibacterium shermanii that is known to synthesize B_{12} [11], may explain the higher concentration of B_{12} in SC as compared to CC. In fact, the present SC was twice as concentrated in B_{12} as CC (32 µg/g vs. 15 ug/g). In this sense, it has to be stated that the mass of B_{12}-containing foodstuff (SC curd) ingested was half of that of CC (780 g vs. 1670 g). This combination of greater concentration and smaller mass implies that the release of B_{12} was proportionally faster in SC. Another important difference in the manufacturing process of these cheeses is the timing of the salting of the curd. For CC, salt is applied prior to the pressuring procedure, whereas for SC it is done after. Salting the curd stimulates the leak of whey that will be lost during pressuring. The lower loss of whey in SC implies that it is richer in plasmin (protease). In fact, Richardson and Pearce [35] reported that SC has 2–3 times more plasmin than CC. This protease preferentially hydrolyzes casein suggesting that links casein-casein or casein-B_{12} would be weaker in SC than in CC. In fact, those authors indicated that the extent of casein degradation in SC was related to plasmin content, whereas little evidence of plasmin degradation was observed in CC. Together with the more B_{12}-concentrated mass in SC, this suggests that the digestion of SC may release B_{12} faster and in a greater amount than CC, saturating B_{12} receptors in the ileum and losing a higher proportion of B_{12} (unabsorbed) downstream in the intestinal lumen (Figure 1). For CC, the more gradual release of B_{12} may have reduced the saturation of the receptors improving the efficiency of B_{12} absorption.

For SC, however, it cannot be ruled out that the greater presence of B_{12}-binding proteins from bacterial origin in SC might have also contributed to differences in bioavailability of B_{12} compared to CC.

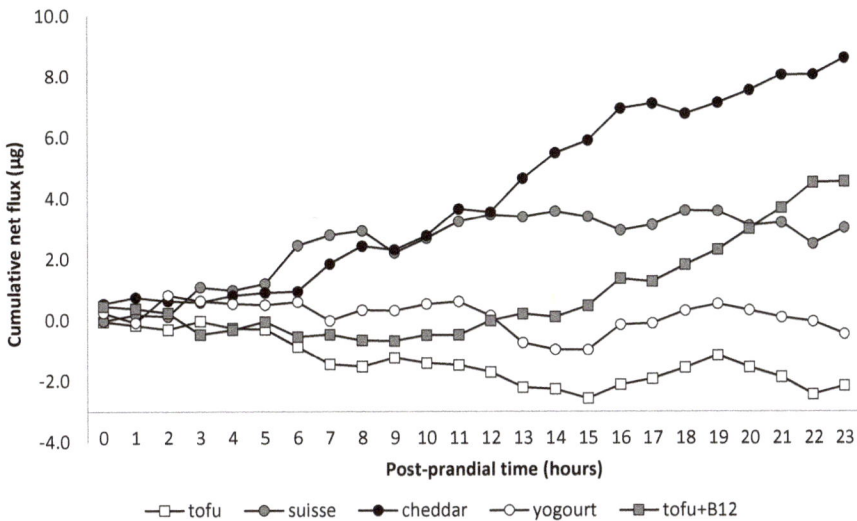

Figure 1. Calculated cumulative net portal-drained viscera flux of B_{12} (µg) by post-prandial time. TF = tofu; SC = Swiss cheese; CC = Cheddar cheese; YG = yogurt; TB_{12} = tofu + vitamin B_{12}.

13. Conclusions

Dairy products can be considered as adequate sources of dietary B_{12}. Among the tested products, CC had the best bioavailability of B_{12} followed by TB_{12} and SC. This might be related to the rate of release of B_{12} from the food matrix leaving the stomach modulating the saturation of B_{12} receptor in the ileum and the efficiency of intestinal absorption of this vitamin.

Further investigations are needed to assess the importance of this phenomenon for B_{12} bioavailability in foodstuffs.

Author Contributions: D.B.D., C.L.G. and J.-J.M. designed the experiment; D.B.D., I.A. and J.-J.M. performed the experiment; D.B.D. and I.A. collected samples and performed laboratory analyses; D.B.D., CL.G. and J.-J.M. analyzed the data. All authors were involved in the preparation of the manuscript.

Funding: This research was funded by Dairy Research Cluster Initiative (Dairy Farmers of Canada, Agriculture and Agri-Food Canada, the Canadian Dairy Network and the Canadian Dairy Commission) grant number CL04-Dairy-Activity N10 30V1.

Acknowledgments: The authors are grateful to S. Daudelin for his technical assistance and to the animal care team under supervision of M. Turcotte.

Conflicts of Interest: The authors declare no conflict of interest.

References

1. Miller, D.R.; Specker, B.L.; Ho, M.L.; Norman, E.J. Vitamin B_{12} status in a macrobiotic community. *Am. J. Clin. Nutr.* **1991**, *53*, 524–529. [CrossRef] [PubMed]
2. Tucker, K.L.; Rich, S.; Rosenberg, I.H.; Jacques, P.; Dallal, G.; Wilson, P.W.; Selhub, J. Plasma vitamin B_{12} concentrations relate to intake source in the Framingham offspring study. *Am. J. Clin. Nutr.* **2000**, *71*, 514–522. [CrossRef] [PubMed]
3. Vogiatzoglou, A.; Smith, A.D.; Nurk, E.; Berstad, P.; Drevon, C.A.; Ueland, P.M.; Vollset, S.E.; Tell, G.S.; Refsum, H. Dietary sources of vitamin B_{12} and their association with plasma vitamin B_{12} concentrations in the general population: The Hordaland Homocysteine Study. *Am. J. Clin. Nutr.* **2009**, *89*, 1078–1087. [CrossRef] [PubMed]

4. Matte, J.J.; Guay, F.; Christiane, L. Bioavailability of vitamin B$_{12}$ in cows' milk. *Brit. J. Nutr.* **2012**, *107*, 61–66. [CrossRef] [PubMed]

5. Farquharson, J.; Adams, J.F. The forms of vitamin B$_{12}$ in foods. *Br. J. Nutr.* **1976**, *36*, 127–136. [CrossRef] [PubMed]

6. Ball, G.F.M. *Vitamins in Foods: Analysis, Bioavailability, and Stability*; CRC Press: Boca Raton, FL, USA, 2006.

7. Gardner, N.; Champagne, C.P. Production of *Propionibacterium shermanii* biomass and vitamin B$_{12}$ on spent media. *J. Appl. Microbiol.* **2005**, *99*, 1236–1245. [CrossRef] [PubMed]

8. Arkbage, K.; Witthoft, C.; Fondén, R.; Jägerstad, M. Retention of vitamin B$_{12}$ during manufacture of six fermented dairy products using a validated radio protein-binding assay. *Int. Dairy J.* **2003**, *13*, 101–109. [CrossRef]

9. Canadian Council on Animal Care. *Guide to the Care and Use of Experimental Animals*; Canadian Council on Animal Care: Ottawa, ON, Canada, 2009.

10. National Farm Animal Care Council. *Code of Practice for the Care and Handling of Pigs*; Agriculture Canada: Ottawa, ON, Canada, 2014.

11. Martens, J.-H.; Barg, H.; Warren, M.J.; Jahn, D. Microbial production of vitamin B$_{12}$. *Appl. Microbiol. Biotechnol.* **2002**, *58*, 275–285. [CrossRef] [PubMed]

12. Matte, J.J.; Guay, F.; Le Floc'h, N.; Girard, C.L. Bioavailability of dietary cyanocobalamin (vitamin B$_{12}$) in growing pigs. *J. Anim. Sci.* **2010**, *88*, 3936–3944. [CrossRef] [PubMed]

13. Flohr, J.R.; DeRouchey, J.M.; Woodworth, J.C.; Tokach, M.D.; Goodband, R.D.; Dritz, S.S. A survey of current feeding regimens for vitamins and trace minerals in the US swine industry. *J. Swine Health Prod.* **2016**, *24*, 290–303.

14. Hooda, S.; Matte, J.J.; Wilkinson, C.W.; Zijlstra, R.T. Technical note: An improved surgical model for the long-term studies of kinetics and quantification of nutrient absorption in swine. *J. Anim. Sci.* **2009**, *87*, 2013–2019. [CrossRef] [PubMed]

15. Manet, L. Techniques usuelles de biologie clinique. In *Hématologie*; Editions Medicales Flammarion: Paris, France, 1969.

16. Girard, C.L.; Lapierre, H.; Desrochers, A.; Benchaar, C.; Matte, J.J.; Rémond, D. Net flux of folates and vitamin B$_{12}$ through the gastrointestinal tract and the liver of lactating dairy cows. *Br. J. Nutr.* **2001**, *86*, 707–715. [CrossRef] [PubMed]

17. SAS Institute. *SAS/STAT User's Guide*; SAS Inst. Inc.: Cary, NC, USA, 2004.

18. Guilloteau, P.; Zabielski, R.; Hammon, H.M.; Metges, C.C. Nutritional programming of gastrointestinal tract development. Is pig a good model for man? *Nutr. Res. Rev.* **2010**, *23*, 4–22. [CrossRef] [PubMed]

19. Schneider, Z.; Stroinski, A. *Comprehensive B$_{12}$: Chemistry, Biochemistry, Nutrition, Ecology, Medicine*; Walter de Gruyter: Berlin, Germany, 1987.

20. Combs, G.F., Jr. *The Vitamins: Fundamental Aspects in Nutrition and Health*, 4th ed.; Academic Press: San Diego, CA, USA, 2012.

21. Wardener, H.E.; He, F.; Macgregor, G.A. Plasma sodium and hypertension. *Kidney Int.* **2004**, *66*, 2454–2466. [CrossRef] [PubMed]

22. Siregar, H.; Chou, C.C. Relative contribution of fat, protein, carbohydrate, and ethanol to intestinal hyperemia. *Am. J. Physiol.* **1982**, *242*, 27–31. [CrossRef] [PubMed]

23. Chou, C.C.; Coatney, R.W. Nutrient-induced changes in intestinal blood flow in the dog. *Br. Vet. J.* **1994**, *150*, 423–437. [CrossRef]

24. Greibe, E. Nutritional and biochemical aspects of cobalamin throughout life. In *Vitamin B$_{12}$: Advances and Insights*; CRC Press: Boca Raton, FL, USA, 2017.

25. Artegoitia, V.M.; De Veth, M.J.; Harte, F.; Ouellet, D.R.; Girard, C.L. Casein hydrolysate and whey proteins as excipients for cyancobalamin to increase intestinal absorption in the lactating dairy cow. *J. Dairy Sci.* **2015**, *98*, 8128–8132. [CrossRef] [PubMed]

26. Burn-Murdoch, R.A.; Fisher, M.A.; Hunt, J.H. The slowing of gastric emptying by proteins in test meals. *J. Physiol.* **1978**, *274*, 477–485. [CrossRef] [PubMed]

27. Gizis, E.; Kim, Y.P.; Brunner, J.R.; Schweigert, B.S. Vitamin B$_{12}$ content and binding capacity of cow's milk proteins. *J. Nutr.* **1965**, *87*, 349–352. [CrossRef] [PubMed]

28. Dalziel, J.E.; Young, W.; McKenzie, C.M.; Haggarty, N.W.; Roy, N.C. Gastric emptying and gastrointestinal transit compared among native and hydrolyzed whey and casein milk proteins in an aged rat model. *Nutrients* **2017**, *9*, 1351. [CrossRef] [PubMed]

29. Bender, D.A. *Nutritional Biochemistry of the Vitamins*; Cambridge University Press: Cambridge, UK, 2003.

30. Adams, J.F.; Ross, S.K.; Mervyn, L.; Boddy, K.; King, P. Absorption of cyanocobalamin, coenzyme B_{12}, methylcobalamin, and hydroxocobalamin at different dose levels. *Scand. J. Gastroenter.* **1971**, *6*, 249–252. [CrossRef]

31. Webb, B.H.; Johnson, A.H.; Alford, J.A. *Fundamentals of Dairy Chemistry*, 2nd ed.; Avi Publishing CO Inc.: Westport, MA, USA, 1974.

32. Jalan, K.N.; Mahalanabis, D.; Maitra, T.K.; Agarwal, S.K. Gastric acid secretion rate and buffer content of the stomach after a rice and a wheat-based meal in normal subjects and patients with duodenal ulcer. *Gut* **1979**, *20*, 389–393. [CrossRef] [PubMed]

33. Fedosov, S.N.; Nexo, E.; Heegaard, C.W. Binding of aquocobalamin to bovine casein and its peptides via coordination to histidine residues. *Int. Dairy J.* **2018**, *76*, 30–39. [CrossRef]

34. Rioux, L.E.; Turgeon, S.L. The ratio of casein to whey protein impacts yogurt digestion in vitro. *Food Dig.* **2012**, *3*, 25–35. [CrossRef]

35. Richardson, B.C.; Pearce, K.N. The determination of plasmin in dairy products. *J. Dairy Sci. Technol.* **1981**, *16*, 209–220.

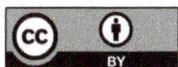

nutrients

MDPI

Review

Food Byproducts as Sustainable Ingredients for Innovative and Healthy Dairy Foods

Maite Iriondo-DeHond [1,2]**, Eugenio Miguel** [1] **and María Dolores del Castillo** [2,*]

[1] Instituto Madrileño de Investigación y Desarrollo Rural, Agrario y Alimentario (IMIDRA), N-II km 38,200, 28800 Alcalá de Henares, Spain; maite.iriondo@madrid.org (M.I.-D.); eugenio.miguel@madrid.org (E.M.)
[2] Instituto de Investigación en Ciencias de la Alimentación (CIAL) (CSIC-UAM), C/ Nicolás Cabrera, 9, Campus de la Universidad Autónoma de Madrid, 28049 Madrid, Spain
*   Correspondence: mdolores.delcastillo@csic.es; Tel.: +34-91-0017900 (ext. 953)

Received: 6 August 2018; Accepted: 21 September 2018; Published: 22 September 2018

Abstract: The valorization of food wastes and byproducts has become a major subject of research to improve the sustainability of the food chain. This narrative review provides an overview of the current trends in the use of food byproducts in the development of dairy foods. We revised the latest data on food loss generation, the group of byproducts most used as ingredients in dairy product development, and their function within the food matrix. We also address the challenges associated with the sensory properties of the new products including ingredients obtained from byproducts, and consumers' attitudes towards these sustainable novel dairy foods. Overall, 50 studies supported the tremendous potential of the application of food byproducts (mainly those from plant-origin) in dairy foods as ingredients. There are promising results for their utilization as food additives for technological purposes, and as sources of bioactive compounds to enhance the health-promoting properties of dairy products. However, food technologists, nutritionists and sensory scientists should work together to face the challenge of improving the palatability and consumer acceptance of these novel and sustainable dairy foods.

Keywords: byproducts; sustainability; functional foods; dairy products

---

1. Introduction

Sustainability presents both an opportunity and a challenge to the dairy sector. It is an opportunity, because the possibility of using food-processing byproducts for bioactive compound and nutrient extraction has created enormous scope for waste reduction and indirect income generation [1]. However, the challenge is to sustainably intensify the global food production system to enhance food security and nutrition without sacrificing the environment, and to render the concept of sustainable functional foods into a marketable product that is acceptable to consumers [2,3].

The development of novel food and/or functional food products is increasingly challenging, as it has to fulfill the consumer's expectations for products that are simultaneously palatable and healthy [4]. Compared to conventional foods, the development of functional components and technological solutions can be demanding and expensive, and needs of a tight strategy between research and business. All this occurs in a context where functional food markets are continuously changing [5,6].

The purpose of this review is to summarize the research findings on the application of various food-processing byproducts used as a source of targeted compounds or as whole ingredients in the manufacturing of dairy foods. So far, most studies available on the valorization of agro-industrial food wastes focus on specific byproducts and their applications in different foods. In this review, the focus is on dairy product development, and how byproducts can be used in their manufacturing to improve their technological and health-promoting properties.

2. Materials and Methods

The present narrative review was conducted by a literature search consulting the PubMed, Web of Science and Scopus databases. The search was limited to English written articles published during the last 18 years, from January 2000 to July 2018. Search terms for general and specific food processing byproducts ("food byproduct", "food waste", "food loss", "vegetable byproduct", "fruit byproduct", "grape pomace", "orange pomace", "coffee byproduct", "cheese whey", "fish byproduct", "meat byproduct"), were combined with search terms for dairy matrices ("dairy", "yogurt", "fermented milk", "milk", "cheese", "butter", "ice-cream"). In addition, references of relevant reviews and original research articles were manually searched to find out more potential eligible studies. Data on legislation were consulted from the Codex Alimentarius guidelines, the United Nations Food and Agriculture Organization (FAO), the European Food Safety Authority (EFSA) and the Food and Drug Administration (FDA). Data from the FAO Food Balance Sheets regarding worldwide production and losses of the different food commodity groups for the most recent year available (2013) were accessed to study the latest state of global food loss generation.

The selection of the papers to be included in the review was performed after a thorough study of their content by the authors. The information extracted from the identified references included first author's name, author affiliation, publication year, dairy product developed, food byproduct used as an ingredient, purpose of adding the food byproduct as an ingredient (technological or health-promoting function) and outcomes. The selection process resulted in the identification of 50 eligible studies which directly addressed the application of a food byproduct as an ingredient in a dairy matrix.

3. Byproducts Used as Novel Ingredients in Dairy Foods

Food loss was redefined by FAO in 2014 as "the decrease in quantity and quality of food". Food waste is considered as part of food loss and refers to discarding or alternative non-food use of food that is safe and nutritious for human consumption along the food chain [7]. Food losses and waste represent an imbalance in the availability and accessibility dimensions in the global food system. Different multifaceted strategies have been proposed by the FAO Committee on Global Food Security to promote the development of a sustainable food system, including food byproduct valorization. In this sense, a reduction in food losses and waste could potentially lead to positive economic, social and environmental outcomes, improving food availability and accessibility, and enhancing a sustainable use of natural resources on which the future production of food depends [8].

The most recent Food Balance Sheets [9] indicate that fruits and vegetables presented the highest values of food losses along the food chain compared to the rest of the commodity groups: cereals, roots and tubers, oilseeds and pulses, meat, fish and seafood, and dairy products. Correspondingly, there has been increasing interest in using fruit and vegetable byproducts as novel ingredients in the development of foods, including dairy products. This focus may be explained by several factors: their impact on the environment, their potential health-promoting phytochemical content, and the fact that plant-derived byproducts and losses mostly occur before household consumption, which makes them still available for reutilization.

Of the studies on the development of innovative and health-promoting dairy products using sustainable ingredients published from 2000 to 2018 (*n* = 50 eligible studies), 88% used side-streams from plant materials. Most studies used byproducts from fruits (43%), followed by the application of winery (19%) and vegetable (13%) byproducts. Among fruit and vegetable byproducts, most research has been carried out using citrus and tomato side-streams as ingredients in dairy formulations (Figure 1), which means that efforts have been made to valorize byproducts from food groups that present some of the largest food losses [9]. In 2013 alone, 13.4 and 6.9 million oranges and tomatoes were lost during storage and transportation [9]. It is evident that the amount of food loss is correlated to the amount of the food item produced, but the ratio of food loss within a production chain for a specific item can also help identify which foods are more susceptible to being lost. As seen in Figure 2, bananas, plantains and pineapples have some of the highest loss rates among fruits and vegetables during storage and transportation. This way, further strategies for food loss and waste reduction could focus on using byproducts from these foods as novel ingredients.

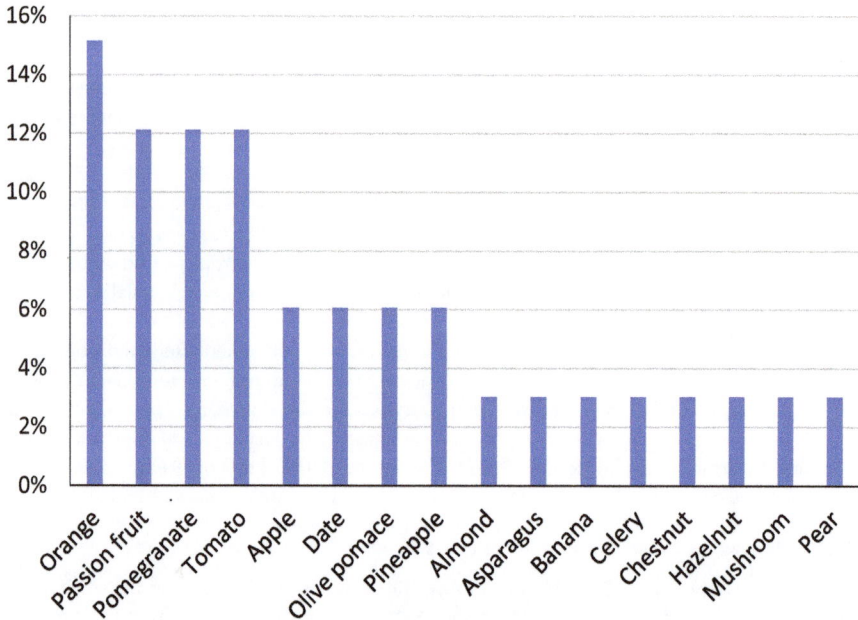

Figure 1. Percentage of research studies that used byproducts from various sources among the fruit and vegetable commodity groups in dairy food manufacturing from 2000 until July 2018 (*n* = 50 studies reviewed).

Byproducts from meat, fish and seafood contain high amounts of protein, which may be less interesting in dairy food manufacturing as they already contain this compound in their matrix. However, when protein has been needed, it has mostly been obtained from cheese whey, which is a saccharide and protein rich waste generated during cheese production [10]. Using a byproduct from the same industry as a food ingredient not only enhances the sustainability within the dairy industry, but also may translate into fewer sensory difficulties when developing the product due to the similarities of the food matrices.

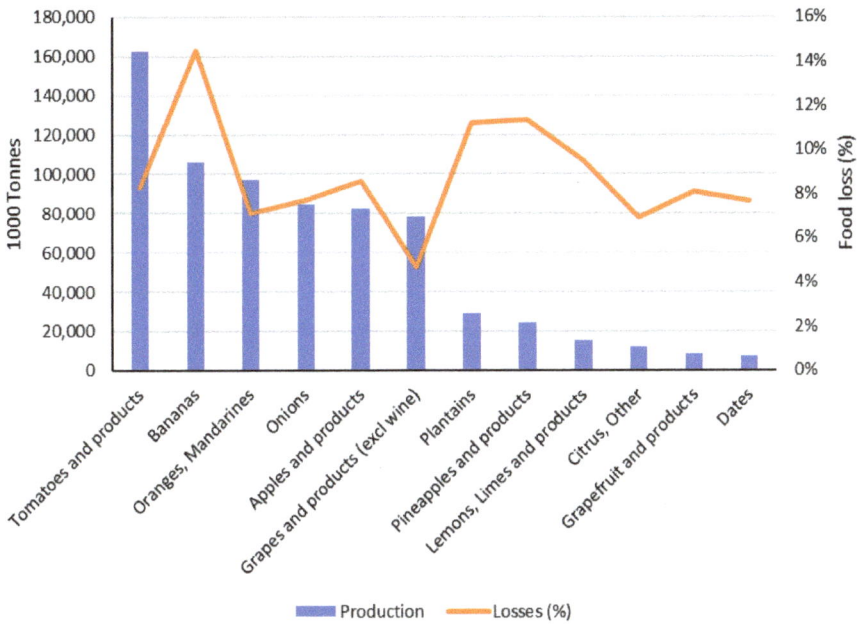

Figure 2. Worldwide food production (1000 tonnes) and its corresponding food loss (%) generated during storage and transportation within the fruit and vegetable commodity groups in 2013. Data obtained from the latest Food Balance Sheets, accessed in 2018 [9].

4. Approaches in the Application of Food Byproducts in the Dairy Industry

The exploitation of byproducts generated during food processing or discarded produce as a source of functional compounds and their application in other foods is very much desirable as part of a waste management system [11]. In this review, we divide the applications of food byproducts in dairy foods in two categories: those with technical purposes, which include the improvement of shelf life, safety, stability, sensory quality, etc.; and those with biological purposes, which aim to enhance health-promoting effects for their conversion into functional foods. A summary of the applications so far proposed is shown in Table 1.

Table 1. Dairy foods found in the literature (from 2000 to July 2018, $n = 49$) developed using food processing byproducts as sustainable ingredients.

Dairy Product	Food Industry	Byproduct	Doses	Function	Reference
Dairy beverage	Vegetable	Mushroom residue	1, 2 and 3 g/kg	Technological (antioxidant) Health-promoting (source of phenols)	Vital et al., 2017 [12]
		Olive vegetable water	100 mg/L to 200 mg/L	Health-promoting (source of phenols, probiotic protection)	Servili et al., 2011 [13]
	Cereal	Rice bran	1% to 3%	Health-promoting (source of fiber and phenols, probiotic protection)	Demirci et al., 2017 [14]
	Dairy	Whey protein	2%	Technological (texturizing agent) Health-promoting (source of protein)	Akalin et al., 2012 [15]
		Whey protein and buttermilk	0% to 100% replacement of skim milk powder	Technological (texturizing agent) Health-promoting (source of protein)	Saffon et al., 2013 [16]
		Whey protein	8% to 14%	Technological (texturizing agent) Health-promoting (source of protein, probiotic protection)	Zhang et al., 2015 [17]
Fermented milk		Chestnut flour	2%	Health-promoting (source of phenols, probiotic protection)	Ozcan et al., 2016 [18]
		Apple	1%	Health-promoting (source of fiber, probiotic protection)	Do Espírito Santo et al., 2012 [19]
		Apple pomace	2.5% to 10%	Health-promoting (source of fiber)	Issar et al., 2016 [20]
	Fruit	Banana	1%	Health-promoting (source of fiber, probiotic protection)	Do Espírito Santo et al., 2012 [19]
		Pineapple peel powder	1%	Technological (texturizing agent)	Sah et al., 2016 [21]
		Pineapple peel powder	1%	Health-promoting (probiotic protection)	Sah et al., 2015 [22]
		Passion fruit peels	1%	Technological (texturizing agent)	Espírito-Santo et al., 2012 [23]
		Passion fruit peels	0.7%	Health-promoting (source of fiber)	Do Espírito Santo et al., 2012 [24]
		Passion fruit	1%	Health-promoting (source of fiber, probiotic protection)	Do Espírito Santo et al., 2012 [19]
		Passion fruit peels	1%	Health-promoting (source of fiber)	Perina et al., 2015 [25]
	Vegetable	Okara	3% to 10%	Health-promoting (source of fiber)	Chen et al., 2010 [26]
		Olive pomace	100 mg/L TPC	Health-promoting (source of phenols, probiotic protection)	Aliakbarian et al., 2015 [27]

Table 1. *Cont.*

Dairy Product	Food Industry	Byproduct	Doses	Function	Reference
	Winery	Wine pomace extract	100 mg/L TPC	Health-promoting (source of phenols, probiotic protection)	Aliakbarian et al., 2015 [27]
		Grape marc flour	10, 20 and 50 g/L	Health-promoting (source of phenols, probiotic protection)	Aliakbarian et al., 2013 [28]
		Wine pomace extract and flour	1% to 3% 1% to 2%	Technological (antioxidant, colorant) Health-promoting (source of fiber and phenols)	Tseng and Zhao 2013 [29]
		Wine pomace extract	788 mg GAE/100 g	Health-promoting (source of phenols, probiotic protection)	Dos Santos et al., 2017 [30]
		Wine pomace flour	10, 20 and 50 g/L	Health-promoting (source of phenols, probiotic protection)	Frumento et al., 2013 [28]
	Cereal	Wheat bran	1.5%	Health-promoting (source of fiber)	Hashim et al., 2009 [31]
		Rice bran	0.2% to 0.6%	Technological (colorant)	Nontasan et al. 2012 [32]
	Dairy	Whey protein	3.3, 5 and 10 g/L	Technological (texturizing agent) Health-promoting (source of protein)	Sandoval-Castilla et al., 2004 [33]
		Date byproducts	1.5% to 4.5%	Health-promoting (source of fiber)	Hashim et al., 2009 [31]
		Orange peels, pulp, seed powders	1% to 3%	Technological (texturizing agent)	Yi et al., 2014 [34]
	Fruit	Orange byproducts	0.2 to 1 g/mL	Technological (texturizing agent)	Sendra et al., 2010 [35]
		Orange albedo, flavedo and pulp powders	0.6% to 1%	Health-promoting (source of fiber)	García-Pérez et al., 2005 [36]
Yogurt		Pomegranate peel extract	5% to 35%	Health-promoting (source of phenols)	El Said et al., 2014 [37]
		Hazelnut skin powder	3% to 6%	Health-promoting (source of fiber)	Bertolino et al., 2015 [38]
		Pomegranate seed	25 mg/L	Technological (antioxidant)	Ersöz et al., 2011 [39]
	Marine	Fish oil	15 mL/100 g	Health-promoting (source of omega-3)	Ghorbanzade et al., 2017 [40]
		Fish oil	13 g/100 g	Health-promoting (source of omega-3)	Zhong et al., 2018 [41]
	Vegetable	Asparagus byproducts	1%	Health-promoting (source of fiber)	Sanz et al., 2008 [42]
		Grape seed extract	100 mg/150 g	Health-promoting (source of phenols)	Chouchouli et al., 2013 [43]
	Winery	Grape skin flour	0.167 to 1 g/100 g	Health-promoting (source of phenols)	Karnopp et al., 2017 [44]
		Grape skin flour	60 g/kg	Health-promoting (source of phenols)	Marchiani et al., 2016 [45]
		Grape seed	25 mg/L	Technological (antioxidant)	Ersöz et al., 2011 [39]
Dairy dessert	Fruit	Date byproduct	0.5, 1 and 2 ratio dried date powder/date syrup	Technological (texturizing agent) Health-promoting (source of phenols)	Jridi et al., 2015 [46]
	Vegetable	Okara	3% to 10%	Health-promoting (source of fiber)	Chen et al., 2010 [26]

Table 1. *Cont.*

Dairy Product	Food Industry	Byproduct	Doses	Function	Reference
Ice-cream	Fruit	Orange peels, pulp, seed powders	1% to 1.5%	Technological (texturizing agent)	Crizel et al., 2014 [47]
		Pomegranate peels	0.1% and 0.4%	Health-promoting (source of phenols)	Çam et al., 2013 [48]
	Vegetable	Lycopene from tomato byproducts	70 mg/kg	Technological (antioxidant, colorant, antimicrobial)	Kaur et al., 2011 [11]
		Carotenoids from tomato peels	1% to 5%	Technological (antioxidant, colorant)	Rizk et al., 2014 [49]
	Winery	Grape wine lees	50, 100 and 150 g/kg	Health-promoting (source of phenols)	Hwang et al., 2009 [50]
	Fruit	Almond peel extract	100 ppm to 400 ppm	Technological (antioxidant)	Nadeem et al., 2014 [51]
Butter	Vegetable	Lycopene from tomato byproducts	20 mg/kg	Technological (antioxidant, colorant, antimicrobial)	Kaur et al., 2011 [11]
		Tomato processing byproduct	400 and 800 mg/kg	Technological (antioxidant)	Abid et al., 2017 [52]
Cheese	Cereal	Corn bran	5%	Health-promoting (source of phenols)	Lucera et al., 2018 [53]
		Wheat bran	10 g/500g	Health-promoting (probiotic protection)	Terpou et al., 2018 [54]
	Dairy	Fluid whey	Water substitution	Technological (texturizing agent)	Erbay et al., 2015 [55]
	Fruit	Pomegranate peel	100 mL/25 g	Technological (antioxidant, antimicrobial)	Shan et al., 2011 [56]
		Orange byproduct fibers	3% to 5%	Technological (texturizing agent)	Saraç and Dogan 2016 [57]
		Pear stones	3% to 5%	Technological (texturizing agent)	Saraç and Dogan 2016 [57]
		Spinach	3% to 5%	Technological (texturizing agent)	Saraç and Dogan 2016 [57]
		Celery byproduct fibers	3% to 5%	Technological (texturizing agent)	Saraç and Dogan 2016 [57]
	Vegetable	Okara	1% to 4%	Health-promoting (source of fiber)	Chen et al., 2010 [26]
		Tomato peels	5%	Health-promoting (source of phenols)	Lucera et al., 2018 [53]
		Broccoli stems and leaves	5%	Health-promoting (source of phenols)	Lucera et al., 2018 [53]
		Artichoke external leaves	5%	Health-promoting (source of phenols)	Lucera et al., 2018 [53]
	Winery	Grape seed	100 mL/25 g	Technological (antioxidant, antimicrobial)	Shan et al., 2011 [56]
		Wine pomace, skin and seed extracts	0.1, 0.2 and 0.3 wt/vol	Health-promoting (source of phenols)	Da Silva et al., 2015 [58]
		Wine pomace flour	0.8 and 1.6 w/w	Health-promoting (source of phenols)	Marchiani et al., 2015 [59]
		Grape pomace	5%	Health-promoting (source of phenols)	Lucera et al., 2018 [53]

4.1. Technological Applications of Food Byproducts in Dairy Formulations

One of the major emerging technologies is the application of food byproducts as natural additives. The implementation of this approach could serve a double purpose. As a waste reduction measure, it would enhance sustainability and increase industrial profitability. In addition, it would be possible to fulfill the requirements of consumers concerned about chemical residues in their foods that look for clean-label and naturally-preserved healthy foods [60].

The addition of food additives is regulated under Codex Alimentarius guidelines. Therefore, food byproducts used as natural additives must consider current regulations and undertake proper authorization if necessary. In this section, we summarize the ongoing research carried out to apply food byproducts as additives in dairy products.

4.1.1. Use of Byproducts as Antioxidants

The Codex General Standard for Food Additives defines antioxidants as food additives which prolong the shelf-life of foods by protecting against deterioration caused by oxidation [61]. In dairy products, lipid oxidation produces fatty acid hydroperoxides, an intermediary tasteless and odorless compound which can further react with fatty acids leading to the formation of secondary lipid oxidation products and protein damage [62]. These reactions result in the production of off-flavors in milk and dairy products, which are described as cardboardy and metallic [63]. These off-flavors can be detected in raw or pasteurized milk, in any dairy product that has not been flavored, and especially in high-fat products such as butter or ice-cream. Therefore, changes in the properties and palatability of these products can lead to a decrease of consumer acceptability and confidence in dairy products [12].

The susceptibility of milk lipids to oxidation depends on several factors: intrinsic factors, extrinsic factors and their interrelation [62]. Intrinsic factors include the composition of the milk system, which is constituted by a complex mixture of pro-oxidants (transition metals) and antioxidants (tocopherols, uric acid, ascorbic acid), whose relative concentration in milk are related to seasonal, physiological and nutritional effects on the cow [64]. Extrinsic factors that affect lipid oxidation refer to environmental and physical factors (light exposure, temperature, pH, water activity, etc.), and to changes that occur during processing and storage (homogenization, heat treatment, fermentation, proteolysis) [65].

This way, the addition of antioxidants in milk is one of the main methods used for preventing and retarding lipid oxidation. The most commonly applied antioxidants in dairy foods, when their use is not explicitly excluded by legislation, are ascorbates and tocopherols [66].

As an alternative to conventional antioxidants, different bioactive compounds recovered from food byproducts have been used to prevent lipid oxidation of dairy foods and increase their shelf life. These efforts have been made especially in high-fat content dairy foods, such as cheese and butter, but also in yogurts and other dairy products such as milk drinks fortified in omega-3 fatty acids, which have a higher risk of lipid deterioration. *Agaricus blazei* mushroom residue has been added to milk fortified in omega-3 fatty acids, which decreased lipid oxidation when subjected to photooxidation [12]. Wine grape pomace also proved to delay lipid oxidation in yogurt [29], whereas grape seed and pomegranate peel extracts have been applied effectively to protect against lipid oxidation in cheese during storage [56].

Butter contains the largest amount of fat among dairy foods (approximately 80%) and can be kept well for at least 20 days if correctly stored at 10 °C, protecting it from moisture evaporation and light induced photooxidation. However, during cold storage, autoxidation is the main cause of deterioration, which depends on the copper present in the product [67]. Antioxidants from tomato processing byproducts were used as agents against lipid peroxidation in conventional and traditional Tunisian butter, showing a protective action during 4 months of cold storage [11,52]. A protective effect against lipid oxidation during 3 months of cold storage was also shown by adding almond peel extract in whey butter, which contains a higher concentration of unsaturated fatty acids that are more vulnerable to oxidative breakdown [51]. The addition of almond peel extract allowed whey butter storage up to 3 months which showed no significant differences in acceptability scores against milk butter [51].

It is relevant to consider the dosage of the extract added to the food product, as it can affect both the antioxidant behavior of the extract and the final sensory acceptability of the food. The effectiveness of tomato processing byproducts as antioxidants in butter was found to be dose dependent: lower amounts of the extract (400 mg tomato processing byproduct/kg butter) considerably inhibited the formation of oxidation products, extending the shelf life of the product up to two months; whereas greater concentrations of tomato processing byproducts (800 mg tomato processing byproduct/kg butter) showed pro-oxidant properties with detrimental effects on the stability of the butter [52]. This change in the antioxidant/pro-oxidant capacity of certain compounds was also described in other studies [68], which observed that extracts with high concentrations of b-carotene lost their antioxidant effect becoming pro-oxidant, possibly due to long-chain-oxidized products of the carotenoid.

The addition of byproduct extracts can lead to either positive or negative effects on the sensory properties of the final product, depending on the dosage, the type of recovered byproduct compounds and the food matrix in which it is incorporated. In ice-cream, the addition of tomato peel carotenoid concentrations of 4% or higher lowered acceptance scores for flavor, texture, melting quality and color [49]. Tomato byproducts used in a different matrix, butter, significantly improved the product's appearance after 4 months of cold storage compared to the control butter [11]. Different byproduct extracts, such as grape and pomegranate seed extracts, decreased fat deterioration in sheep yogurt, but their sensory profile was significantly less acceptable than the control samples immediately after yogurt manufacture and after 14 days of storage [39].

4.1.2. Use of Byproducts as Antimicrobials

Preservatives are food additives that prolong food shelf life by protecting against deterioration caused by microorganisms. Different types of preservatives include: antimicrobial antimould antirope and antimycotic agents, antimicrobial synergists, bacteriophage control agents and fungistatic agents [61]. Food byproducts have been used as preservative agents with antimicrobial activity to ensure that manufactured dairy foods remain unspoiled and safe during their whole shelf-life.

Several studies have shown that food byproducts can be used against spoilage and pathogenic bacteria without interfering with the viability of starter cultures and other microorganisms involved in fermentation processes, ensuring that the quality of the developed products is maintained. The bacterial concentrations required in yogurts and fermented milks by the Codex Alimentarius (10^7 CFU/g) were still met when different byproducts were added into the food matrix (grape pomace flour and extracts, grape skin and seeds, hazelnut skins, pineapple peels, pomegranate seeds, passion peels, etc.) [22,24,27,28,38,39,45]. In cheese, there is less information on the effect of byproduct addition on molds, yeasts and bacteria during ripening, even though they are essential for the correct development of cheese flavor and texture [69,70]. Winemaking byproducts have been added in Toma-like and cheddar cheese products, showing that their addition did not interfere with starter and nonstarter bacteria nor with cheese proteolysis [59]. Therefore, there is an opportunity to study whether the addition of recovered compounds interferes during ripening in other cheese types that involve the growth of different molds in the cheese rind (soft cheese, natural rind cheese, etc.).

4.1.3. Action Against Dairy Food Spoilage Microorganisms

Milk spoilage is primarily due to the growth of psychrophilic microorganisms that trigger lipolysis and proteolysis reactions of milk fatty acids and proteins, respectively [71]. Lipolysis of milk lipids to free fatty acids and partial glycerides contributes to the desirable flavor of milk and other dairy products, but when present in high concentrations, it can lead to the development of off-flavors. These are described as rancid, butyric, bitter, unclean, soapy and astringent [72]. Once lipolysis produces detectable off-flavors it is not possible to remove them from the product [73]. In addition, the hydrolysis of milk proteins produced by proteases from *Pseudomonads, Aeromonads, Serratia* and *Bacillus* spp. also result in the release of off-flavors due to the production of bitter peptides and milk gelation and coagulation [74–76].

Milk spoilage is mediated by lipases that are naturally present in milk (lipoprotein lipase) or by lipases and proteases from psychrophilic bacterial contamination occurring during milking, storage and transportation that result in the destabilization of milk during cold storage [62,77]. One of the most important properties of these bacterial enzymes is their heat stability. This is because most of them can retain at least some of their activity after pasteurization or ultra-high temperature (UHT) treatment, even though bacteria are destroyed [63,78]. Therefore, it is important to develop good practices and strategies to minimize the risk, such as achieving a low microbial count in milk before pasteurization as the action of the residual enzymes during storage will shorten the milk's shelf life [74].

Quality issues and defects associated with excessive lipolysis in dairy products include rancid flavors and poor foaming capacity in pasteurized milk, rancid flavor due to increasing free fatty acids in UHT milk, and spoilage of milk powder during storage. Flavor defects in cheese and butter can be caused by lipolysis before or after manufacture, whereas yogurt is less susceptible to lipolysis defects due to a combination of factors such as low pH, low storage temperature and short shelf life [73].

Although different applications of recovered food byproducts are being studied to valorize them as novel food ingredients, there is a lack of information on the effect of the addition of these extracts in the lipolysis or proteolysis of dairy foods. This should be considered, as some additives, such as pepper, promote lipase activity in cheese, producing soapy and rancid off-flavors [73]. To our knowledge, there is only one study that described the effect of byproducts on the hydrolysis of lipids in dairy foods. Tomato processing byproducts were used in butter and ice-cream to prevent lipolysis during 4 months in refrigerated storage [11]. A significant decrease in the liberation of free fatty acids was observed in lycopene added butter after 3 months compared to control butter, suggesting that this extract may exert a protective action against lipolysis.

4.1.4. Action Against Foodborne Pathogens in Dairy Foods

The milk matrix is an ideal media for microorganism proliferation. This also includes pathogenic bacteria, where mycobacteria, *Brucella sp., Listeria monocytogenes, Staphylococcus aureus* and enterobacteria (including toxigenic *Escherichia coli* and *Salmonella*) are the most frequently found pathogenic bacteria in dairy foods [76]. The origin of pathogen proliferation can be either endogenous (from udder infection) or exogenous (contact with contaminated environment) [79]. Therefore, implementation of Hazard Analysis and Critical Control Points (HACCP) and quality assurance programs through European Union (EU) directives (2004/41/EC, EU 605/2010) on milk hygiene and public health conditions have been put into practice to ensure food safety [80].

Milk heat treatment, such as pasteurization or UHT processes, kill pathogenic bacteria. However, inadequate pasteurization or post-pasteurization contamination can cause milk re-contamination if sanitation measures in the processing plant are not sufficient, leading to food poisoning incidences [74]. Outbreaks of food-borne illnesses have been mainly linked to the consumption of raw milk or products made of unpasteurized milk such as raw milk cheeses, whose consumption is continuously growing [81]. Besides not using heat treatment, traditional raw milk cheese producers may not use starter cultures in their elaboration process, which increases the risk of pathogen multiplication as the competitive activity of the lactic acid starter is eliminated [82]. In this sense, the addition of preservatives to dairy products is principally used in cheese. Preservatives may be added during cheese production and ripening to all the edible part of the cheese or only for rind treatment [66,83].

The number of dairy food infection outbreaks due to pathogen contamination of other dairy foods is less common, although some cases have been reported for yogurt and fermented milks [84]. In these products the acidity of the matrix acts as a barrier to bacterial growth. However, milk must be pasteurized as some pathogens, such as *E. coli* 0157:H7, can be tolerant to the acid environment [85].

Many studies have analyzed the antimicrobial and antimycotic *in vitro* properties of extracts recovered from food byproducts. The antimicrobial action against foodborne pathogens has been associated with the polyphenols of plant based byproducts, which may penetrate the cell wall causing membrane disruption, damage of membrane proteins and enzymes, and structural changes that lead to bacterial death [86–88].

The number of studies analyzing the efficacy of byproduct polyphenolic extracts included in the dairy food matrix on food pathogen control is still limited. Pomegranate peel and grape seed extracts proved to be effective natural preservatives against *Listeria monocytogenes, Staphylococcus aureus* and *Salmonella enterica* in cheese [56]. Pathogen counts in cheese significantly decreased with the byproduct extract treatments. However, the cheese matrix required higher concentrations of the byproduct extracts to efficiently deliver the antibacterial effect compared to the *in vitro* analyses performed in the culture medium. This could be explained by the effect of the micro-architecture of the food matrix. Microbial growth occurs in the aqueous phase of food and is affected by food structure which can restrict the mobility of bacteria. In cheese, which is a gelled emulsion, fat and protein content together with low water content may act as a protective barrier between the bacteria and the extracts, requiring higher concentrations of preservatives to control the growth of pathogens [89].

The addition of herbs and spices in cheese has been part of the cheese culture in many countries for centuries. Some examples include the French Banon covered in chestnut leaves, or the Spanish Majorero cheese with sweet pepper. In this sense, the antimicrobial effect of herbs and spices and their application as cheese preservatives has been more commonly studied [90,91]. This tradition could be used as a cultural advantage for the application of plant-based byproducts as preservative and flavoring agents in innovative cheese developments. As consumers already feel familiar with this type of cheese products, it could increase product acceptability and facilitate its introduction into the market.

4.1.5. Use of Byproducts as Colorants

Colorants are food additives that add or restore color in foods [61]. Their role is involved in the improvement of the appearance and color of foods, and in the maintenance of their natural color during processing and storage [92]. Color stands as one of the most important quality attributes for the food industry, as it directly affects consumers' acceptance and food selection [93].

Current market trends include the substitution of synthetic colorants for natural compounds, which has been motivated by consumers' concern about the safety of synthetic food dyes (side effects, toxicity and allergic reactions), and by the possible health-promoting benefits of natural pigments [94].

Fruit and vegetable byproducts have become an important source of natural pigments as they are colored by green chlorophylls, yellow-orange-red carotenoids, red-blue-purple anthocyanins and red betanins [95].

Anthocyanins have been widely extracted from various plant based foods and byproducts, such as radishes, red potatoes, red cabbage, black carrots, purple sweet potatoes, coffee husks, berries, winery byproducts, etc. [96–98]. However, their use as food colorants has been limited. The list of anthocyanin colorants in the Codex Alimentarius includes only grape skin extract (E163), and in the FDA, "grape color extract" and "grape skin extract" (enocyanin) [61,99].

Anthocyanin application in dairy foods comes with a range of unique coloring challenges, as their stability is affected by changes in pH, fat content in the dairy matrix and manufacturing and storage conditions including extreme temperature and light exposure [97]. Moreover, their use may add specific flavors associated with phenolic compounds. This is the case in some studies where the addition of wine byproducts in yogurt and fermented milks for polyphenol enrichment and color improvement resulted in a decrease in overall liking due to a predominant astringent sensation [29,44,45]. This problem is solved by adding sucrose or other ingredients to the basal recipe to eliminate the astringency. Higher sensory scores in flavor and overall acceptability were reported in wine pomace-fortified fermented milks compared to control samples [30]. The greater acceptability of the polyphenol-fortified samples was probably due to the influence of the intensified color on the perception of taste. Other satisfactory applications of food byproducts as colorants have been reported using anthocyanins from grapes and beetroot betalains. The coloring compounds proved to be stable in semisolid petit-suisse-like cheese probably due to its low water content, slightly acid pH and the low temperature and light-impermeable packaging during storage [100].

Carotenoids stand as the major group of compounds used as coloring agents. Their use is widely extended, and the number of authorized carotenoids used as colorants varies depending on each country. Most commercial carotenoids are produced synthetically (β-carotene, astaxanthin, canthaxanthin and zeaxanthin), although some are obtained from natural sources (annatto, paprika, saffron, marigold, tomato, algae) and microbial fermentation [95]. Extraction of lycopene from tomato processing byproducts has been optimized and registered as the food color "E160d" in Europe [61]. In dairy foods, lycopene from tomato byproducts has been applied in the coloring of butter and ice-cream showing a stable reddish color for up to 4 months [11,49].

4.1.6. Use of Byproducts as Texturizing Agents

Texturizing agents are used to add or modify the overall texture and mouth feel of food products by providing creaminess, thickness, viscosity or a stable structure. This category comprises a wide range of food additives including emulsifiers, stabilizers, thickeners and bulking agents [61]. Texturizing agents are commonly used in dairy products. Hydrocolloids are used for stabilizing and thickening purposes in fermented milks, milk drinks, dairy desserts, cream and ice-cream. Phosphates and coagulation agents are also permitted as stabilizers and to aid in the curdling of milk in cheese production, respectively [66,101].

Most hydrocolloids used in dairy foods come from natural origin as they are manufactured by isolation from seaweeds and plant cells [102]. Moreover, many of these hydrocolloids are extracted from plant food wastes, such as pectin, which is commonly isolated from apple pomace and citrus peels, as well as from other fruit and vegetable byproducts such as passion fruit peels, rapeseed cake, olive pomace, grape pomace, onion hulls, etc. [103–106]. Their application in dairy foods as isolated ingredients is increasing which is a step forward in valorizing underused fractions. However, the isolation of specific compounds generates once again other byproducts. To improve economic and environmental sustainability within the food chain, newer approaches trying to use byproducts as whole ingredients without further processing should be developed. This represents a harder challenge as byproducts used as ingredients comprise a much more complicated matrix than an isolated compound, which could lead to problems associated with product stability and unwanted interaction with other compounds.

In this sense, fewer studies have reported the use of food byproducts as whole ingredients with texturizing purposes. Some examples include the use of liquid fluid whey instead of the generally used powdered form, which showed promising results on the physical quality of white cheese powder [55]. Dietary fiber from orange byproducts was used to maintain the texture of lemon ice-cream when reducing its fat content by 50% [47], and as fat replacers in low-fat yogurt [34]. The authors showed that reducing particle size of the orange dietary fibers by micronization increased their water and oil holding capacities, which are also important functional properties in relation to the facilitation of digestion and absorption of nutrients in the body.

Texture, rheological parameters and the microstructure of yogurt gels have been analyzed when adding different fibers. A gel structure with large pores and reduced cross-linking between casein micelles in yogurts was observed with 1% of pineapple peel powders, which was associated with lower yogurt firmness and weak rheological properties due to the incompatibility between milk proteins and polysaccharides from the pineapple peel powders [21]. Although the presence of fiber particles always alters yogurt structure, high amounts of passion fruit peel powders or orange byproduct fibers counterbalanced this negative effect and strengthened the casein network possibly due to the water absorption capacity of the fibers [23,35]. This effect of fiber dose and fiber type was also observed in the firmness and spreadability parameters of butter fortified with fibers (from 3% to 5%) from vegetal and fruit wastes: stone pear, celery roots and leaves, spinach and orange albedo [57].

4.2. Health-Promoting Applications of Food Byproducts in Dairy Formulations

Advances in nutrition and medical science have shown that both nutrients and non-nutrient components of foods are important for maintaining good health. This, together with the increasing knowledge of the biochemical structure and functions of bioactive compounds and their effects on the human body, have led to the rise in popularity of functional foods [1]. Although there is no universally accepted definition of functional foods, they can be described as foods that claim to have health benefits beyond basic nutrition [107]. Functional foods are an increasing market segment aimed at consumers who are taking greater responsibility for their own health and well-being [108]. Simultaneously, diet-related illnesses, such as cardiometabolic diseases including coronary heart disease, stroke, type 2 diabetes and obesity stand as one of the greatest global health and economic burdens of our times, accounting for 31% of all deaths worldwide [109,110]. As part of a healthy dietary pattern and lifestyle, functional foods stand as a promising strategy in non-communicable disease prevention.

Within a scope of food waste reduction, much progress has been made using food byproducts as sources of bioactive compounds or as functional ingredients by themselves for the development of dairy functional products. It must be noted that new food ingredients developed from food byproducts that have not been used for human consumption within the EU prior to 1997 must be subjected to official review and approval according to the European Regulation on Novel Foods and Novel Food Ingredients (258/97). This section summarizes the research that has been carried out using byproducts in the manufacture of health-promoting dairy foods.

4.2.1. Use of Byproducts in the Development of Functional Dairy Foods Containing Polyphenols

Polyphenols are secondary metabolites that are synthesized during normal plant development and in response to stress conditions [111]. Plant phenolics include phenolic acid and its derivatives, flavonoids, lignans and stilbenes [112]. Although phenolic compounds are not considered nutrients, several biological and pharmacological activities have been attributed to dietary polyphenols, including antioxidant, anti-allergic, anti-inflammatory, anti-viral, anti-microbial and anti-carcinogenic effects [113]. These properties play a relevant role in the prevention of several major chronic diseases associated with oxidative stress, such as cardiovascular diseases, cancers, type II diabetes, neurodegenerative diseases and osteoporosis [114]. In this sense, the health-protecting capacity of plant phenolics has become of great interest for researchers, the food industry and consumers.

Peels, husks, hulls, pods and bran are major processing byproducts of the fruit, vegetable and cereal industry that are considered sources of polyphenols. They have mostly been applied for polyphenol fortification in yogurt and fermented milks. Namely, winemaking byproducts have been used as the main source of polyphenols, including different flours and extracts from grape pomace and other selective fractions, such as grape skins and seeds. This could be justified both by the fact that black grapes stand among the richest dietary sources of polyphenols [115,116] and by the high amount of grape losses generated during processing and conversion into wine, storage and transportation, which reached 3.6 million in 2013 [9]. Other byproducts from fruits, nuts, vegetables and cereals have also been used as sources of polyphenols for the development of fermented milks and yogurts. These byproducts included pomegranate seeds and peels, almond peels, hazelnut skins, olive pomace and rice bran [12,14,18,37–39].

The addition of polyphenols to dairy foods other than yogurt and fermented milks has received less attention. Wine pomace byproducts have also been the major source of polyphenols used to formulate cheese [53,56,58,59] and ice-cream [50], although other phenol byproduct sources have recently been studied in spreadable cheese (tomato peels, broccoli stems and leaves, corn bran and artichoke external leaves) [53]. The application of broccoli stems in spreadable cheese is particularly interesting, as it could increase glucosinolate content in the product, which are compounds also associated with beneficial health properties [117].

Wine pomace flours have been directly used as ingredients in fermented milk and yogurt development [28,29,45]. The advantage of using powders instead of extracts from the byproducts is that less processing is required, which is a more sustainable approach as it consumes less energy and does not generate secondary byproducts. On the other hand, the disadvantage of using powders is that higher doses are needed to achieve significant polyphenol fortification levels, which penalizes the organoleptic properties of the products. That is why many studies have switched towards using extracts from wine pomace [27,30,39,43].

In this sense, product formulations with a compromise between functional properties and sensory acceptance need to be developed. In foods, polyphenols may contribute to the bitterness, astringency, color, flavor and odor of the products [118]. Polyphenols are associated with the precipitation of salivary glycoproteins and mucopolysaccharides on the tongue, resulting in roughness and dryness on the palate [119]. This is why several studies have reported an inverse relation between polyphenol dosage and consumer acceptance in dairy products [29,38,44,59]. A decrease in the overall acceptance of yogurts with 6% added polyphenols from grape skin flours [45] and of yogurts with 1% and 2% grape pomace powders [120] was observed compared to yogurt formulations with lower doses due to flavor, texture and consistency parameters.

In order to mask the negative sensory effects of polyphenols, several researchers have evaluated their use together with other ingredients. In yogurt and fermented milk fortification with wine pomace byproducts, the best acceptance scores were obtained when polyphenols were added in combination with sucrose (5%), oligofructose (0.5% to 0.667%) or grape juice (0.167% to 0.5% and 15%) [30,44].

Besides the sensory and quality challenges associated with the addition of polyphenols in the dairy matrix, the bioaccessibility and bioavailability of the bioactive compounds should be taken into consideration to truly establish whether the wanted biological health effects are being met. Evidence suggests that polyphenols are absorbed in a relatively low amount. Most polyphenols are poorly absorbed in the gastrointestinal track, reaching the colon where they are metabolized by colonic microbiota. These metabolites are responsible for the biological activities associated with polyphenols [121]. The resulting bioactivity will depend both on the interactions between polyphenols and other macromolecules (lipids, proteins and carbohydrates), which will affect their bioaccessibility and bioavailability, and on the specific microbiota present in each individual's colon, which can give rise to different phenolic metabolites [117,122]. Therefore, further knowledge on the food matrix and food interaction together with the role of gut microbiota on the metabolism and activation of the dietary constituents, will provide original ideas for the development of new functional foods, in which a combination of plant-derived food ingredients with the appropriate bacterial strains will lead to improved biological activity for a specific food product [117].

4.2.2. Use of Byproducts in the Development of Functional Dairy Foods Containing Dietary Fiber

Plant-derived byproducts, such as seed, skins, pods, peels, pomace, hulls, husks, cores, stores, etc., are known sources of bioactive compounds and nutrients including dietary fiber [1,123], whose caloric value has been estimated at 2 kcal per g (FDA, 2018). The European Food Safety Authority (2010) [124] defines this nutrient as non-digestible carbohydrates, including non-starch polysaccharides, resistant starch and oligosaccharides, and lignin. A terminology often encountered is the classification of dietary fiber as "soluble" or "insoluble" [125]. Therefore, the physicochemical properties of the different dietary fibers can be determinant when selecting their applications.

Worldwide and country-specific governmental institutions confirmed that there is evidence of health benefits associated with consumption of diets rich in fiber-containing foods, and recommendations on the intake of dietary fiber range between 25 g to 38 g per day [126]. Health benefits have been related to a reduced risk of coronary heart disease, intestinal disorders, type 2 diabetes and improved weight maintenance [127–129].

Product innovations have been focused on increasing the fiber content of dairy foods with two purposes: to help consumers achieve the daily recommended intake of dietary fiber, and as a marketing strategy to add a nutritional claim on the food package. The European Parliament and Council, (2006) (Regulation No. 1924/2006) [130] stated that the nutritional claim "source of fiber" or "high in fiber" can only be made when the product contains at least 3% (or 1.5 g of fiber per 100 kcal) or 6% (or 3 g of fiber per 100 kcal) dietary fiber, respectively. Bearing this in mind, several researchers have used dietary fiber concentrations ranging from 2.5% to 10% to evaluate its feasibility as an ingredient in dairy products, as an increase in concentrations of dietary fiber in foods can lead to changes in the resultant nutritional, textural, rheological, and sensory properties of the developed products [131].

Development of dairy foods fortified with high contents of dietary fiber have mostly been carried out in yogurt and fermented milks. Available studies have used a wide variety of plant-origin sources derived from fruit and vegetable industry byproducts. Water soluble soybean polysaccharides from okara, which is the byproduct of tofu, soymilk and soybean protein isolate, were used in the development of ice-cream, pudding and a milk-based beverage [26]. Optimal sensory acceptance of products was achieved in milk beverages and pudding with 4% dietary fiber, and in ice-cream with 2% dietary fiber. Higher dietary fiber doses were rejected as consumers considered the foods too thick when evaluated using Just About Right (JAR) scales. In fermented milks and yogurts, fiber from apple pomace (3% to 10%), date byproducts (1.5% to 4.5%) and hazelnut skins (3% to 6%) were used in the development of dietary fiber-fortified foods [20,31,38]. In these cases, optimal sensory acceptance of the products was obtained at 3% fiber addition from hazelnut skins and dates, and 5% fiber addition from apple pomace.

These examples demonstrate that it is possible to increase the doses of dietary fiber for the development of dairy products with optimal sensory acceptance that could be labeled as "source of fiber" on their package. Achieving a "high in fiber" label may be more problematic both from a technological and biological point of view, as textures may be too thick, and consumption of high content dietary fiber products may cause potential secondary effects from carbohydrate fermentation including bloating, distension, flatulence, loose stools and increased stool frequency [132].

Other studies have successfully fortified yogurts and fermented milks with dietary fiber from other byproduct sources, such as orange, passion fruit and asparagus byproducts, but in lower doses (0.6%–1%), which also contribute to increasing the daily intake of dietary fiber in consumers' diets and potentially promote associated health benefits, but do not achieve a nutritional claim [24,25,36,42].

Lower doses of dietary fiber from food byproducts have also been used in the development of fermented milks to protect probiotics and enhance their viability. It is well documented that probiotic bacteria grow slowly in milk because they are devoid of proteolytic enzymes [133]. Therefore, milk solids supplementation is a good practice to improve probiotic growth during fermentation and favor their viability in the product [134]. Rice bran, olive and wine pomace, cheese whey, pineapple, apple, banana and chestnut byproducts have been used for probiotic protection in fermented milks [13,14,17–19,22,27,28,30]. To our knowledge, the only attempt to use byproducts to promote probiotic viability in a different dairy matrix has been using wheat bran in cheese [54].

In addition to enhancing probiotic viability, probiotic strains can act synergistically with specific types of fiber during fermentation to improve the fatty acid composition in fermented milks. This is because some strains of bacteria are able to change the fatty acid profile of milk during fermentation and produce functional fatty acids, including conjugated fatty acids, as the result of their growth and metabolism [135]. Moreover, the addition of other ingredients into the milk, such as prebiotics, can further increase the content of functional fatty acids in fermented milks [136]. In a study using *Lactobacillus acidophilus* and *Bifidobacterium animals* subsp. *lactis* strains, the addition of banana fiber significantly increased α-linoleic acid content, whereas passion fruit fiber promoted the increase of conjugated linoleic acids in probiotic yogurts [19]. Therefore, further studies should focus on the probiotic-fiber synergistic effect to improve the nutritional quality of dairy products, as the application of dietary fiber from fruit byproducts could be a more cost-effective and sustainable option than the addition of conjugated linoleic acids precursors and commercial soluble fiber that are normally used to improve the fatty acid profile of yogurts.

4.2.3. Use of Animal Origin Byproducts in the Development of Functional Dairy Foods

Ingredients derived from animal origin byproducts have been used in the development of dairy foods fortified in omega-3 fatty acids and dairy foods with a high protein content. Fish oil extracted from fish wastes is an excellent source of many unsaturated fatty acids, including long chain omega-3 cis-5,8,11,15,17-eicosapentaenoic acid (EPA) and cis-4,7,10,13,16,19-docosahexaenoic acid (DHA) [137]. However, its application in food formulations fortified in omega-3 is limited because of its easy oxidation and strong odor [41]. Successful attempts to develop yogurts containing omega-3 that had sensory attributes similar to plain yogurt were obtained by encapsulating fish oil in nano-liposomes [40], and adding a fish oil/γ-oryzanol nanoemulsion to yogurt [41].

Functional dairy foods using whey proteins obtained from cheese processing have been widely used as fat replacers and in the development of dairy foods with the nutritional claim "source of protein" or "high in protein" that are already commercially available. Problems associated with using whey proteins and sodium caseinate as fat replacers in yogurt included powdery taste, excessive acid development from lactose fermentation, higher syneresis, excessive firmness and grainy texture [33]. Improved texture parameters have been achieved in low fat yogurts and low fat probiotic yogurts with added whey-buttermilk protein aggregates, whey protein concentrate and heat-treated whey protein concentrates [15–17].

5. Sensory Challenges and Consumer Perspective of Using Byproducts in Dairy Foods

Towards the end of the nineties, consumer acceptance was both referred to as the key success factor for functional foods and the top priority for further research [138]. Since then, several authors have tried to cover this research gap, focusing on sensory and consumer science of functional foods. The latest findings have shown that the perceived importance of food for health is still increasing, but that consumers' critical attitude towards functional foods is also increasing, which translates into lower willingness to compromise on taste for health [139].

The current approach to the development of functional foods using byproducts as novel ingredients has focused on selecting specific concentrations of the byproducts to improve the technological and health-promoting properties of the products, and afterwards, evaluating their sensory acceptance. Not all studies included sensory or consumer analyses of the developed product, and when done, many studies were short on the number of volunteers to achieve significant conclusions. This context reflects that the gap in sensory and consumer research is still present, and that further analyses in this field need to be included in the academic and industry sectors to respond to the good-tasting functional food demand.

The challenge of developing good-tasting functional foods within the dairy industry increases when using food byproducts. Several authors have reported organoleptic issues associated with the use of byproducts in dairy foods, mainly due to the acrid, astringent, bitter or salty off-flavors inherent to plant-based phytonutrients [29,45,140]. In addition, there is a lack of information on the consumer's perspective of using food byproducts as ingredients in other foods. The possible concerns regarding food quality and safety that may arise, as well as the importance of sustainability as a driver in food choice should be investigated.

Bearing in mind that the functional food segment is a highly competitive and continuously changing market, using food byproducts as ingredients could be regarded as an opportunity for product differentiation. Further research should focus on the development of innovative flavors and textures to achieve more palatable foods, as well as on suitable marketing strategies to place these healthy and sustainable products in the market.

6. Conclusions

The applications described in this review show the high potential of valorizing food byproducts for the development of innovative and healthy dairy foods. Byproducts used as sustainable ingredients or sources of bioactive compounds have been shown to be effective for a wide range of technological and nutritional purposes in dairy product manufacture. This approach not only takes a step forward to waste reduction in the food chain, but also offers new ways to diversify the production of dairy foods, creating the possibility of satisfying a market niche based on functional and sustainable products. It is crucial that food technologists, nutritionists and sensory scientists work together to face the challenge of developing more palatable and well accepted foods. Moreover, it is necessary to analyze the consumer's perception and potential food safety concerns on the use of byproducts in food formulations, and specifically, for the dairy food segment.

Author Contributions: M.I-D. and M.D.d.C. selected the topics and designed the review. M.I-D. conducted the literature search and wrote the manuscript. All authors reviewed and agreed on the final version.

Funding: The authors would like to thank the projects FPLACT16 and SUSCOFFEE (AGL2014-57239-R) for the financial support. The grant of M. Iriondo-DeHond was funded by the Instituto Madrileño de Investigación y Desarrollo Rural, Agrario y Alimentario (IMIDRA).

Conflicts of Interest: The authors declare no conflict of interest.

References

1. Sharma, S.K.; Bansal, S.; Mangal, M.; Dixit, A.K.; Gupta, R.K.; Mangal, A.K. Utilization of food processing by-products as dietary, functional, and novel fiber: A review. *Crit. Rev. Food Sci. Nutr.* **2015**, *56*, 1647–1661. [CrossRef] [PubMed]
2. Godfray, H.C.J.; Beddington, J.R.; Crute, I.R.; Haddad, L.; Lawrence, D.; Muir, J.F.; Pretty, J.; Robinson, S.; Thomas, S.M.; Toulmin, C. Food security: The challenge of feeding 9 billion people. *Science* **2010**, *327*, 812–818. [CrossRef] [PubMed]
3. Fan, S.; Brzeska, J. Sustainable food security and nutrition: Demystifying conventional beliefs. *Glob. Food Sec.* **2016**, *11*, 11–16. [CrossRef]
4. Granato, D.; Branco, G.F.; Cruz, A.G.; de Faria, J.A.F.; Shah, N.P. Probiotic dairy products as functional foods. *Compr. Rev. Food Sci. Food Saf.* **2010**, *9*, 455–470. [CrossRef]
5. Menrad, K. Market and marketing of functional food in Europe. *J. Food Eng.* **2003**, *56*, 181–188. [CrossRef]
6. Urala, N.; Lähteenmäki, L. Consumers' changing attitudes towards functional foods. *Food Qual. Prefer.* **2007**, *18*, 1–12. [CrossRef]
7. FAO. *Definitional Framework of Food Loss*; Working Paper; Food and Agriculture Organization of the United Nations: Rome, Italy, 2014; pp. 1–18.
8. *A Report by the High Level Panel of Experts on Food Security and Nutrition of the Committee on World Food Security: HLPE Food Losses and Waste in the Context of Sustainable Food Systems*; Hlpe Report: Rome, Italy, 2014.
9. FAO FAOSTAT. Available online: http://www.fao.org/faostat (accessed on 18 December 2017).
10. Pasotti, L.; Zucca, S.; Casanova, M.; Micoli, G.; Cusella De Angelis, M.G.; Magni, P. Fermentation of lactose to ethanol in cheese whey permeate and concentrated permeate by engineered Escherichia coli. *BMC Biotechnol.* **2017**, *17*, 1–12. [CrossRef] [PubMed]
11. Kaur, D.; Wani, A.A.; Singh, D.P.; Sogi, D.S. Shelf Life Enhancement of Butter, Ice-Cream, and Mayonnaise by Addition of Lycopene. *Int. J. Food Prop.* **2011**, *14*, 1217–1231. [CrossRef]
12. Vital, A.C.P.; Croge, C.; Gomes-da-Costa, S.M.; Matumoto-Pintro, P.T. Effect of addition of Agaricus blazei mushroom residue to milk enriched with Omega-3 on the prevention of lipid oxidation and bioavailability of bioactive compounds after *in vitro* gastrointestinal digestion. *Int. J. Food Sci. Technol.* **2017**, *52*, 1483–1490. [CrossRef]
13. Servili, M.; Rizzello, C.G.; Taticchi, A.; Esposto, S.; Urbani, S.; Mazzacane, F.; Di Maio, I.; Selvaggini, R.; Gobbetti, M.; Di Cagno, R. Functional milk beverage fortified with phenolic compounds extracted from olive

vegetation water, and fermented with functional lactic acid bacteria. *Int. J. Food Microbiol.* **2011**, *147*, 45–52. [CrossRef] [PubMed]

14.   Demirci, T.; Aktaş, K.; Sözeri, D.; Öztürk, H.İ.; Akın, N. Rice bran improve probiotic viability in yoghurt and provide added antioxidative benefits. *J. Funct. Foods* **2017**, *36*, 396–403. [CrossRef]

15.   Akalın, A.S.; Unal, G.; Dinkci, N.; Hayaloglu, A.A. Microstructural, textural, and sensory characteristics of probiotic yogurts fortified with sodium calcium caseinate or whey protein concentrate. *J. Dairy Sci.* **2012**, *95*, 3617–3628. [CrossRef] [PubMed]

16.   Saffon, M.; Richard, V.; Jiménez-Flores, R.; Gauthier, S.; Britten, M.; Pouliot, Y. Behavior of heat-denatured whey:buttermilk protein aggregates during the yogurt-making process and their influence on set-type yogurt properties. *Foods* **2013**, *2*, 444–459. [CrossRef] [PubMed]

17.   Zhang, T.; Mccarthy, J.; Wang, G.; Liu, Y.; Guo, M. Physiochemical properties, microstructure, and probiotic survivability of nonfat goats' milk yogurt using heat-treated whey protein concentrate as fat replacer. *J. Food Sci.* **2015**, *80*, M788–M794. [CrossRef] [PubMed]

18.   Ozcan, T.; Yilmaz-Ersan, L.; Akpinar-Bayizit, A.; Delikanli, B. Antioxidant properties of probiotic fermented milk supplemented with chestnut flour (*C astanea sativa* Mill). *J. Food Process. Preserv.* **2016**. [CrossRef]

19.   Do Espírito Santo, A.P.; Cartolano, N.S.; Silva, T.F.; Soares, F.A.; Gioielli, L.A.; Perego, P.; Converti, A.; Oliveira, M.N. Fibers from fruit by-products enhance probiotic viability and fatty acid profile and increase CLA content in yoghurts. *Int. J. Food Microbiol.* **2012**, *154*, 135–144. [CrossRef] [PubMed]

20.   Issar, K.; Sharma, P.C.; Gupta, A. Utilization of apple pomace in the preparation of fiber-enriched acidophilus yoghurt. *J. Food Process. Preserv.* **2016**. [CrossRef]

21.   Sah, B.N.; Vasiljevic, T.; McKechnie, S.; Donkor, O.N. Physicochemical, textural and rheological properties of probiotic yogurt fortified with fibre-rich pineapple peel powder during refrigerated storage. *LWT-Food Sci. Technol.* **2016**, *65*, 978–986. [CrossRef]

22.   Sah, B.N.; Vasiljevic, T.; McKechnie, S.; Donkor, O.N. Effect of refrigerated storage on probiotic viability and the production and stability of antimutagenic and antioxidant peptides in yogurt supplemented with pineapple peel. *J. Dairy Sci.* **2015**, *98*, 5905–5916. [CrossRef] [PubMed]

23.   Espírito-Santo, A.P.; Lagazzo, A.; Sousa, A.L.O.P.; Perego, P.; Converti, A.; Oliveira, M.N. Rheology, spontaneous whey separation, microstructure and sensorial characteristics of probiotic yoghurts enriched with passion fruit fiber. *Food Res. Int.* **2013**, *50*, 224–231. [CrossRef]

24.   Do Espírito Santo, A.P.; Perego, P.; Converti, A.; Oliveira, M.N. Influence of milk type and addition of passion fruit peel powder on fermentation kinetics, texture profile and bacterial viability in probiotic yoghurts. *LWT-Food Sci. Technol.* **2012**, *47*, 393–399. [CrossRef]

25.   Perina, N.P.; Granato, D.; Hirota, C.; Cruz, A.G.; Bogsan, C.S.B.; Oliveira, M.N. Effect of vegetal-oil emulsion and passion fruit peel-powder on sensory acceptance of functional yogurt. *Food Res. Int.* **2015**, *70*, 134–141. [CrossRef]

26.   Chen, W.; Duizer, L.; Corredig, M.; Goff, H.D. Addition of soluble soybean polysaccharides to dairy products as a source of dietary fiber. *J. Food Sci.* **2010**, *75*, 478–484. [CrossRef] [PubMed]

27.   Aliakbarian, B.; Casale, M.; Paini, M.; Casazza, A.; Lanteri, S.; Perego, P. Production of a novel fermented milk fortified with natural antioxidants and its analysis by NIR spectroscopy. *Food Sci. Technol. Int.* **2015**, *62*, 376–383. [CrossRef]

28.   Frumento, D.; do Espirito Santo, A.P.; Aliakbarian, B.; Casazza, A.A.; Gallo, M.; Converti, A.; Perego, P. Development of milk fermented with Lactobacillus acidophilus fortified with Vitis vinifera marc flour. *Food Technol. Biotechnol.* **2013**, *51*, 370–375.

29.   Tseng, A.; Zhao, Y. Wine grape pomace as antioxidant dietary fibre for enhancing nutritional value and improving storability of yogurt and salad dressing. *Food Chem.* **2013**, *138*, 356–365. [CrossRef] [PubMed]

30.   Dos Santos, K.M.O.; de Oliveira, I.C.; Lopes, M.A.C.; Cruz, A.P.G.; Buriti, F.C.A.; Cabral, L.M. Addition of grape pomace extract to probiotic fermented goat milk: The effect on phenolic content, probiotic viability and sensory acceptability. *J. Sci. Food Agric.* **2017**, *97*, 1108–1115. [CrossRef] [PubMed]

31.   Hashim, I.B.; Khalil, A.H.; Afifi, H.S. Quality characteristics and consumer acceptance of yogurt fortified with date fiber. *J. Dairy Sci.* **2009**, *92*, 5403–5407. [CrossRef] [PubMed]

32.   Nontasan, S.; Moongngarm, A.; Deeseenthum, S. Application of Functional Colorant Prepared from Black Rice Bran in Yogurt. *APCBEE Procedia* **2012**, *2*, 62–67. [CrossRef]

33. Sandoval-Castilla, O.; Lobato-Calleros, C.; Aguirre-Mandujano, E.; Vernon-Carter, E.J. Microstructure and texture of yogurt as influenced by fat replacers. *Int. Dairy J.* **2004**, *14*, 151–159. [CrossRef]

34. Yi, T.; Huang, X.; Pan, S.; Wang, L. Physicochemical and functional properties of micronized jincheng orange by-products (Citrus sinensis Osbeck) dietary fiber and its application as a fat replacer in yogurt. *Int. J. Food* **2014**, *86*, 565–572. [CrossRef] [PubMed]

35. Sendra, E.; Kuri, V.; Fernández-López, J.; Sayas-Barberá, E.; Navarro, C.; Pérez-Alvarez, J.A. Viscoelastic properties of orange fiber enriched yogurt as a function of fiber dose, size and thermal treatment. *LWT-Food Sci. Technol.* **2010**, *43*, 708–714. [CrossRef]

36. García-Pérez, F.J.; Lario, Y.; Fernández-López, J.; Sayas, E.; Pérez-Alvarez, J.A.; Sendra, E. Effect of orange fiber addition on yogurt color during fermentation and cold storage. *Color. Res. Appl.* **2005**, *30*, 457–463. [CrossRef]

37. El-Said, M.M.; Haggag, H.F.; Fakhr El-Din, H.M.; Gad, A.S.; Farahat, A.M. Antioxidant activities and physical properties of stirred yoghurt fortified with pomegranate peel extracts. *Ann. Agric. Sci.* **2014**, *59*, 207–212. [CrossRef]

38. Bertolino, M.; Belviso, S.; Dal Bello, B.; Ghirardello, D.; Giordano, M.; Rolle, L.; Gerbi, V.; Zeppa, G. Influence of the addition of different hazelnut skins on the physicochemical, antioxidant, polyphenol and sensory properties of yogurt. *LWT-Food Sci. Technol.* **2015**, *63*, 1145–1154. [CrossRef]

39. Ersöz, E.; Kınık, Ö.; Yerlikaya, O.; Açu, M. Effect of phenolic compounds on characteristics of strained yoghurts produced from sheep milk. *Afr. J. Agric. Res.* **2011**, *6*, 5351–5359. [CrossRef]

40. Ghorbanzade, T.; Jafari, S.M.; Akhavan, S.; Hadavi, R. Nano-encapsulation of fish oil in nano-liposomes and its application in fortification of yogurt. *Food Chem.* **2017**, *216*, 146–152. [CrossRef] [PubMed]

41. Zhong, J.; Yang, R.; Cao, X.; Liu, X.; Qin, X. Improved physicochemical properties of yogurt fortified with fish oil/γ-oryzanol by nanoemulsion technology. *Molecules* **2018**, *23*, 56. [CrossRef] [PubMed]

42. Sanz, T.; Salvador, A.; Jiménez, A.; Fiszman, S.M. Yogurt enrichment with functional asparagus fibre. Effect fibre extraction method on rheological properties, colour, and sensory acceptance. *Eur. Food Res. Technol.* **2008**, *227*, 1515–1521. [CrossRef]

43. Chouchouli, V.; Kalogeropoulos, N.; Konteles, S.J.; Karvela, E.; Makris, D.P.; Karathanos, V.T. Fortification of yoghurts with grape (Vitis vinifera) seed extracts. *LWT-Food Sci. Technol.* **2013**, *53*, 522–529. [CrossRef]

44. Karnopp, A.R.; Oliveira, K.G.; de Andrade, E.F.; Postingher, B.M.; Granato, D. Optimization of an organic yogurt based on sensorial, nutritional, and functional perspectives. *Food Chem.* **2017**, *233*, 401–411. [CrossRef] [PubMed]

45. Marchiani, R.; Bertolino, M.; Belviso, S.; Giordano, M.; Ghirardello, D.; Torri, L.; Piochi, M.; Zeppa, G. Yogurt enrichment with grape pomace: Effect of grape cultivar on physicochemical, microbiological and sensory properties. *J. Food Qual.* **2016**, *39*, 77–89. [CrossRef]

46. Jridi, M.; Souissi, N.; Salem, M.B.; Ayadi, M.A.; Nasri, M.; Azabou, S. Tunisian date (Phoenix dactylifera L.) by-products: Characterization and potential effects on sensory, textural and antioxidant properties of dairy desserts. *Food Chem.* **2015**, *188*, 8–15. [CrossRef] [PubMed]

47. Crizel, T. de M.; Araujo, R.R. de; Rios, A. de O.; Rech, R.; Flôres, S.H. Orange fiber as a novel fat replacer in lemon ice cream. *Food Sci. Technol.* **2014**, *34*, 332–340. [CrossRef]

48. Çam, M.; Erdoğan, F.; Aslan, D.; Dinç, M. Enrichment of functional properties of ice cream with pomegranate by-products. *J. Food Sci.* **2013**, *78*, 1543–1550. [CrossRef]

49. Rizk, E.M.; El-Kady, A.T.; El-Bialy, A.R. Charactrization of carotenoids (lyco-red) extracted from tomato peels and its uses as natural colorants and antioxidants of ice cream. *Ann. Agric. Sci.* **2014**, *59*, 53–61. [CrossRef]

50. Hwang, J.Y.; Shyu, Y.S.; Hsu, C.K. Grape wine lees improves the rheological and adds antioxidant properties to ice cream. *LWT-Food Sci. Technol.* **2009**, *42*, 312–318. [CrossRef]

51. Nadeem, M.; Mahud, A.; Imran, M.; Khalique, A. Enhancement of the oxidative stability of whey butter through almond (Prunus dulcis) peel extract. *J. Food Process. Preserv.* **2014**, *39*, 591–598. [CrossRef]

52. Abid, Y.; Azabou, S.; Jridi, M.; Khemakhem, I.; Bouaziz, M.; Attia, H. Storage stability of traditional Tunisian butter enriched with antioxidant extract from tomato processing by-products. *Food Chem.* **2017**, *233*, 476–482. [CrossRef] [PubMed]

53. Lucera, A.; Costa, C.; Marinelli, V.; Saccotelli, M.A.; Alessandro, M.; Nobile, D.; Conte, A. Fruit and vegetable by-products to fortify spreadable cheese. *Antioxidants* **2018**. [CrossRef] [PubMed]

54. Terpou, A.; Bekatorou, A.; Bosnea, L.; Kanellaki, M.; Ganatsios, V.; Koutinas, A.A. Wheat bran as prebiotic cell immobilisation carrier for industrial functional Feta-type cheese making: Chemical, microbial and sensory evaluation. *Biocatal. Agric. Biotechnol.* **2018**, *13*, 75–83. [CrossRef]

55. Erbay, Z.; Koca, N. Effects of whey or maltodextrin addition during production on physical quality of white cheese powder during storage. *J. Dairy Sci.* **2015**, *98*, 8391–8404. [CrossRef] [PubMed]

56. Shan, B.; Cai, Y.-Z.; Brooks, J.D.; Corke, H. Potential application of spice and herb extracts as natural preservatives in cheese. *J. Med. Food* **2011**, *14*, 284–290. [CrossRef] [PubMed]

57. Göksel Saraç, M.; Dogan, M. Incorporation of dietary fiber concentrates from fruit and vegetable wastes in butter: Effects on physicochemical, textural, and sensory properties. *Eur. Food Res. Technol.* **2016**, *242*, 1331–1342. [CrossRef]

58. Felix da Silva, D.; Matumoto-Pintro, P.T.; Bazinet, L.; Couillard, C.; Britten, M. Effect of commercial grape extracts on the cheese-making properties of milk. *J. Dairy Sci.* **2015**, *98*, 1552–1562. [CrossRef] [PubMed]

59. Marchiani, R.; Bertolino, M.; Ghirardello, D.; McSweeney, P.L.H.; Zeppa, G. Physicochemical and nutritional qualities of grape pomace powder-fortified semi-hard cheeses. *J. Food Sci. Technol.* **2015**, *53*, 1585–1596. [CrossRef] [PubMed]

60. Ayala-Zavala, J.F.; Vega-Vega, V.; Rosas-Domínguez, C.; Palafox-Carlos, H.; Villa-Rodriguez, J.A.; Siddiqui, M.W.; Dávila-Aviña, J.E.; González-Aguilar, G.A. Agro-industrial potential of exotic fruit byproducts as a source of food additives. *Food Res. Int.* **2011**, *44*, 1866–1874. [CrossRef]

61. *Codex Alimentarius General Standard for Food Additives Codex Stan 192–1995*; Food and Agriculture Organization of the United Nations: Rome, Italy, 2017.

62. Serra, M.; Trujillo, A.J.; Pereda, J.; Guamis, B.; Ferragut, V. Quantification of lipolysis and lipid oxidation during cold storage of yogurts produced from milk treated by ultra-high pressure homogenization. *J. Food Eng.* **2008**, *89*, 99–104. [CrossRef]

63. Marsili, R. Flavors and off-flavors in dairy foods. In *Encyclopedia of Dairy Sciences*, 2nd ed.; Fuquay, J.W., Fox, P.F., McSweeney, P.L.H., Eds.; Elsevier Ltd.: Atlanta, GA, USA, 2011; pp. 533–551.

64. Grażyna, C.; Hanna, C.; Adam, A.; Magdalena, B.M. Natural antioxidants in milk and dairy products. *Int. J. Dairy Technol.* **2017**, *70*, 165–178. [CrossRef]

65. Hedegaard, R.V.; Kristensen, D.; Nielsen, J.H.; Frøst, M.B.; Østdal, H.; Hermansen, J.E.; Kröger-Ohlsen, M.; Skibsted, L.H. Comparison of descriptive sensory analysis and chemical analysis for oxidative changes in milk. *J. Dairy Sci.* **2006**, *89*, 495–504. [CrossRef]

66. Herr, B. Types and functions of additives in dairy products. In *Encyclopedia of Dairy Sciences*; Fuquay, J.W., Fox, P.F., McSweeney, P.L.H., Eds.; Elsevier Ltd.: Atlanta, GA, USA, 2011; pp. 34–40. ISBN 978-0-12-374407-4.

67. Frede, E. Properties and analysis. In *Encyclopedia of Dairy Sciences*; Fuquay, J.W., Fox, P.F., McSweeney, P.L.H., Eds.; Elsevier Ltd.: Rockford, IL, USA, 2011; pp. 506–514.

68. Phan-Thi, H.; Durand, P.; Prost, M.; Prost, E.; Wach??, Y. Effect of heat-processing on the antioxidant and prooxidant activities of b-carotene from natural and synthetic origins on red blood cells. *Food Chem.* **2016**, *190*, 1137–1144. [CrossRef] [PubMed]

69. McSweeney, P.L.H.; Sousa, M.J. Biochemical pathways for the production of flavour compounds in cheeses during ripening: A review. *Lait* **2000**, *80*, 293–324. [CrossRef]

70. Fox, P.F. Proteolysis During Cheese Manufacture and Ripening. *J. Dairy Sci.* **1989**, *72*, 1379–1400. [CrossRef]

71. Ribeiro Júnior, J.C.; de Oliveira, A.M.; Silva, F.D.G.; Tamanini, R.; de Oliveira, A.L.M.; Beloti, V. The main spoilage-related psychrotrophic bacteria in refrigerated raw milk. *J. Dairy Sci.* **2018**, *101*, 75–83. [CrossRef] [PubMed]

72. Deeth, H.; Fitz-Gerald, C.H. Lipolytic enzymes and hydrolitic rancidity in milk and milk products. In *Advanced Dairy Chemistry Vol 2: Lipids*; Fox, P.F., McSweeney, P.L.H., Eds.; Springer: New York, NY, USA, 2006; pp. 481–556.

73. Deeth, H.C. Lipolysis and Hydrolitic Rancidity. In *Encyclopedia of Dairy Sciences*; Fuquay, J.W., Fox, P.F., McSweeney, P.L.H., Eds.; Elsevier Ltd.: Atlanta, GA, USA, 2011; pp. 721–726.

74. Forsythe, S.J. *The Microbiology of Safe Food*, 2nd ed.; Wiley Blackwell: Hoboken, NJ, USA, 2010.

75. Baglinière, F.; Jardin, J.; Gaucheron, F.; de Carvalho, A.F.; Vanetti, M.C.D. Proteolysis of casein micelles by heat-stable protease secreted by Serratia liquefaciens leads to the destabilisation of UHT milk during its storage. *Int. Dairy J.* **2017**, *68*, 38–45. [CrossRef]

76. Lu, M.; Wang, N.S. Spoilage of milk and dairy products. In *The Microbiological Quality of Food-Foodborne Spoilers*; Bevilacqua, A., Corbo, M.R., Milena, S., Eds.; Woodhead Publishing Limited: Cambridge, UK, 2017; pp. 151–178.

77. Baglinière, F.; Tanguy, G.; Salgado, R.L.; Jardin, J.; Rousseau, F.; Robert, B.; Harel-Oger, M.; Vanetti, M.C.D.; Gaucheron, F. Ser2 from Serratia liquefaciens L53: A new heat stable protease able to destabilize UHT milk during its storage. *Food Chem.* **2017**, *229*, 104–110. [CrossRef] [PubMed]

78. Rehman, S.U.; Farkye, N.Y. Phosphatases. In *Encyclopedia of Dairy Sciences*; Fuquay, J.W., Fox, P.F., McSweeney, P.L.H., Eds.; Elsevier Ltd.: Atlanta, GA, USA, 2011; pp. 314–318.

79. Brisabois, A.; Lafarge, V.; Brouillaud, A.; de Buyser, M.L.; Collette, C.; Garin-Bastuji, B.; Thorel, M.F. Pathogenic organisms in milk and milk products: The situation in France and in Europe. *Rev. Sci. Tech.* **1997**, *16*, 467–471.

80. De Buyser, M.L.; Dufour, B.; Maire, M.; Lafarge, V. Implication of milk and milk products in food-borne diseases in France and in different industrialised countries. *Int. J. Food Microbiol.* **2001**, *67*, 1–17. [CrossRef]

81. Yoon, Y.; Lee, S.; Choi, K.H. Microbial benefits and risks of raw milk cheese. *Food Control.* **2016**, *63*, 201–215. [CrossRef]

82. Donnelly, C.W. Growth and survival or microbial pathogens in cheese. In *Cheese: Chemistry, Physics and Microbiology*; Fox, P.F., McSweeney, P.L.H., Cogan, M.T., Guinee, T.P., Eds.; Elsevier: Atlanta, GA, USA, 2004; pp. 541–559.

83. Fuselli, F.; Guarino, C. Preservatives in cheeses. In *Handbook of Cheese in Health: Production, Nutrition and Medical Sciences*; Human Health Handbooks no. 6; Preedy, V.R., Watson, R.R., Patel, V.B., Eds.; Wageningen Academic Publishers: Wageningen, The Netherlands, 2013.

84. Morgan, D.; Newman, C.P.; Hutchinson, D.N.; Walker, A.M.; Rowe, B.; Majid, F. Verotoxin producing Escherichia coli 0 157 infections associated with the consumption of yoghurt. *Epidemiol. Infect.* **1993**, *111*, 181–187. [CrossRef] [PubMed]

85. Cheng, H.Y.; Yu, R.C.; Chou, C.C. Increased acid tolerance of Escherichia coli O157:H7 as affected by acid adaptation time and conditions of acid challenge. *Food Res. Int.* **2003**, *36*, 49–56. [CrossRef]

86. Ultee, A.; Bennik, M.H.J.; Moezelaar, R. The phenolic hydroxyl group of carvacrol is essential for action against the food-borne pathogen Bacillus cereus. *Appl. Environ. Microbiol.* **2002**, *68*, 1561–1568. [CrossRef] [PubMed]

87. Daglia, M. Polyphenols as antimicrobial agents. *Curr. Opin. Biotechnol.* **2012**, *23*, 174–181. [CrossRef] [PubMed]

88. Cowan, M.M. Plant products as antimicrobial agents. *Clin. Microbiol. Rev.* **1999**, *12*, 564–582. [CrossRef] [PubMed]

89. Wilson, P.D.; Brocklehurst, T.F.; Arino, S.; Thuault, D.; Jakobsen, M.; Lange, M.; Farkas, J.; Wimpenny, J.W.T.; Van Impe, J.F. Modelling microbial growth in structured foods: Towards a unified approach. *Int. J. Food Microbiol.* **2002**, *73*, 275–289. [CrossRef]

90. Tayel, A.A.; Hussein, H.; Sorour, N.M.; El-Tras, W.F. Foodborne pathogens prevention and sensory attributes enhancement in processed cheese via flavoring with plant extracts. *J. Food Sci.* **2015**, *80*, M2886–M2891. [CrossRef] [PubMed]

91. Marinho, M.T.; Zielinski, A.A.; Demiate, I.M.; dos Bersot, L.S.; Granato, D.; Nogueira, A. Ripened semihard cheese covered with lard and dehydrated rosemary (*Rosmarinus officinalis* L.) leaves: Processing, characterization, and quality traits. *J. Food Sci.* **2015**, *80*, 2045–2054. [CrossRef] [PubMed]

92. Llamas, N.E.; Garrido, M.; Di Nezio, M.S.; Band, B.S.F. Second order advantage in the determination of amaranth, sunset yellow FCF and tartrazine by UV-vis and multivariate curve resolution-alternating least squares. *Anal. Chim. Acta* **2009**, *655*, 38–42. [CrossRef] [PubMed]

93. Martins, N.; Roriz, C.L.; Morales, P.; Barros, L.; Ferreira, I.C.F.R. Food colorants: Challenges, opportunities and current desires of agro-industries to ensure consumer expectations and regulatory practices. *Trends Food Sci. Technol.* **2016**, *52*, 1–15. [CrossRef]

94. Santos-Buelga, C.; Mateus, N.; De Freitas, V. Anthocyanins. Plant pigments and beyond. *J. Agric. Food Chem.* **2014**, *62*, 6879–6884. [CrossRef] [PubMed]

95. Rodriguez-Amaya, D.B. Natural food pigments and colorants. *Curr. Opin. Food Sci.* **2016**, *7*, 20–26. [CrossRef]

96. Teixeira, A.; Baenas, N.; Dominguez-Perles, R.; Barros, A.; Rosa, E.; Moreno, D.A.; Garcia-Viguera, C. Natural bioactive compounds from winery by-products as health promoters: A review. *Int. J. Mol. Sci.* **2014**, *15*, 15638–15678. [CrossRef] [PubMed]

97. Giusti, M.M.; Wrolstad, R.E. Acylated anthocyanins from edible sources and their applications in food systems. *Biochem. Eng. J.* **2003**, *14*, 217–225. [CrossRef]

98. Prata, E.R.; Oliveira, L.S. Fresh coffee husks as potential sources of anthocyanins. *LWT-Food Sci. Technol.* **2007**, *40*, 1555–1560. [CrossRef]

99. FDA Color Additives Listed for Use in Food. Available online: https://www.fda.gov/ForIndustry/ ColorAdditives/ColorAdditivesinSpecificProducts/InFood/ucm130054.htm (accessed on 26 June 2018).

100. Prudencio, I.D.; Prudêncio, E.S.; Gris, E.F.; Tomazi, T.; Bordignon-Luiz, M.T. Petit suisse manufactured with cheese whey retentate and application of betalains and anthocyanins. *LWT-Food Sci. Technol.* **2008**, *41*, 905–910. [CrossRef]

101. Saunders, A.B. Dairy desserts. In *Encyclopedia of Dairy Sciences*, 2nd ed.; Fuquay, J., Fox, P.F., McSweeney, P.L., Eds.; Elsevier Ltd.: Atlanta, GA, USA, 2011; pp. 905–912.

102. Krog, N. Emulsifiers. In *Encyclopedia of Dairy Sciences*, 2nd ed.; Fuquay, J., Fox, P.F., McSweeney, P.L.H., Eds.; Elsevier Ltd.: Atlanta, GA, USA, 2011; pp. 61–71.

103. Müller-Maatsch, J.; Bencivenni, M.; Caligiani, A.; Tedeschi, T.; Bruggeman, G.; Bosch, M.; Petrusan, J.; Van Droogenbroeck, B.; Elst, K.; Sforza, S. Pectin content and composition from different food waste streams in memory. *Food Chem.* **2016**, *201*, 37–45. [CrossRef] [PubMed]

104. De Oliveira, C.F.; Giordani, D.; Gurak, P.D.; Cladera-Olivera, F.; Marczak, L.D.F. Extraction of pectin from passion fruit peel using moderate electric field and conventional heating extraction methods. *Innov. Food Sci. Emerg. Technol.* **2015**, *29*, 201–208. [CrossRef]

105. Min, B.; Lim, J.; Ko, S.; Lee, K.G.; Lee, S.H.; Lee, S. Environmentally friendly preparation of pectins from agricultural byproducts and their structural/rheological characterization. *Bioresour. Technol.* **2011**, *102*, 3855–3860. [CrossRef] [PubMed]

106. Jeong, H.S.; Kim, H.Y.; Ahn, S.H.; Oh, S.C.; Yang, I.; Choi, I.G. Optimization of enzymatic hydrolysis conditions for extraction of pectin from rapeseed cake (*Brassica napus* L.) using commercial enzymes. *Food Chem.* **2014**, *157*, 332–338. [CrossRef] [PubMed]

107. US General Accounting Office Food Safety. Improvements needed in overseeing the safety of dietary supplements and "functional foods". Available online: https://www.gao.gov/products/GAO/RCED-00-156 (accessed on 31 July 2018).

108. Hasler, C.M. Functional foods: Benefits, concerns and challenges—A position paper from the American Council on Science and Health. *J. Nutr.* **2002**, *132*, 3772–3781. [CrossRef] [PubMed]

109. Mozaffarian, D. Dietary and policy priorities for cardiovascular disease, diabetes, and obesity—A comprehensive review. *Circulation* **2016**, *133*, 187–225. [CrossRef] [PubMed]

110. World Health Organization Cardiovascular Disease. Available online: http://www.who.int/cardiovascular_ diseases/en/ (accessed on 31 July 2018).

111. Naczk, M.; Shahidi, F. Extraction and analysis of phenolics in food. *J. Chromatogr. A* **2004**, *1054*, 95–111. [CrossRef]

112. Costa, C.; Tsatsakis, A.; Mamoulakis, C.; Teodoro, M.; Briguglio, G.; Caruso, E.; Tsoukalas, D.; Margina, D.; Dardiotis, E.; Kouretas, D.; et al. Current evidence on the effect of dietary polyphenols intake on chronic diseases. *Food Chem. Toxicol.* **2017**, *110*, 286–299. [CrossRef] [PubMed]

113. Bahadoran, Z.; Mirmiran, P.; Azizi, F. Dietary polyphenols as potential neutraceuticals in management of diabetes: A review. *J. Diabetes Metab. Disord.* **2013**, *12*, 43. [CrossRef] [PubMed]

114. Scalbert, A.; Manach, C.; Morand, C.; Rémésy, C.; Jiménez, L. Dietary polyphenols and the prevention of diseases. *Crit. Rev. Food Sci. Nutr.* **2005**, *45*, 287–306. [CrossRef] [PubMed]

115. Pérez-Jiménez, J.; Neveu, V.; Vos, F.; Scalbert, A. Identification of the 100 richest dietary sources of polyphenols: An application of the Phenol-Explorer database. *Eur. J. Clin. Nutr.* **2010**, *64*, S112–S120. [CrossRef] [PubMed]

116. Boskou, D. Sources of natural phenolic antioxidants. *Trends Food Sci. Technol.* **2006**, *17*, 505–512. [CrossRef]

117. Tomas-Barberan, F.; Gil-Izquierdo, A.; Moreno, D. Bioavailability and metabolism of phenolic compounds and glucosinolates. In *Designing Functional Foods*; Elsevier: Atlanta, GA, USA, 2009; pp. 194–229. ISBN 978-1-84569-432-6.

118. Shahidi, F.; Naczk, M. *Phenolics in Food and Nutraceuticals*; CRC Press: Boca Raton, FL, USA, 2006; ISBN 0203508734.

119. Haslam, E.; Lilley, T.H. Natural astringency in foodstuffs—A molecular interpretation. *Crit. Rev. Food Sci. Nutr. Nat.* **1988**, 37–41. [CrossRef]

120. Tseng, A.; Zhao, Y. Effect of different drying methods and storage time on the retention of bioactive compounds and antibacterial activity of wine grape pomace (Pinot Noir and Merlot). *J. Food Sci.* **2012**, *77*, 1–10. [CrossRef] [PubMed]

121. Del Rio, D.; Costa, L.G.; Lean, M.E.J.; Crozier, A. Polyphenols and health: What compounds are involved? *Nutr. Metab. Cardiovasc. Dis.* **2010**, *20*, 1–6. [CrossRef] [PubMed]

122. Jakobek, L. Interactions of polyphenols with carbohydrates, lipids and proteins. *Food Chem.* **2015**, *175*, 556–567. [CrossRef] [PubMed]

123. McKee, L.H.; Latner, T.A. Underutilized sources of dietary fiber: A review. *Plant. Foods Hum. Nutr.* **2000**, *55*, 285–304. [CrossRef] [PubMed]

124. European Food Safety Authority Scientific opinion on dietary reference values for carbohydrates and dietary fibre. *EFSA J.* **2010**, *8*, 1–77. [CrossRef]

125. Álvarez, E.E.; González, P. La fibra dietética. *Nutr. Hosp.* **2006**, *21*, 61–72.

126. AECOSAN Report of the Scientific Committee of the Spanish Agency for Consumer Affairs, Food Safety and Nutrition (AECOSAN) about objectives as well as nutritional and physical activity recommendations to tackle obesity in the framework of the NAOS Strategy. *Rev. Com. Cient.* **2014**, *19*, 95–209.

127. Pereira, M.; O'Reilly, E.; Augustsson, K.; Fraser, G.; Goldbourt, U.; Heitmann, B.; Hallmans, G.; Knekt, P.; Liu, S.; Pietinen, P.; et al. Dietary Fiber and Risk of Coronary Heart Disease. *Arch. Intern. Med.* **2004**, *164*, 370–376. [CrossRef] [PubMed]

128. Lindström, J.; Peltonen, M.; Eriksson, J.G.; Louheranta, A.; Fogelholm, M.; Uusitupa, M.; Tuomilehto, J. High-fibre, low-fat diet predicts long-term weight loss and decreased type 2 diabetes risk: The Finnish Diabetes Prevention Study. *Diabetologia* **2006**, *49*, 912–920. [CrossRef] [PubMed]

129. Peters, U.; Sinha, R.; Chatterjee, N.; Subar, A.F.; Ziegler, R.G.; Kulldorff, M.; Bresalier, R.; Weissfeld, J.L.; Flood, A.; Schatzkin, A.; et al. Dietary fibre and colorectal adenoma in a colorectal cancer early detection programme. *Lancet* **2003**, *361*, 1491–1495. [CrossRef]

130. European Parliament and Council Regulation (EC) No 1924/2006 on Nutrition and Health Claims Made on Foods. 2006. Available online: https://eur-lex.europa.eu/LexUriServ/LexUriServ.do?uri=OJ:L:2007:012:0003:0018:EN:PDF (accessed on 31 July 2018).

131. Guillon, F.; Champ, M. Structural and physical properties of dietary fibres, and consequences of processing on human physiology. *Food Res. Int.* **2000**, *33*, 233–245. [CrossRef]

132. Grabitske, H.A.; Slavin, J.L. Gastrointestinal effects of low-digestible carbohydrates. *Crit. Rev. Food Sci. Nutr.* **2009**, *49*, 327–360. [CrossRef] [PubMed]

133. Marafon, A.P.; Sumi, A.; Alcântara, M.R.; Tamime, A.Y.; Nogueira de Oliveira, M. Optimization of the rheological properties of probiotic yoghurts supplemented with milk proteins. *LWT-Food Sci. Technol.* **2011**, *44*, 511–519. [CrossRef]

134. Sodini, I.; Lucas, A.; Tissier, J.P.; Corrieu, G. Physical properties and microstructure of yoghurts supplemented with milk protein hydrolysates. *Int. Dairy J.* **2005**, *15*, 29–35. [CrossRef]

135. Yadav, H.; Jain, S.; Sinha, P.R. Production of free fatty acids and conjugated linoleic acid in probiotic dahi containing Lactobacillus acidophilus and Lactobacillus casei during fermentation and storage. *Int. Dairy J.* **2007**, *17*, 1006–1010. [CrossRef]

136. Do Espírito Santo, A.P.; Silva, R.C.; Soares, F.A.S.M.; Anjos, D.; Gioielli, L.A.; Oliveira, M.N. Açai pulp addition improves fatty acid profile and probiotic viability in yoghurt. *Int. Dairy J.* **2010**, *20*, 415–422. [CrossRef]

137. Jayathilakan, K.; Sultana, K.; Radhakrishna, K.; Bawa, A.S. Utilization of byproducts and waste materials from meat, poultry and fish processing industries: A review. *J. Food Sci. Technol.* **2012**, *49*, 278–293. [CrossRef] [PubMed]

138. Childs, N.M.; Childs, N.M.; Poryzees, G.H. Foods that help prevent disease: Consumer attitudes and public policy implications. *J. Consum. Mark.* **1997**, *14*, 433–447. [CrossRef]

139. Verbeke, W. Functional foods: Consumer willingness to compromise on taste for health? *Food Qual. Prefer.* **2006**, *17*, 126–131. [CrossRef]
140. Urala, N.; Liisa, L. Attitudes behind consumers' willingness to use functional foods. *Food Qual. Prefer.* **2004**, *15*, 793–803. [CrossRef]

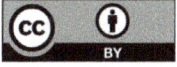

![nutrients logo] *nutrients*

MDPI

Article

Induction of Trained Innate Immunity in Human Monocytes by Bovine Milk and Milk-Derived Immunoglobulin G

Marloes van Splunter [1], Thijs L. J. van Osch [1], Sylvia Brugman [1], Huub F. J. Savelkoul [1], Leo A. B. Joosten [2], Mihai G. Netea [2,3] and R. J. Joost van Neerven [1,4,*]

[1] Cell Biology and Immunology, Wageningen University, Wageningen, P.O. Box 338, 6708 WD Wageningen, The Netherlands; marloes.vansplunter@gmail.com (M.v.S.); thijsvanosch@live.nl (T.L.J.v.O.); sylvia.brugman@wur.nl (S.B.); huub.savelkoul@wur.nl (H.F.J.S.)

[2] Department of Internal Medicine and Radboud Center for Infectious Diseases (RCI), Radboud University Medical Center, 6525 GA Nijmegen, The Netherlands; Leo.Joosten@radboudumc.nl (L.A.B.J.); Mihai.Netea@radboudumc.nl (M.G.N.)

[3] Department for Genomics & Immunoregulation, Life and Medical Sciences Institute (LIMES), University of Bonn, 53115 Bonn, Germany

[4] FrieslandCampina, 3818 LE Amersfoort, The Netherlands

* Correspondence: joost.vanneerven@wur.nl; Tel.: +31-623-537-129

Received: 2 August 2018; Accepted: 21 September 2018; Published: 27 September 2018

Abstract: Innate immune memory, also termed "trained immunity" in vertebrates, has been recently described in a large variety of plants and animals. In most cases, trained innate immunity is induced by pathogens or pathogen-associated molecular patterns (PAMPs), and is associated with long-term epigenetic, metabolic, and functional reprogramming. Interestingly, recent findings indicate that food components can mimic PAMPs effects and induce trained immunity. The aim of this study was to investigate whether bovine milk or its components can induce trained immunity in human monocytes. To this aim, monocytes were exposed for 24 h to β-glucan, Toll-like receptor (TLR)-ligands, bovine milk, milk fractions, bovine lactoferrin (bLF), and bovine Immunoglobulin G (bIgG). After washing away the stimulus and a resting period of five days, the cells were re-stimulated with TLR ligands and Tumor necrosis factor (TNF-) and interleukin (IL)-6 production was measured. Training with β-glucan resulted in higher cytokine production after TLR1/2, TLR4, and TLR7/8 stimulation. When monocytes trained with raw milk were re-stimulated with TLR1/2 ligand Pam3CSK4, trained cells produced more IL-6 compared to non-trained cells. Training with bIgG resulted in higher cytokine production after TLR4 and TLR7/8 stimulation. These results show that bovine milk and bIgG can induce trained immunity in human monocytes. This confirms the hypothesis that diet components can influence the long-term responsiveness of the innate immune system.

Keywords: innate immune memory; trained immunity; raw bovine milk; bovine IgG; bovine lactoferrin; dietary compounds; monocytes

---

1. Introduction

The immune system is divided into two arms, the innate immune system and the adaptive immune system, of which only the latter is known to build long-lasting immune memory in T and B cells. However, recent observations have revealed that the innate immune system can also adapt to previous insults and develop a non-specific memory after infections, a process termed "trained innate immunity" [1,2]. The concept of trained immunity is based on the observation that after a primary infection, an enhanced innate immune response is induced in response to secondary infection or stimulation. In contrast to adaptive immune memory, this enhanced secondary response of trained innate immune cells is not only specific for the antigen that induced the primary response, but is rather a non-specific enhanced response to heterologous stimuli [1]. It is known that invertebrates respond better towards secondary infections, both to the same pathogen as well as towards other unrelated infections. It has been shown that in plants and invertebrates, processes termed "systemic acquired resistance" and "immune priming" occur widely in organisms that possess only an innate immune system [3–9]. Interesting from an evolutionary perspective, among vertebrates there are indications that trained immunity occurs in teleost fish, which are the first vertebrates having a functioning adaptive and innate immune system, as reviewed by Petit and Wiegertjes [10].

In humans, evidence for the existence of trained immunity first emerged from epidemiological studies on vaccination responses, which have indicated that vaccination induces protection not only against the target disease, but also cross-protection against other pathogens [11]. The best known example of this cross-protection is seen after Bacillus Camette-Guérin (BCG) vaccination against *Mycobacterium tuberculosis*, which was shown to protect against all-cause mortality by reducing neonatal sepsis, respiratory infection, and fever [12]. Furthermore, it was shown that BCG vaccination in humans induced trained immunity in both monocytes and Natural killer (NK) cells three months after vaccination, which was mediated by increased H3K4 trimethylation in monocytes [13,14].

The mechanism of trained immunity was first described by Quintin et al., who showed that mice survived when treated first with a sublethal dose of *Candida albicans* followed by a secondary lethal *C. albicans* infection [15]. This outcome was found both in wild-type mice and in T/B-cell defective (Rag 1-deficient) mice, indicating that the adaptive immune system was not involved in the induction of trained immunity. Subsequently, it was shown that β-glucan derived from *C. albicans* could induce trained immunity in purified human monocytes [15]. Some types of β-glucans are present in the cell wall of *C. albicans*, while other types are also present in food as mushrooms, baker's and brewer's yeast, and the cell walls of plants including wheat and oat, as reviewed by Meena et al. [16]. These dietary β-glucans may induce trained immunity as well, although this remains to be demonstrated.

Low-density lipoprotein (oxLDL) particles, induced in blood as a result of Western diets, are known to induce trained immunity in human cells in vitro [17]. A Western diet resulted in transient systemic inflammatory responses in mice, yet at the same time induce long-lived epigenetic and transcriptomic reprogramming of granulocyte–monocyte progenitor cells, leading to trained immunity by monocytes [18]. It can thus be concluded that not only infections by pathogens or vaccination can induce trained immunity, but also dietary components.

Epidemiological studies have revealed that children growing up on a farm and consuming (raw) farm milk have a reduced incidence of asthma, atopy, hay fever, respiratory tract infections (RTI), and otitis media compared to children that consumed heat-treated milk [19–21]. The components that may cause the reduction of allergy and infections in children are thus milk processing-sensitive, and are therefore thought to be heat-sensitive milk proteins. These findings indicate that raw milk or its components can modify immune responses in vivo.

More than 400 components have been identified in bovine milk, and these can be subdivided in multiple fractions [22]. Bovine milk is composed of water (87%), lactose (4–5%), protein (whey and casein) (3%), lipids and fat (3–4%), minerals (0.8%), and vitamins (0.1%) [23–26]. Whey proteins make up 20% of protein concentration of milk, whereas caseins represent 80% of milk proteins [27]. The most abundant whey proteins are β-lactoglobulin, α-lactalbumin, immunoglobulins, such as bovine Immunoglobulin G (bIgG), serum albumin, and lactoferrin (bLF) [27]. Immunologically, the best studied whey proteins are bovine IgG and lactoferrin [28–31].

The aim of this study was to study whether raw bovine milk, milk fractions, or milk proteins such as lactoferrin and IgG can induce trained immunity in human monocytes.

2. Materials and Methods

2.1. Blood Samples and Monocyte Purification

Buffy coats were collected from healthy blood donors at the Sanquin Blood Supply in Nijmegen, the Netherlands. Human peripheral blood mononuclear cells (PBMCs) were isolated from buffy coats using Ficoll plaque plus (17-1440-02, GE Healthcare Life Sciences, Uppsala, Sweden). Monocytes were enriched from freshly isolated PBMCs using negative selection with an Easysep human mono-enrichment kit, according to manufacturer's protocol (19359, Stemcell Technologies, Köln, Germany). Purity was tested by flow cytometry staining isolated cells with α-CD14 (555397, BD Pharmingen, Franklin Lakes, NJ, USA), α-CD3 (555334, BD Pharmingen, Franklin Lakes, NJ, USA), α-CD19 (562947 BD Horizon, Franklin Lakes, NJ, USA), α-CD56 (555516, BD Pharmingen), and fixable viability dye eFluor 450 (65-0863-14, eBioscience, San Diego, CA, USA). Stained cells were measured on FACS CANTO II. Monocytes isolated from subjects used for analysis all had a purity of >70% CD14$^+$ monocytes and <4% CD3$^+$ T cells (see Supplementary Figure S1).

2.2. Trained Immunity Model in Human Monocytes

The trained immunity model in human monocytes was performed as previously described [32,33] with some adjustments, and is depicted in Figure 1. This in-vitro model is widely accepted as reflecting trained immunity in macrophages [1–6]. Isolated monocytes were transferred into a 96-well plate (1×10^5 monocytes/well) (Costar3596, Washington, DC, USA), and the training stimulation or culture medium Roswell Park Memorial Institute (RPMI) 1640 Dutch modifications from Sigma-Aldrich (St. Louis, MO, USA), supplemented with 1% gentamicin, 1% L-glutamine, and 1% pyruvate (Life Technologies, Nieuwerkerk, The Netherlands), but without serum, was added in a total volume of 200 μL for 24 h at 37 °C. For the different training stimuli and their concentrations, see Section 2.3. After 24 h, the plates were washed twice with warm Phosphate-buffered saline (PBS), and RPMI medium +10% human pooled serum was added for five days and refreshed after two to three days. In these five days, monocytes differentiated towards macrophages, and at day six macrophages were stimulated in the presence or absence of TLR-ligands Pam3CSK4 10 μg/mL (L2000; EMC microcollections, Tübingen, Germany) Ultra-pure lipopolysaccharide (LPS) 0.1 μg/mL (3pelps, Invivogen, San Diego, CA, USA) and R848 10 μg/mL (TLRL-R848-5, Invivogen). After 24 h of secondary stimulation, the supernatant was collected and stored at −80 °C.

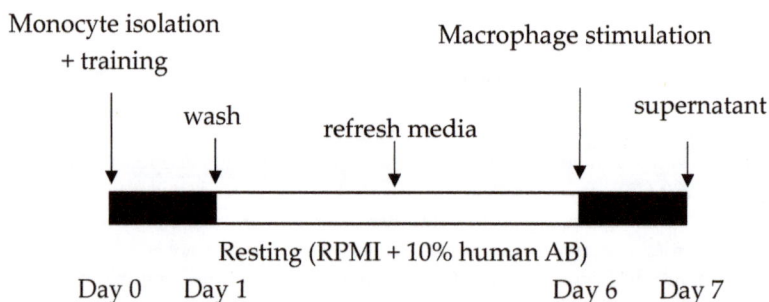

Figure 1. Trained immunity model in human monocytes. At day 0, peripheral blood mononuclear cells (PBMCs) were isolated from buffy coats, and monocytes were isolated by negative selection. Monocytes were stimulated (trained) for 24 h, after which the stimulus was washed away and monocytes differentiated towards macrophages during a five-day resting period. At day six, macrophages were re-stimulated with Toll-like receptor (TLR)-ligands, and after 24 h the supernatant was collected and measured for cytokines.

2.3. Reagents

Candida albicans β-glucan (1 µg/mL) was a kind gift of Prof. David Williams (East Tennessee State University), and was isolated and purified as previously described [34]. Pooled human serum was collected in serum tubes and heat inactivated for 30 min at 56 °C. Afterwards, the serum was aliquoted and stored −80 °C until use. For every refreshment of the medium, freshly pooled serum was thawed.

Raw bovine milk (1:100), bovine lactoferrin (100 µg/mL), bovine IgG (200 µg/mL), lactose (463 µg/mL), whey protein (liquid SPC 1:100), casein (264 µg/mL), cream serum (3.6 µg/mL), and anhydrous milk fat (458.9 µg/mL) were obtained from FrieslandCampina, Wageningen, The Netherlands. As bLF and bIgG contained some endotoxin, they were treated with Triton-X114 to remove LPS, as described by Teodorowicz et al. [35]. After LPS removal, bIgG and bLF contained less than 10 pg/mL LPS at the dilutions used for all experiments. Endotoxin levels were measured using an Endozyme recombinatant Factor C assay (Hyglos, Bernried, Germany).

2.4. Cytokine Measurement

In the supernatant, the production of interleukin (IL)-6 (558276, BD Pharmingen, Franklin Lakes, NJ, USA) and Tumor necrosis factor (TNF)-α (560112, BD Pharmingen) was measured using cytometric bead array on the FACS CANTO II, according to manufacturer's protocol.

2.5. Statistical Analysis

IBM SPSS Statistics software, version 23, Armonk, NY, USA, was used to perform statistical analysis. All experiments with β-glucan, raw bovine milk, bovine lactoferrin and bovine IgG were performed at least five times, with monocytes isolated from PBMC, with a minimum of eleven volunteers in total. In order to assess the training effect of a specific ligand upon a secondary stimulation, non-trained cells stimulated with Pam3CSK4, LPS or R848 were compared with trained cells re-stimulated with Pam3CSK4, LPS, or R848. Differences between the groups were analyzed using the Wilcoxon signed-rank test, and were considered statistically significant at a p value of <0.05. On the screening experiments of the training stimuli (Figure 2 and Supplementary Figure S2), statistical analysis was performed using a paired T-test, after checking the measurements for being normally distributed using a Shapiro Wilk test.

3. Results

3.1. Screening of Bovine Milk and Milk Fractions for the Induction of Trained Immunity

To determine if milk and its major components can induce trained immunity, we screened the effects of raw milk, whey proteins, casein, milk fat, cream, and lactose, which were tested on monocytes using the experimental set-up, as depicted in Figure 1 (based on [32,33]). β-glucans were included as a positive control, as were TLR ligands as components that induce tolerance in this model system (see Supplementary Figure S2). As raw milk added directly to human monocytes reduced cell viability, raw milk's major components were tested at the equivalent concentrations present in raw milk (casein, milk fat, cream, and lactose).

Supplementary Figure S2 shows that monocytes stimulated with β-glucans acted as a positive control, and when re-stimulated with R848, produced higher IL-6 and TNF-α levels compared to control cells (non-trained cells in culture medium). The same induction of IL-6 and TNF-α was also seen when cells trained with β-glucans were re-stimulated with Pam3CSK4 (Pam) and LPS. In contrast, training with TLR-ligands Pam, LPS, and R848 induced tolerance to re-stimulation, as published elsewhere [32,33], and was not due to cell death.

When raw milk and milk components were tested for their ability to induce trained immunity, raw milk induced variable production of IL-6 and TNF-α for different secondary stimulations, while inducing non-significant elevated levels of IL-6 upon Pam, LPS, and R848 stimulation compared to non-trained cells (Figure 2A). Whey proteins and cream induced trained immunity when re-stimulated with R848 (Figure 2A,B). This was also seen after stimulation with Pam and LPS. Milk fat was dissolved in Dimethyl sulfoxide (DMSO), which inhibited cytokine production in the assay. No additional induction of tolerance was observed by the milk fat diluted in DMSO, therefore it was not included in further experiments. As whey proteins induced trained immunity comparable to β-glucan for both IL-6 and TNF-α, the effect of three prominent immune-related whey proteins was investigated. LPS-free, isolated bovine lactoferrin (bLF) and bovine IgG (bIgG), but not Transforming Growth Factor (TGF)-β, seem to induce trained immunity. Bovine milk proteins are thus able to induce trained immunity.

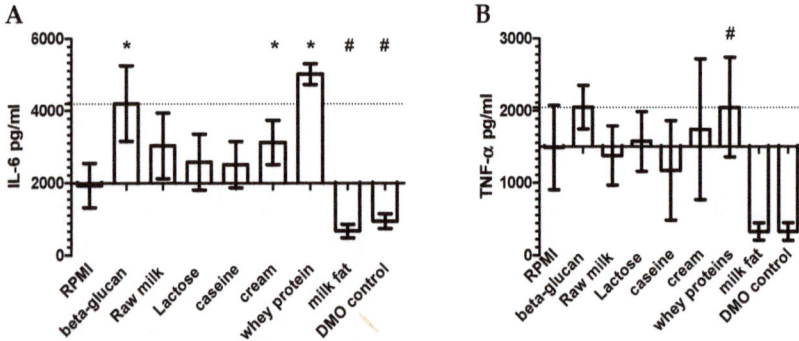

Figure 2. Selection of bovine milk fractions that can induce trained immunity. Monocytes were stimulated 24 h in the presence or absence of β-glucan (1 µg/mL), raw milk (1:100), lactose (463 µg/mL), casein (264 µg/mL), cream (3.6 µg/mL), whey protein (liquid serum protein concentrate (SPC) 1:100), milk fat dissolved in Dimethyl sulfoxide (DMSO) (458.9 µg/mL), and DMSO (1.8 uL/mL, the same concentration as used for milk fat). After five days of rest, the differentiated macrophages were stimulated for 24 h with R848 (10 µg/mL). After stimulation with R848, the produced IL-6 and Tumor necrosis factor (TNF)-α (pg/mL) were measured in supernatant. Data shown as mean ± standard error of mean (SEM), with the IL-6 and TNF-α production of non-trained cells (Roswell Park Memorial Institute (RPMI) medium) as the x-axis and the cytokine production by β-glucan trained cells (positive control) as dotted lines. RPMI, Beta-glucan, raw milk, lactose: $n = 5$; all other stimuli: $n = 3$. Statistical analysis was done by performing a paired T-test. * $p < 0.05$, # $p < 0.10$.

3.2. Induction of Trained Immunity by Raw Milk and Bovine Immunoglobulin G

To extend and statistically analyse our initial observations, we studied the induction of trained immunity by raw milk, bIgG, and bLF in a number of additional individuals. β-glucan was included as a positive control. Stimulation of isolated monocytes with β-glucans consistently resulted in higher IL-6 production compared to non-trained monocytes upon re-stimulation with TLR-ligands Pam, LPS, and R848 (Supplementary Figure S3). Also, a higher TNF-α production by β-glucan trained monocytes was observed for LPS and R848 re-stimulated macrophages, but not for Pam re-stimulated macrophages.

Figure 3 shows that only upon re-stimulation with Pam, training with raw bovine milk is able to induce higher production of IL-6 compared to non-trained (RPMI) monocytes. This effect is not observed for IL-6 production after re-stimulation with other TLR-ligands, and not for TNF-α production after stimulation with any TLR-ligand (see also Supplementary Figure S4B).

In contrast to the screening experiment, bLF did not consistently induce trained immunity when more subjects were tested (see Figure 4). Supplementary Figure S4 and Supplementary Table S1 show that donors respond to bLF training in a very heterogeneous manner, in which only some donors show increased training by bLF, resulting in no statistically significant effect overall.

In line with the selection experiment and raw bovine milk, bovine IgG was able to consistently induce trained immunity (Figure 5). When monocytes were stimulated with bIgG and re-stimulated with R848, the cells produced more IL-6 and TNF-α and more TNF-α upon LPS stimulation compared to non-trained cells (RPMI). Upon re-stimulation with Pam, bIgG tended to increase the production of IL-6 and TNF-α, albeit not significantly (Supplementary Figure S4).

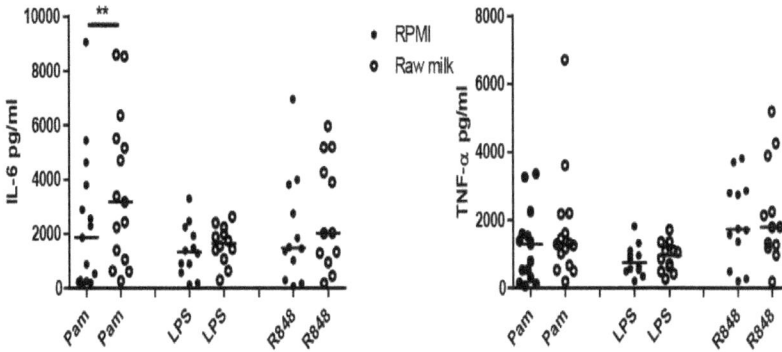

Figure 3. Induction of trained immunity by raw bovine milk. Monocytes were stimulated 24 h in the presence or absence of raw bovine milk (1:100); after five days of rest, the differentiated macrophages were re-stimulated for 24 h with Pam3Cysk4 (Pam) (10 µg/mL), Ultra-pure lipopolysaccharide (LPS) (0.1 µg/mL), or R848 (10 µg/mL). After stimulation with R848, the produced IL-6 and TNF-α (pg/mL) was measured in supernatant. In 5–6 independent experiments, $n = 15$ (Pam) or $n = 12$ (LPS, R848) Data shown as dot plot with median. Statistics was done by performing a Wilcoxon signed rank test between raw bovine milk and RPMI for every secondary stimulation (Pam, LPS, R848). ** $p < 0.01$.

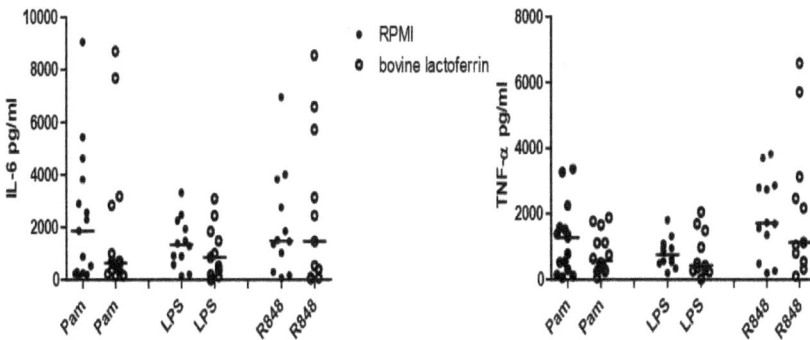

Figure 4. Bovine lactoferrin does not induce trained immunity. Monocytes were stimulated 24 h in the presence or absence of bovine lactoferrin (bLF) (100 µg/mL); after five days of rest, the differentiated macrophages were re-stimulated for 24 h with Pam3Cysk4 (10 µg/mL), LPS (0.1 µg/mL), or R848 (10 µg/mL). After stimulation with R848, the produced IL-6 and TNF-α (pg/mL) was measured in supernatant. In 5–6 independent experiments, $n = 15$ (Pam) or $n = 11$ (LPS, R848). Data shown as dot plot with median. Statistics was done by performing a Wilcoxon signed rank test between bLF and RPMI for every secondary stimulation (Pam, LPS, R848). No significant differences were observed.

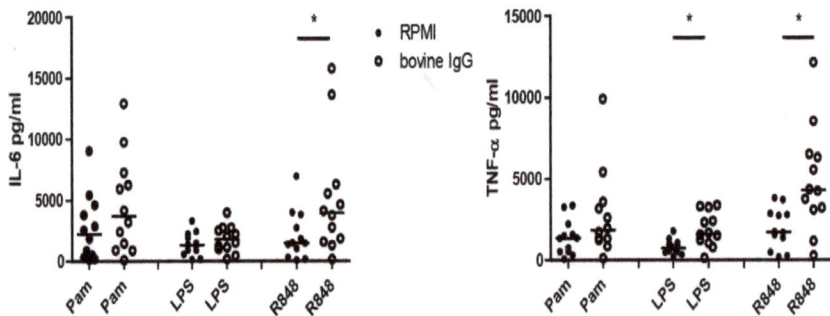

Figure 5. Induction of trained immunity by bovine IgG. Monocytes were stimulated 24 h in the presence or absence of bovine IgG (200 µg/mL); after five days of rest, the differentiated macrophages were re-stimulated for 24 h with Pam3Cysk4 (Pam) (10 µg/mL), LPS (0.1 µg/mL), or R848 (10 µg/mL). After stimulation with R848, the produced IL-6 and TNF-α (pg/mL) was measured in supernatant. In 5 independent experiments, $n = 12$. Data shown as dot plot with median. Statistics were done by performing a Wilcoxon signed rank test between bovine IgG and RPMI for every secondary stimulation (Pam, LPS, R848). * $p < 0.05$.

4. Discussion

Here we show that bIgG and raw bovine milk can induce trained immunity in human monocytes. These findings confirm the hypothesis that dietary components can modulate the responsiveness of the innate immune system to pathogen-related stimuli.

One of the first components that was shown to induce trained immunity was β-1, 3-(D)-glucan derived from *C. albicans*, which exerted this effect via epigenetic changes in trimethylation of H3K4, induced after binding to Dectin-1 [15]. Epigenomic profile analysis revealed changes in H3K4m1, H3K4me3, and H3K27ac when comparing a β-glucan trained compared to non-trained macrophages [33]. Based on these studies β-1, 3-(D)-glucan derived from *C. albicans* has become a model compound to study the mechanisms of trained immunity.

Cell metabolism is important in monocyte-to-macrophage differentiation, and also for M1 versus M2 functions [36]. Resting and tolerant macrophages use oxidative phosphorylation to generate ATP, while activated (trained) macrophages shift to aerobic glycolysis (Warburg effect) via the dectin-1-Akt-mTOR and HIF-1α pathway [33,37]. Resting macrophages have a functional tricarboxylic acid (TCA) cycle that, together with glycolysis, enhances membrane synthesis and induces TLR-mediated activation in dendritic cells [33]. Two other metabolic pathways that are important in vitro and in vivo for trained immunity induction are glutaminolysis and the cholesterol synthesis pathway [38,39]. β-glucan-induced trained immunity via the dectin-1 pathway also effects the TCA cycle, as glycolysis inhibitors (rapamycin) also inhibit β-glucan-mediated trained immunity [38]. This indicates that β-glucan-induced trained immunity also effects the TCA cycle, and does not only signal via the dectin-1 pathway. This links cell metabolism, metabolites, and epigenetic mechanisms, suggesting that β-glucan induces trained immunity by modifying cell metabolism.

In our hands, β-glucan induced higher levels of IL-6 compared to non-trained cells when trained macrophages were re-stimulated with ligands for TLR1/2 (Pam), TLR4 (LPS), and TLR7/8 (R848). TNF-α production was increased after LPS and R848 re-stimulation. Unexpectedly, TNF-α production was not increased after Pam re-stimulation, which is in contrast to Ifrim et al., albeit using the same concentration and same supplier of Pam3CSK4 [32].

Until now, it has not been clear if dietary components can also induce immune training in humans after nutritional intervention. In a pilot study in humans, where baker's yeast (*S. cerevisiae*)-derived β-glucans (1000 mg/day) were used as a food supplement for seven days, no trained immunity effects were observed [40]. In contrast, it was recently shown that diets high in fat can also induce trained immunity in vivo in mice, and oxLDL can induce immune training in human monocytes in vitro [17,18], suggesting that nutrition may indeed directly affect innate immune function.

As breast milk and bovine milk contain many immune-modulating components [22], we set out to study whether (raw) bovine milk or milk components can induce trained immunity in human monocytes as well. A trained immunity effect was observed for IL-6 production by raw bovine milk when stimulated with TLR1/2 ligand PamCSK4, but not for stimulation through TLR4 or TLR7/8 (Figure 4). In contrast, treatment with bIgG induced trained immunity after stimulation of TLR4 (LPS) and TLR7/8 (R848), but not after TLR1/2 stimulation. This indicates that the training effect of raw milk (for TLR1/2) is not mediated via bLF or bovine IgG, as no effect was observed for training with bLF and bIgG after TLR1/2 stimulation. Furthermore, as undiluted and low dilutions of milk compromised viability of the monocytes, raw milk was tested at a 100-fold dilution, whereas bIgG was tested at the levels present in raw milk. This can explain why raw milk does not induce trained immunity via TLR7/8.

It is not clear which component in raw milk is responsible for this training effect. One possibility is that bovine miRNAs in extracellular vesicles (exosomes) may do this. These vesicles are described to induced higher production of IL-6, but not higher TNF-α production, in LPS stimulated RAW264.7 cells [41].

In our initial screen of raw milk and the major milk components, the clearest training effect after TLR7/8 stimulation was seen for whey proteins (Figure 2), as well as for the isolated whey proteins bLF and bIgG (data not shown). The whey proteins were a liquid whey fraction that contained 60% protein, and as with the raw milk, was used at a 100-fold dilution. However, it should be stated that this preparation also contained some casein and lactose. As these did not have an effect on innate immune training, we assume the effect seen using this whey proteins was the result of the presence of bIgG, and possibly also of bLF. Next to whey proteins, lipid-rich cream—but not milk fat (triglycerides)—induced a small training effect. This indicates that either the lipids or the intact milk fat globular membranes present in cream serum, but not the triglycerides, may induce trained immunity to some extent.

For bIgG a consistent trained immunity effect was observed for re-stimulation with TLR7/8. However, this was not seen for bLF; bLF could induce trained immunity in some donors (Supplementary Table S1, Supplementary Figure S4C), but the overall response was not significant (Figure 4). The lack of training induced by bLF in most donors was not due to cell death. Besides, in Supplementary Table S1 it can be observed that subjects in which no training for bLF is seen, trained immunity induction by other training-stimuli is possible. It can be thus concluded that the variability of trained immunity responses depends on the training stimulus, and the mechanisms responsible for this effect remain to be elucidated in future studies. Furthermore, we have recently observed that a three peripheral blood mononuclear cells—week dietary intervention with bLF could enhance the response of pDC of elderly women to TLR7/8 (van Splunter, unpublished observations), and future studies should determine the involvement of trained immunity in this effect.

BLF can be taken up by human cells via three different receptors: intelectin [42], low-density-lipoprotein (CD91) [43], and CXCR4 [43]. Most likely, bovine lactoferrin (LF) can also bind to soluble CD14 and TLR4, as human LF is 69% homologous to bovine LF and can bind sCD14 [44] and TLR4 [45], which are expressed by monocytes [46]. In a human study in which subjects received 200 mg bLF and 100 mg Ig-rich whey proteins twice per day, a significant reduction in rhinovirus induced common cold was observed [47]. This protective effect of bLF and bIgG on rhinovirus infections that are recognized by the immune system via TLR2 and TLR7/8 might thus be linked to trained immunity [48].

In addition to the effect shown after TLR7/8 re-stimulation, bIgG was also able to induce trained immunity when re-stimulated with TLR4, but not with TLR1/2. Bovine Immunoglobulin G is known to bind to human monocytes, macrophages, and monocyte-derived dendritic cells via FcγRII (CD32 receptor) [49]. Den Hartog et al. showed that bIgG could bind to human airway pathogens,

Nutrients **2018**, *10*, 1378

such as respiratory syncytial virus (RSV), *haemophilus influenzae* type b (Hib) and influenza virus [49]. These pathogens can activate TLR2 and TLR4 (Hib and RSV), TLR7 (RSV and influenza) and TLR8 (RSV) [49–51].

We propose that the mechanism for the trained immunity induction by bIgG occurs via binding to FcγRII (CD32). In murine macrophages, crosslinking of FcγRII/III leads to activation of mitogen-activated protein (MAP) kinase family members p38 and JNK [52]. In human monocytes, inhibiting p38 and JNK abolished trained immunity induced by flagellin (TLR5) after re-stimulating through TLR4 [32]. TLR induced signaling via MyD88 or TIR-domain-containing adapter-inducing interferon-β (TRIF) leads to pro-inflammatory cytokine production, and is partly regulated by the p38MAPK/MK2 pathway [53,54]. Furthermore, in trained immunity epigenetic changes (e.g., H3K4 trimethylation) on the promotor of pro-inflammatory cytokine genes (IL-6, TNF-α) are induced by training stimuli, resulting in increased cytokine production [15]. Therefore, altogether, we hypothesize that bIgG can exert a trained immunity effect in macrophages by activating the MAP kinase pathway via FcγRII, thereby inducing epigenetic changes on the promotors of IL-6 and TNF-α genes, leading to enhanced NF-κB-dependent TLR-mediated responses.

5. Conclusions

In summary, our data show that raw bovine milk and bIgG isolated from raw colostrum can induce trained immunity in human monocytes. This strengthens the hypothesis that diet can influence the responsiveness of the innate immune system. Important to underline however is that the trained immunity program induced by milk, and milk components are very likely different from those induced by other dietary components, such as the Western-type diet. This can be concluded by the deleterious effects of Western-diet-induced trained immunity on atherosclerosis, whereas no such effects have been reported for milk. Future whole-genome transcriptome and epigenome studies should describe the trained immunity activation program induced by milk, fully describing the impact of dairy milk on long-term reprogramming of innate immunity.

Supplementary Materials: The following are available online at http://www.mdpi.com/2072-6643/10/10/1378/s1. Table S1: Trained immunity induced per training stimulus, compared to non-trained cells. after TLR7/8 (R848) stimulation (IL-6 production), Figure S1: Gating strategy and purity of isolated monocytes (84.6%). Staining was performed with live/death staining, CD3 and CD14, Figure S2: Induction of trained immunity or tolerance is dependent on the training of monocytes. Monocytes were stimulated 24 h in the presence or absence of β-glucan (1 µg/mL); Pam3Cysk4 (10 µg/mL), LPS (0.1 µg/mL) or R848 (10 µg/mL), after 5 days of rest the differentiated macrophages were stimulated for 24 h with R848 (10 µg/mL). After stimulation with R848 the produced IL-6 and TNF-α (pg/mL) was measured in supernatant. Data shown as mean ± SEM, with the IL-6 and TNF-α production of non-trained cells (RPMI) as *x*-axis. RPMI and β-glucan $n = 5$; TLR stimuli $n = 3$. Data was statistically analysed using a paired *t*-test. * $p < 0.05$, Figure S3: Induction of trained immunity by β-glucan. Monocytes were stimulated 24 h in the presence or absence of β-glucan (1 µg/mL), after 5 days of rest the differentiated macrophages were re-stimulated for 24 h with Pam3Cysk4 (Pam) (10 µg/mL), LPS (0.1 µg/mL) or R848 (10 µg/mL). After stimulation with R848 the produced IL-6 and TNF-α (pg/mL) was measured in supernatant. $n = 15$ (Pam) or $n = 12$ (LPS, R848) in 5–6 independent experiments. Data shown as dot plot with median. Statistics was done by performing a Wilcoxon signed rank test between beta-glucan and RPMI for every secondary stimulation (Pam, LPS, R848). * $p < 0.05$; ** $p < 0.01$, Figure S4; Paired analysis plots of monocytes trained with β-glucan, raw milk, bLF and bIgG and re-stimulated with Pam, LPS or R848 at day 6. In supernatant of day 7 IL-6 (pg/mL) was measured.

Author Contributions: R.J.J.v.N., M.G.N., L.A.B.J., S.B., H.F.J.S., and M.v.S. designed the experiments. M.v.S. and T.L.J.v.O. performed the experiments. Data analysis was done by M.v.S. R.J.J.v.N., M.G.N., L.A.B.J., S.B., H.F.J.S., and M.v.S. edited and contributed to drafts of the manuscript. All authors approved the final form of the manuscript.

Funding: This study was financed in part by FrieslandCampina. M.G.N. was supported by a Spinoza grant of the Netherlands Organization for Scientific Research.

Acknowledgments: We would like to thank Trees Jansen and Liesbeth Jacobs for their willingness to practice the trained immunity protocol at Radboudumc.

Conflicts of Interest: R.J.J.v.N. is employed by FrieslandCampina, and M.v.S. is supported by an unrestricted grant from FrieslandCampina.

References

1. Netea, M.G.; Quintin, J.; Van Der Meer, J.W.M. Trained immunity: A memory for innate host defense. *Cell Host Microbe* **2011**, *9*, 355–361. [CrossRef] [PubMed]
2. Netea, M.G.; van der Meer, J.W.M. Trained Immunity: An Ancient Way of Remembering. *Cell Host Microbe* **2017**, *21*, 297–300. [CrossRef] [PubMed]
3. Durrant, W.E.; Dong, X. Systemic Acquired Resistance. *Annu. Rev. Phytopathol.* **2004**, *42*, 185–209. [CrossRef] [PubMed]
4. Gao, Q.-M.; Zhu, S.; Kachroo, P.; Kachroo, A. Signal regulators of systemic acquired resistance. *Front. Plant Sci.* **2015**, *6*, 228. [CrossRef] [PubMed]
5. Reimer-Michalski, E.M.; Conrath, U. Innate immune memory in plants. *Semin. Immunol.* **2016**, *28*, 319–327. [CrossRef] [PubMed]
6. Tate, A.T.; Andolfatto, P.; Demuth, J.P.; Graham, A.L. The within-host dynamics of infection in trans-generationally primed flour beetles. *Mol. Ecol.* **2017**, *26*, 3794–3807. [CrossRef] [PubMed]
7. Green, T.J.; Helbig, K.; Speck, P.; Raftos, D.A. Primed for success: Oyster parents treated with poly(I:C) produce offspring with enhanced protection against Ostreid herpesvirus type I infection. *Mol. Immunol.* **2016**, *78*, 113–120. [CrossRef] [PubMed]
8. Kurtz, J. Specific memory within innate immune systems. *Trends Immunol.* **2005**, *26*, 186–192. [CrossRef] [PubMed]
9. Pham, L.N.; Dionne, M.S.; Shirasu-Hiza, M.; Schneider, D.S. A specific primed immune response in Drosophila is dependent on phagocytes. *PLoS Pathog.* **2007**, *3*, e26. [CrossRef] [PubMed]
10. Petit, J.; Wiegertjes, G.F. Long-lived effects of administering β-glucans: Indications for trained immunity in fish. *Dev. Comp. Immunol.* **2016**, *64*, 93–102. [CrossRef] [PubMed]
11. Benn, C.S.; Netea, M.G.; Selin, L.K.; Aaby, P. A Small Jab—A Big Effect: Nonspecific Immunomodulation by Vaccines. *Trends Immunol.* **2013**, *34*, 431–439. [CrossRef] [PubMed]
12. Aaby, P.; Roth, A.; Ravn, H.; Napirna, B.M.; Rodrigues, A.; Lisse, I.M.; Stensballe, L.; Diness, B.R.; Lausch, K.R.; Lund, N.; et al. Randomized trial of BCG vaccination at birth to low-birth-weight children: Beneficial nonspecific effects in the neonatal period? *J. Infect. Dis.* **2011**, *204*, 245–252. [CrossRef] [PubMed]
13. Kleinnijenhuis, J.; Quintin, J.; Preijers, F.; Joosten, L.A.B.; Ifrim, D.C.; Saeed, S.; Jacobs, C.; van Loenhout, J.; de Jong, D.; Stunnenberg, H.G.; et al. Bacille Calmette-Guerin induces NOD2-dependent nonspecific protection from reinfection via epigenetic reprogramming of monocytes. *Proc. Natl. Acad. Sci. USA* **2012**, *109*, 17537–17542. [CrossRef] [PubMed]
14. Kleinnijenhuis, J.; Quintin, J.; Preijers, F.; Joosten, L.A.B.; Jacobs, C.; Xavier, R.J.; van der Meer, J.W.M.; van Crevel, R.; Netea, M.G. BCG-induced trained immunity in NK cells: Role for non-specific protection to infection. *Clin. Immunol.* **2014**, *155*, 213–219. [CrossRef] [PubMed]
15. Quintin, J.; Saeed, S.; Martens, J.H.A.; Giamarellos-Bourboulis, E.J.; Ifrim, D.C.; Logie, C.; Jacobs, L.; Jansen, T.; Kullberg, B.-J.; Wijmenga, C.; et al. Candida albicans infection affords protection against reinfection vai functional reprogramming of monocytes. *Cell Host Microbe* **2012**, *16*, 123–128. [CrossRef]
16. Meena, D.K.; Das, P.; Kumar, S.; Mandal, S.C.; Prusty, A.K.; Singh, S.K.; Akhtar, M.S.; Behera, B.K.; Kumar, K.; Pal, A.K.; et al. Beta-glucan: An ideal immunostimulant in aquaculture (a review). *Fish Physiol. Biochem.* **2013**, *39*, 431–457. [CrossRef] [PubMed]
17. Bekkering, S.; Quintin, J.; Joosten, L.A.B.; Van Der Meer, J.W.M.; Netea, M.G.; Riksen, N.P. Oxidized low-density lipoprotein induces long-term proinflammatory cytokine production and foam cell formation via epigenetic reprogramming of monocytes. *Arterioscler. Thromb. Vasc. Biol.* **2014**, *34*, 1731–1738. [CrossRef] [PubMed]
18. Christ, A.; Günther, P.; Lauterbach, M.A.R.; Duewell, P.; Biswas, D.; Pelka, K.; Scholz, C.J.; Oosting, M.; Haendler, K.; Baßler, K.; et al. Western Diet Triggers NLRP3-Dependent Innate Immune Reprogramming. *Cell* **2018**, *172*, 162–175. [CrossRef] [PubMed]
19. Loss, G.; Apprich, S.; Waser, M.; Kneifel, W.; Genuneit, J.; Büchele, G.; Weber, J.; Sozanska, B.; Danielewicz, H.; Horak, E.; et al. The protective effect of farm milk consumption on childhood asthma and atopy: The GABRIELA study. *J. Allergy Clin. Immunol.* **2011**, *128*, 766–773. [CrossRef] [PubMed]

20. Loss, G.; Depner, M.; Ulfman, L.H.; van Neerven, R.J.J.; Hose, A.J.; Genuneit, J.; Karvonen, A.M.; Hyvärinen, A.; Kaulek, V.; Roduit, C.; et al. Consumption of unprocessed cow's milk protects infants from common respiratory infections. *J. Allergy Clin. Immunol.* **2015**, *135*, 56–62. [CrossRef] [PubMed]

21. Waser, M.; Michels, K.B.; Bieli, C.; Flöistrup, H.; Pershagen, G.; Von Mutius, E.; Ege, M.; Riedler, J.; Schram-Bijkerk, D.; Brunekreef, B.; et al. Inverse association of farm milk consumption with asthma and allergy in rural and suburban populations across Europe. *Clin. Exp. Allergy* **2006**, *37*, 661–670. [CrossRef] [PubMed]

22. Van Neerven, R.J.J.; Knol, E.F.; Heck, J.M.L.; Savelkoul, H.F.J. Which factors in raw cow's milk contribute to protection against allergies? *J. Allergy Clin. Immunol.* **2012**, *130*, 853–858. [CrossRef] [PubMed]

23. Haug, A.; Høstmark, A.T.; Harstad, O.M. Bovine milk in human nutrition—A review. *Lipids Health Dis.* **2007**, *6*, 25. [CrossRef] [PubMed]

24. Lindmark-Månsson, H.; Fondén, R.; Pettersson, H.E. Composition of Swedish dairy milk. *Int. Dairy J.* **2003**, *13*, 409–425. [CrossRef]

25. Gaucheron, F. The minerals of milk. *Reprod. Nutr. Dev.* **2005**, *45*, 473–483. [CrossRef] [PubMed]

26. Heck, J.M.L.; van Valenberg, H.J.F.; Dijkstra, J.; van Hooijdonk, A.C.M. Seasonal variation in the Dutch bovine raw milk composition. *J. Dairy Sci.* **2009**, *92*, 4745–4755. [CrossRef] [PubMed]

27. Pereira, P.C. Milk nutritional composition and its role in human health. *Nutrition* **2014**, *30*, 619–627. [CrossRef] [PubMed]

28. Lönnerdal, B. Nutritional roles of lactoferrin. *Curr. Opin. Clin. Nutr. Metab. Care* **2009**, *12*, 293–297. [CrossRef] [PubMed]

29. Ochoa, T.J.; Pezo, A.; Cruz, K.; Chea-Woo, E.; Cleary, T.G. Clinical studies of lactoferrin in children. *Biochem. Cell Biol.* **2012**, *90*, 457–467. [CrossRef] [PubMed]

30. Korhonen, H.; Marnila, P.; Gill, H.S. Bovine milk antibodies for health. *Br. J. Nutr.* **2000**, *84* (Suppl. S1), S135–S146. [CrossRef]

31. Ulfman, L.; Leusen, J.H.W.; Savelkoul, H.F.J.; Warner, J.O.; van Neerven, R.J.J. Effects of bovine immunoglobulins on immune function, allergy and infection. *Front. Nutr.* **2018**, *5*, 52. [CrossRef] [PubMed]

32. Ifrim, D.C.; Quintin, J.; Joosten, L.A.B.; Jacobs, C.; Jansen, T.; Jacobs, L.; Gow, N.A.R.; Williams, D.L.; van der Meer, J.W.M.; Netea, M.G. Trained Immunity or Tolerance: Opposing Functional Programs Induced in Human Monocytes after Engagement of Various Pattern Recognition Receptors. *Clin. Vaccine Immunol.* **2014**, *21*, 534–545. [CrossRef] [PubMed]

33. Saeed, S.; Quintin, J.; Kerstens, H.H.D.; Rao, N.A.; Aghajanirefah, A.; Matarese, F.; Cheng, S.-C.; Ratter, J.; Berentsen, K.; van der Ent, M.A.; et al. Epigenetic programming of monocyte-to-macrophage differentiation and trained innate immunity. *Science* **2014**, *345*, 1251086. [CrossRef] [PubMed]

34. Müller, A.; Rice, P.J.; Ensley, H.E.; Coogan, P.S.; Kalbfleish, J.H.; Kelley, J.L.; Love, E.J.; Portera, C.A.; Ha, T.; Browder, I.W.; et al. Receptor binding and internalization of a water-soluble (1,3)-beta-D-glucan biologic response modifier in two monocyte/macrophage cell lines. *J. Immunol.* **1996**, *156*, 3418–3425. [PubMed]

35. Teodorowicz, M.; Perdijk, O.; Verhoek, I.; Govers, C.; Savelkoul, H.F.J.; Tang, Y.; Wichers, H.; Broersen, K. Optimized triton X-114 assisted lipopolysaccharide (LPS) removal method reveals the immunomodulatory effect of food proteins. *PLoS ONE* **2017**, *12*, e0173778. [CrossRef] [PubMed]

36. O'Neill, L.A.J.; Grahame Hardie, D. Metabolism of inflammation limited by AMPK and pseudo-starvation. *Nature* **2013**, *493*, 346–355. [CrossRef] [PubMed]

37. Cheng, S.C.; Quintin, J.; Cramer, R.A.; Shepardson, K.M.; Saeed, S.; Kumar, V.; Giamarellos-Bourboulis, E.J.; Martens, J.H.A.; Rao, N.A.; Aghajanirefah, A.; et al. MTOR- and HIF-1α-mediated aerobic glycolysis as metabolic basis for trained immunity. *Science* **2014**, *345*, 1250684. [CrossRef] [PubMed]

38. Arts, R.J.W.; Novakovic, B.; ter Horst, R.; Carvalho, A.; Bekkering, S.; Lachmandas, E.; Rodrigues, F.; Silvestre, R.; Cheng, S.C.; Wang, S.Y.; et al. Glutaminolysis and Fumarate Accumulation Integrate Immunometabolic and Epigenetic Programs in Trained Immunity. *Cell Metab.* **2016**, *24*, 807–819. [CrossRef] [PubMed]

39. Bekkering, S.; Arts, R.J.W.; Novakovic, B.; Kourtzelis, I.; van der Heijden, C.D.C.C.; Li, Y.; Popa, C.D.; ter Horst, R.; van Tuijl, J.; Netea-Maier, R.T.; et al. Metabolic Induction of Trained Immunity through the Mevalonate Pathway. *Cell* **2018**, *172*, 135–146. [CrossRef] [PubMed]

40. Leentjens, J.; Quintin, J.; Gerretsen, J.; Kox, M.; Pickkers, P.; Netea, M.G. The effects of orally administered beta-glucan on innate immune responses in humans, a randomized open-label intervention pilot-study. *PLoS ONE* **2014**, *9*, e108794. [CrossRef] [PubMed]

41. Sun, Q.; Chen, X.; Yu, J.; Zen, K.; Zhang, C.Y.; Li, L. Immune modulatory function of abundant immune-related microRNAs in microvesicles from bovine colostrum. *Protein Cell* **2013**, *4*, 197–210. [CrossRef] [PubMed]

42. Lönnerdal, B.; Jiang, R.; Du, X. Bovine Lactoferrin Can Be Taken Up by the Human Intestinal Lactoferrin Receptor and Exert Bioactivities. *J. Pediatr. Gastroenterol. Nutr.* **2011**, *53*, 606–614. [CrossRef] [PubMed]

43. Takayama, Y.; Aoki, R.; Uchida, R.; Tajima, A.; Aoki-Yoshida, A. Role of CXC chemokine receptor type 4 as a lactoferrin receptor. *Biochem. Cell Biol.* **2017**, *95*, 57–63. [CrossRef] [PubMed]

44. Baveye, S.; Elass, E.; Fernig, D.G.; Blanquart, C.; Mazurier, J.; Legrand, D. Human lactoferrin interacts with soluble CD14 and inhibits expression of endothelial adhesion molecules, E-selectin and ICAM-1, induced by the CD14-lipopolysaccharide complex. *Infect. Immun.* **2000**, *68*, 6519–6525. [CrossRef] [PubMed]

45. Ando, K.; Hasegawa, K.; Shindo, K.I.; Furusawa, T.; Fujino, T.; Kikugawa, K.; Nakano, H.; Takeuchi, O.; Akira, S.; Akiyama, T.; et al. Human lactoferrin activates NF-κB through the Toll-like receptor 4 pathway while it interferes with the lipopolysaccharide-stimulated TLR4 signaling. *FEBS J.* **2010**, *277*, 2051–2066. [CrossRef] [PubMed]

46. Verschoor, C.P.; Kohli, V. Cryopreserved whole blood for the quantification of monocyte, T-cell and NK-cell subsets, and monocyte receptor expression by multi-color flow cytometry: A methodological study based on participants from the Canadian longitudinal study on aging. *Cytometry Part A* **2018**, *93*, 548–555. [CrossRef] [PubMed]

47. Vitetta, L.; Coulson, S.; Beck, S.L.; Gramotnev, H.; Du, S.; Lewis, S. The clinical efficacy of a bovine lactoferrin/whey protein Ig-rich fraction (Lf/IgF) for the common cold: A double blind randomized study. *Complement. Ther. Med.* **2013**, *21*, 164–171. [CrossRef] [PubMed]

48. Triantafilou, K.; Vakakis, E.; Richer, E.A.J.; Evans, G.L.; Villiers, J.P.; Triantafilou, M. Human rhinovirus recognition in non-immune cells is mediated by Toll-like receptors and MDA-5, which trigger a synergetic pro-inflammatory immune response. *Virulence* **2011**, *2*, 22–29. [CrossRef] [PubMed]

49. den Hartog, G.; Jacobino, S.; Bont, L.; Cox, L.; Ulfman, L.H.; Leusen, J.H.W.; van Neerven, R.J.J. Specificity and Effector Functions of Human RSV-Specific IgG from Bovine Milk. *PLoS ONE* **2014**, *9*, e112047. [CrossRef] [PubMed]

50. Mogensen, T.H.; Paludan, S.R.; Kilian, M.; Ostergaard, L. Live Streptococcus pneumoniae, Haemophilus influenzae, and Neisseria meningitidis activate the inflammatory response through Toll-like receptors 2, 4, and 9 in species-specific patterns. *J. Leuk. Biol.* **2006**, *80*, 267–277. [CrossRef] [PubMed]

51. Schijf, M.A.; Lukens, M.V.; Kruijsen, D.; Van Uden, N.O.P.; Garssen, J.; Coenjaerts, F.E.J.; Van't Land, B.; Van Bleek, G.M. Respiratory syncytial virus induced type I IFN production by pDC is regulated by RSV-infected airway epithelial cells, RSV-exposed monocytes and virus specific antibodies. *PLoS ONE* **2013**, *8*, e81695. [CrossRef] [PubMed]

52. Rose, D.; Winston, B.; Chan, E.; Riches, D.; Gerwins, P.; Johnson, G.; PM, H. Fc gamma receptor cross-linking activates p42, p38 and JNK/SAPK mitogen-activated protein kinases in murine macrophages: Role for p42MAPK in Fc gamma receptor-stimulated TNF-alpha synthesis. *J. Immunol.* **1977**, *158*, 3433–3438. [CrossRef]

53. Gais, P.; Tiedje, C.; Altmayr, F.; Gaestel, M.; Weighardt, H.; Holzmann, B. TRIF signaling stimulates translation of TNF-alpha mRNA via prolonged activation of MK2. *J. Immunol.* **2010**, *184*, 5842–5848. [CrossRef] [PubMed]

54. Tartey, S.; Takeuchi, O. Pathogen recognition and Toll-like receptor targeted therapeutics in innate immune cells. *Int. Rev. Immunol.* **2017**, *36*, 57–73. [CrossRef] [PubMed]

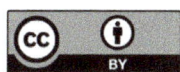

MDPI
St. Alban-Anlage 66
4052 Basel
Switzerland
Tel. +41 61 683 77 34
Fax +41 61 302 89 18
www.mdpi.com

Nutrients Editorial Office
E-mail: nutrients@mdpi.com
www.mdpi.com/journal/nutrients

www.ingramcontent.com/pod-product-compliance
Lightning Source LLC
Chambersburg PA
CBHW051847210326
41597CB00033B/5804